GENETIC MEDICINE

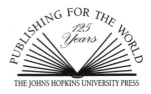

PUBLISHING FOR THE WORLD
125 Years

THE JOHNS HOPKINS UNIVERSITY PRESS

Genetic Medicine

A Logic of Disease

BARTON CHILDS, M.D.
Professor Emeritus of Pediatrics and Biology
The Johns Hopkins University
Baltimore, Maryland

THE JOHNS HOPKINS UNIVERSITY PRESS
Baltimore & London

Johns Hopkins Paperbacks edition, 2003
2 4 6 8 9 7 5 3 1

The Johns Hopkins University Press
2715 North Charles Street
Baltimore, Maryland 21218-4363
www.press.jhu.edu

Library of Congress Cataloging-in-Publication Data will be found at the end
of this book.
A catalog record for this book is available from the British Library.

ISBN 0-8018-7442-4 (pbk.)

To my wife

Contents

Preface

This is a book about medical thinking. It is about the ideas that direct the human enterprise of medicine along paths that accord with both physicians and the people they serve. Research in biology and events in society have made clear that traditional medical thinking is not enough; new ideas are needed. One set of ideas has to do with how medical care is made available and paid for. Another has to do with squaring new procedures and treatments with ethics and social mores. Still another has to do with accommodating the individuality of disease. Information, now accumulating at unprecedented rates, is overwhelming medicine, and there are questions about how to make it useful for medical practitioners and students. It is with how all these ideas affect medical education that this book is most concerned.

Much new information has to do with descriptions of the structure and functions of molecules that govern the properties of cells, organs, and individuals. Among these is the DNA, which specifies and regulates the proteins that do the cells' work and comprises that which is transmitted to offspring and distributed within families and populations in pursuit of the maintenance of species. The rules governing the first of these roles are a property of preclinical teaching, while those governing the second are cited only occasionally in the medical school curriculum. Both are included in genetics, a biological science that, unlike biochemistry and physiology, developed and prospered outside medicine and, until recent decades, overlapped with the latter only in regard to rare diseases. But now genetics is exposing medicine to concepts that provide new ways to think about disease, its causes, and its pathogenesis. We have no choice but to examine how these ideas are influencing medical thinking today, how they should do so, and how we might use them to make medical education more relevant to what is happening in communities no less than in laboratories. In short, we should ask how genetics might be integrated with medicine.

Since the words *genetics* and *medicine* appear again and again in this book, their meanings must be clear. What I mean by *medicine* is defined broadly by *Webster's Second International Unabridged Dictionary* as "the science and art dealing with the maintenance of health and the prevention, alleviation, or cure of disease." Obviously this includes individual encounters of doctor and patient as well as public health and epidemiology, in which the health of populations is at issue. I have also used *medicine* to encompass the whole medical enterprise, including academic medicine and practice, the various colleges, associations, academies, and professional associations, medical schools, and departments of public health. With the phrase *medical thinking* I mean the widely held ideas that inform both the behavior of those engaged in medical care and the expectations of patients, and that figure tacitly and overtly in medical education.

The same dictionary defines *genetics* as "a branch of biology that deals with the heredity and variation of organisms and with the mechanisms by which these are effected." The definition includes both descriptive and analytic components that distinguish genetics from, for example, molecular biology. The characterization of the structure of a gene is the purview of molecular biology; its use in elucidating a step in development is developmental biology. Neither is genetics. But to show how a gene is inherited and how it contributes to variation in individuals and populations is genetics. I also refer to a *genetics enterprise* that has a place in biology and medicine.

Medicine integrated biochemistry and physiology long ago, but genetics taps into aspects of biology outside the province of either. Mendelian segregation and independent assortment, gene action, mutation, mitosis, meiosis and reproduction, polymorphism and the composition of the gene pool, the distribution of genes in families, natural selection, and evolution are the elements of genetics that caused Sewall Wright to call it the "rootstock" of biology, and, as such, medicine cannot afford to be without it (1). Spontaneously and gradually, a synthesis of genetic and medical ideas—or perhaps a "geneticization" of medical thought—is now beginning. It is a wedding of equals, and its offspring affords us a new logic, a new way of examining old questions of the nature of disease and its causes.

This book is devoted to expounding this logic. It may be said that everything in the book is already well known, and so it is when each element is examined separately. But when knitted together, the union of parts engenders an unanticipated whole: a new way of seeing commonplace facts, and one that strengthens medicine's basis in both biology and society. In its position of interface, medicine provides a bridge to unite them. Medical education is up to the minute in developing the biological link but deficient in perceiving both how much the biology of human beings has been defined by the environments in which the species evolved and how modern cultures are influencing that definition. These are deficiencies that genetics can remedy.

Much of the book is written in a historical context. Only within such a context can new ideas be perceived as new. Owsei Temkin observed that "the full meaning of a concept can be grasped as little without its history as the adult body can be understood without its ontogeny and phylogeny. . . . Ideas develop in analogy to the formation of ever-higher species and the development of their foetuses. In all of them the modified surviving characteristics of more primitive stages can be recognized" (2). What could be a more pointed testimonial to these observations than the continuing presence of Archibald Garrod's idea of the inborn error, which has been transformed into such distant cousins of alkaptonuria as cancer and congenital anomalies and which in the guise of variations in the unit steps of physiological homeostasis has become a central focus in medicine? Brandt observed that "the study of history is inevitably a dialogue with the present" (3). The history of the inborn error is an example of such a dialogue, and so is that of the concept of the gene, which, beginning with the abstractions of Mendel, Galton, and the drosophilists, gradually took on functional, structural, and molecular dimensions. All of these definitions are in use in medicine today, and we will continue to need them as long as our analysis proceeds from phenotype to gene.

Ideally this book should have been written by a paleo-physiological-biochemical-molecular biological-medical-genetical-historical philosopher. If genetics is the rootstock of biology and the gene is at the heart of genetics, then the gene must also be at the heart of disease. If so, medical thinking and medical teaching must be transformed to include the implications of genetics, which touch on all of the disciplines mentioned. Of course, the book could have been written by a committee that included at least one contributor from all the relevant disciplines, but the product of a consortium risks failing to attain the synthesis and integration needed to focus a diversity of viewpoints on the needs of any one of them. I am a pediatrician with experience in human genetics. While my credentials scarcely qualify me as an authority in any of the disciplines named, they may be enough to allow me to advance an argument favoring a synthesis of genetic and medical ideas; the idea of disease in both an ontogenetic and a phylogenetic context is the backbone of the book. No doubt my deficiencies will be easily perceived, but they need not interfere with the main purpose of the book, which is to propose a context within which to teach medicine, the better to accommodate it to the scientific and social changes swirling about us. If the argument has merit, others may be stimulated to rework it, fill in gaps, or perhaps offer alternatives.

Finally, for whom is the book written? Obviously, since its focus is on medical education, it is written for medical educators, including teachers of both basic science and clinical medicine. I hope the book will appeal also to medical geneticists, to physicians interested in public health, and perhaps especially to family physicians—indeed, to all physicians or students interested in examining ideas that could inform and guide their work. Whether the book will appeal to those in the social sciences or other disciplines now pressing their viewpoints on medicine, I cannot guess. I hope that, were they to read it, they would find it worthwhile, because the book will show that medicine can, if it will, embrace both science and society.

Acknowledgments

It is a pleasure to acknowledge the help of friends and colleagues. I owe a special debt to David Valle, with whom I have taught elective courses for graduate students in genetics. Many of the thoughts expressed in the book were generated in those courses, so there is an obligation to those students, too. In addition, Dr. Valle read the entire manuscript and gave me many valuable and illuminating criticisms. Indeed, chapter 14, on defining the gene, owes as much to him as to me. Kirby Smith, Joseph D. McInerney, and John W. Littlefield also read the whole book, to my profit in both principle and detail. I have the same obligation to Alfred Knudson, whose criticisms of the manuscript were both helpful and to the point. I was also stimulated by reading his book, *Genetics and Disease* (McGraw-Hill, 1965), which was an earlier effort to show how medical thought would profit by genetic modification.

Ideas for the book were often generated in conversation with friends. For this, I am particularly grateful to Charles Scriver and Alexander Bearn, as well as for their much-valued encouragement before and during the writing. I also relied on Bearn's biography of Archibald Garrod for insights into Garrod's thinking. Reassuring reports on reading the book were also given by Henry Seidel and Peter Rowe, and over the years Saul Brusilow has been a patient wedding guest to my ancient mariner. Alexander Leaf's encouragement was especially helpful, coming from a nongeneticist interested in preventive medicine. And I owe a long-standing debt to Joshua Lederberg for his interest and help in other projects that led inevitably to this one. I am also very grateful to Janet Smith, who cheerfully typed draft after draft after draft. Finally, I thank McGraw-Hill for permission to use parts of chapter 2 of the seventh edition of *The Metabolic and Molecular Bases of Inherited Disease.*

GENETIC MEDICINE

1

Introduction

War is too important to be left to the military.
—Aristide Briand, letter to David Lloyd George

The necessity to commit so much of his nation's human, material, and financial resources to the pursuit of the 1914–18 war led Briand, then premier of France, to express this opinion in a 1916 letter to the British prime minister. It seemed that the generals were too intent on military objectives to be aware of the war's impact on civilian soldiers, their families, and the whole of society. So civilian authority was imposed on the grand strategy of war. Today the same fate is overtaking medicine, not for any failure (it has been a huge success), but because medicine is being perceived as too important to be left to the doctors.

The list of interested parties is long. In addition to biologists, it includes anthropologists (1–3), economists (4–6), epidemiologists, ethicists (7–9), lawyers (10), sociologists (11–16), humanists (17), social and medical historians (18–22), theologians, philosophers (23–26), politicians and governments, representatives of business and industry, and elements of the population that include lobbying groups and the now very numerous disease-related organizations. All of these bodies have their own ideas about medicine and how, as outsiders, they might influence it. They have observed how encompassing medicine has become, how invasive, and how risky. Many say it is far too expensive, others that it threatens ethical and moral principles. Legal actions abound as never before, and an insatiable need for new technology has generated new businesses.

It was the isolation of the generals of the Great War that excited the attention of civilians. Can it be that medicine has been isolated from its constituencies and did not anticipate their need to participate? Or is it that the tentacles of a highly technological medicine have reached into so many aspects of human life and society that everyone is unavoidably involved in it in some way? Perhaps it is both.

Each of the disciplines listed above relies on some set of time-honored traditions and principles to which it appeals for authority. Medicine has a long tradition, too, dating to the ancients, and it has followed unswervingly its aim of helping the sick. It appeals to science, especially biology, for the information to construct its special knowledge, but it may be unique in that it appeals also to social rules for its practice, and the intensity of the interest in medicine of so many elements of society testifies to its dependence on them. Indeed, medical wisdom is best exemplified in the consonance of the uses of its scientific knowledge with the social milieus in which it is dispensed. The latter includes several levels of society. At the level of the individual, there are intensely personal one-to-one encounters, and as the familial nature of disease becomes more obvious, whole families become the object of scrutiny. Communities, too, are involved in services offered by departments of health, well-baby clinics, immunizations, and programs for testing for specific genes. Health maintenance organizations are community resources, and we are seeing the engagement of state and federal governments in debates about access to and costs of medical care. Governments have long been engaged in regulation and support of research and training.

Cultural impact is also observed in substantial changes in the way people live. Diet, exercise, and disciplined living have all had an impact on health, and industry has not been slow to develop markets for paraphernalia appropriate to new lifestyles. Other debates touching on mores, ethics, and philosophy swirl around such issues as the use of abortion to prevent the birth of babies shown by antenatal tests to be doomed to abnormality. Questions are raised about progress itself: Would a substantial lengthening of the human lifespan be compatible with a culture worth living in? And is medical progress dimming our perception of the necessity to die (7)? In all of these social activities, medicine, as the only repository of knowledge of how human biology is affected by disease, is deeply involved. Some of the agencies formally appointed to represent it, however, concentrate on preserving a historical medical presence and do not always see such issues as within their purview.

But that that presence is being changed anyway is evident in a new language, one that reveals a new public perception. Medicine has become "health care," which is "delivered" to "consumers" by "care givers." "Health maintenance" is provided by "HMOs," which, along with "for profit" hospitals, constitute a "health industry," a phrase that refers to the whole medical enterprise. These nontraditional words and phrases represent the thinking of those to whom medicine in all its forms is a commodity to be packaged and delivered. They constitute an ominous language that should be widely remarked. It omits the humanism of encounters between doctors and patients, the ideas and intellectual energy that went into the development of medicine's laboratory arm, and the clinical and basic research that supports its claim to be a learned profession. And this language is inimical to medicine's identity as a vital element of our culture that contributes both to the humanities and to science and is worthy of its university affiliation.

What about medicine's scientific face? Does scientific medicine have a theoretical base of ultimate appeal? Some would say it is contained in biology, which is itself founded on the rock of evolution. But this is only a partial truth, since medicine has tended to adopt only those aspects of biology that are clearly relevant to the attainment of medicine's conventional aims. The choice of what is considered relevant biology is revealed very early to the medical student, who is taught that knowledge of normal structure and function must precede that of disease, that pathogenesis represents abnormality. This is an unassailable principle but cannot be an adequate basis for understanding disease if it omits details of how "the normal" became the norm, how it varies in both biology and the public perception, and what implications this has for both congruence and incongruence of species and individuals with their physical and cultural environments. That is, an adequate basis for understanding disease must appeal to natural selection and evolution; medical thinking that fails to do so is based on a selective biology.

EDUCATION AND TRAINING

How can medical teaching be based on this limited conception? Is it possible that too little distinction is drawn between education and training? The word *education* derives from the Latin *ducare*, meaning to lead, and the prefix *e,* or *ex,* meaning out of. But what does the educator lead the student out of? Perhaps it is the morass of facts that must be synthesized and integrated to bring out meanings not inherent in the facts themselves. Hence, education deals with ideas that form frameworks within which to work with factual information to form coherent structures of knowledge. Information and knowledge are not the same thing; the former consists of facts and data, the latter includes perception and comprehension. Perhaps information is the thread of which the fabric of knowledge is woven. Thus, it seems possible to be informed but not knowledgeable, let alone wise—wisdom being the capacity to discern relationships, to assign value to knowledge and to use it rationally. The embededness of these concepts was acknowledged with poetic economy by T. S. Eliot in "Choruses from 'The Rock'": "Where is the wisdom we have lost in knowledge? Where is the knowledge we have lost in information?"

Our word *training* also derives from the Latin, this time from *trahere,* meaning to pull or drag. Is there in the contrast between the Latin words for education and training a hint of volition in the former and of coercion in the latter? Perhaps, but while everyone knows that training involves learning the information and processes for actual doing, the best training is to be had under the tutelage of teachers both knowledgeable and wise. So education arms the student for the future; training, for the present. Education leads into adaptive paths; training shows how to do the adapting. Training is leavened by the yeast of education.

Used in this way, *education* raises questions of why things happen and training of how. Answers to the how questions explain pathogenesis and the consequent signs and symptoms and point the way to effective treatments. In contrast, answers to the why questions explain why disease exists at all, why human disorders differ from those of other species, why this person came down with this disease at this time of life while that person came down with another disease at another stage, and perhaps most important, in going beyond the proximate causes to the conditions that engender them, such answers suggest how disease might be prevented. That is, answers to the why questions invoke not only biology but also all those other disciplines that clamor to be heard. For example, if some aspect of how society works is perceived as a remote cause of disease (let us think here of the tobacco industry), then other disciplines are necessarily engaged. The medical student needs to think about how these diverse influences bear on the patients who suffer with each disease, in addition to the measures to be taken to treat and prevent them. In such thinking, the origins of disease in incongruities between human biology and an environment strongly influenced by human culture will become apparent.

Education, as I have used the word here, is synthetic; training, analytic. When the analytic is emphasized at the expense of the synthetic, the cultural and biological origins of the conditions that predispose to the immediate causes of disease may be omitted, and an essential dimension of understanding is compromised. One result is that the biology presented to first-year medical students, while completely coherent within itself, may not correlate well with principles of disease that must encompass both molecular biology and the behavior of whole organisms that bring to the experience of disease a phylogenetic, an ontogenetic, and a cultural identity. The synthesis of medical thinking with principles that express this uniqueness of endowment, development, and experience constitutes a logic of disease. This book is devoted to developing such a logic.

A Logic of Disease

To be comprehensible, a logic of disease requires a language common to biology, medicine, and other disciplines. In fact, there is such a language: that of the DNA. In literature the same language is used to describe in detail an hour in the life of an ordinary citizen and, in the broadest strokes, the rise and collapse of civilizations. But what happened during the hour so minutely scrutinized was unquestionably informed and constrained by the culture of the civilization of which the citizen was a part. At the same time, we know that the fates of civilizations hinge on the actions of their citizens. In like manner, the DNA provides a language that prefigures possibilities and constraints for both the development and the present state of the homeostasis of cells, organs, and individuals, while also encoding their phylogenetic history. So the language of the DNA connects physiology with evolution. It is a language common to biology and medicine, a language useful for describing how and why things work and fail to work, and it is a language with which those other disciplines must be familiar if medicine is to go forward in their company.

A New Infrastructure?

Is medicine ready for such a logic? The literature of medical education suggests that something is needed, while that of medical sociology and economics tells us that substantial changes in medical practice are already upon us. So, if medicine is to retain its authority in the "health industry," it will be because changes in economics and practice are justified by the ideas and principles that constitute a medical "infrastructure." This is a trendy word, entirely consonant with "health industry," but it does define the structure on which some edifice or system is based—that which gives it meaning and unity, and which enables it to function within its boundaries. In ordinary usage, infrastructure includes highways, transportation, communication, waste disposal, public buildings, and the like—the physical apparatus that enables nations, cities, and other communities to work. Schools and universities are also often included as necessary elements of a workable society. What I mean by proposing an overhaul of the medical infrastructure is the establishment of a more comprehensive integration, even a synthesis, of the ideas of medicine and genetics, the better to accommodate not only conventional medical aims but also those of the other clamorous disciplines.

The Gene and Individual Variation

The central feature in the integration of biology and medicine is the idea of the gene, expressed in the language of the DNA. Genes specify the proteins that form the units of which homeostatic devices are composed. The structure and function of these units is the focus of molecular biology. But molecular biology is entirely reductionist, while the idea of the gene leads us not only centrifugally to the ultimate dispersion of our particulate nature but also centripetally to the coherent articulation of those parts into unique, individual, open systems. In addition, the principle of the gene ties both species and individual to their phylogenetic history, to ontogeny, and to the homeostasis of the moment. It is the embodiment of a biological memory as well as a portent of the future. It is the genes that are transmitted from one generation to the next. Then, after providing the organism with an outline for its structure and development and after specifying the molecules that are the engines of cells, organs, and individuals, the genes become the servant of all of these, responding to signals from within and without that promote choices among the options inherent in the outline and that enable uniquely individual open systems to live in congruence with the environment. The indifference of that environment tests the powers of such open systems to reproduce and so to contribute to the variety of the species. Thus, in exercising at once a determining and a responsive role in the characterization of variable phenotypes that are subject to natural selection, the genes are instruments of evolution.

If genes and their products are so central to evolution, development, individuality, and living in congruence with the environment, it is inescapable that variant products, specified by variant genes, must have a cardinal role in living incongruently with the environment—that is, in disease and in the way each individual expresses it. Such genetically determined incongruence is a consequence of the species' need for a sufficient store of variability to preserve its competence to adapt to new environments. So, if the genes are so critical in the making of a human being and in the governance of each unique life, medical education ought, perhaps, to begin with the idea of the genes, their origins, their structure, their variation, and all their works, including as one of the most prominent ideas of medicine their role, by means of variation in the unit steps of homeostasis, in the promotion of individuality. Today, genetics is recognized in the medical curriculum and in practice as "medical genetics," a diminutive branch, even a twig, of the mighty oak of medicine. The phrase suggests that there is a bit of medicine that is genetic, implying a limit to how much disease can be illuminated by genetic principles. But when these words are reversed to read "genetic medicine," no such limitation is suggested, and it is implied that any or all of medicine may be the beneficiary.

Genetic Medicine

Medical genetics was readily accepted as a medical specialty. It fulfills the criteria of disease classification and departmental segregation observed in the organization of medical schools, and, like other specialties, it has an accrediting board and an American college. But how is a genetic medicine to be defined, and how pursued? As the phrase suggests, it is a medicine in which the idea of disease is observed to obey a logic imposed by the qualities of the genes that lay out options for and set limits on the variability of individual human beings. Those genes determine, through the properties of their products, who is vulnerable to which disease to be experienced when in life and as a result of which experiences of the environment.

Diseases are caused by the independent action of neither genes nor experiences, but by the influence of each on the protein products that are unit steps of the homeostasis of specific individuals in whom they coincide for reasons traceable to phylogeny and culture. That is, the qualities of diseases are constrained by human evolution and by the ecological and social organization on which individual open systems depend. This view of disease departs from the conventional definition that fixes on reductionist causes by emphasizing the origins of such causes, deepening thereby our understanding of how diseases are engendered. It is a significant change in medical thinking. But is it likely that such a change will be accepted, especially in view of the manifest success of current medical practices? And if a shift in mentality is feasible, how can such a logic help students and physicians to a better understanding of disease?

Feasibility

As for feasibility, medical thinking has changed before. The nineteenth century saw an association of clinical expressions with morbid anatomy, while in the early twentieth century, the Flexner report marked a move away from morbid anatomy to a physiological and biochemical analysis of the pathogenesis of disease, while today's molecular and genetic explanations mark the era of the analysis of the individual. Physicians are conservative about changes in their thinking, but they do not oppose its evolution. As for the reorientation suggested here, something of the sort is already happening. Every day the journals carry news of the isolation of genes for classical inborn errors and descriptions of new genetic vulnerabilities. The Human Genome Project, whose promise it is to identify all of the tens of thousands of human gene loci, is proceeding apace. So the idea of genes as real entities with variable structures and functions that have palpable influences on the existence and expressions of disease has not only penetrated medical thought but has also begun to pervade its academic reaches. For example, the mutant low-density lipoprotein receptor as a contributor to atherosclerosis in some people is a staple of medical teaching. And if one such variant, why not others? There are others, including genes specifying lipoproteins, endothelins, fibrinogen, angiotensin-converting enzyme, platelet and growth factors, and others too whose variants conspire to contribute to atherosclerosis and coronary artery disease. High blood pressure, diabetes, and schizophrenia are other disorders that are yielding to the pursuit of the gene hunters. But the aggregated mass of newly discovered genes will contribute to a babel of voices unless coherence is imposed by some logic. So it is not a matter of feasibility, it is a matter of necessity.

Uses of the Logic

How will a logic of disease serve students, practitioners, patients, and society? Answering these questions is what this book is about.

A medical mentality that embraces an idea of disease based on the gene and its relationship to ontogeny, phylogeny, culture, and society as well as to natural selection and evolution offers several advantages. First, the same logic would underlie the search for causes and pathogenesis of all diseases. The logic applies across all classes. Second, in the logic, diseases are perceived as stemming from incongruities between the unit steps of homeostasis, each specified by a gene that is itself a product of phylogeny, and aspects of the environment, including those related to the organization of societies and cultures. It is these remote causes that determine who gets sick, when, and in what way, and that set the stage for the action of the proximate provocations of disease. Third, since evolution is a consequence of descent with modification, the logic emphasizes the individuality of the patients who have diseases that are outcomes of the mutations that account for that modification. Each patient is a unique version of the disease, with unique needs for management. Fourth, since genetic vulnerabilities lead to incongruence with aspects of the environment, logic requires the same energy and zeal in the search for preventive environments as for treatments. Indeed, as the list of human genes and their mutants expands, prevention could even attain a position of primacy in medical thinking. And since the vulnerabilities are genetic and familial, it is likely that such preventive duties will fall to primary care physicians. Fifth, by giving medical students a view of the cosmos along with the facts, relationships among disciplines within medicine are likely to be clarified. If medicine is to chart its own destiny in a political world, its various compartments must be unified by a common mentality. The medical specialties, preventive medicine, and public health are each perceived as separate enterprises, but all are informed by the principle of the human species composed of genetically unique open systems, each a novel test of selective pressures exerted by nature and society.

Finally, the logic offers an intellectual framework in which to think about medicine's inner coherence and how it relates to the cultures and societies of this world. Given such a logic, medicine can participate with authority in debates about social issues that touch on the health of individuals, species, and the planet. An example is the International Physicians for the Prevention of Nuclear War, who were awarded the Nobel Peace Prize for their advocacy of control over nuclear weapons. No doubt they were acting as informed citizens, but they were no less agents of medicine. Are they not an example to us all?

I
Medical Thinking

The introductory chapter proposed a logic of disease arising from a synthesis of conventional medical thinking and principles expressing the uniqueness of human beings. This section of the book is devoted to providing the basis for that logic.

In chapter 2, alternative medical mentalities are contrasted in the ideas of William Osler and Archibald Garrod, leaders in setting the agenda for medical thinking at different times. The contrast lies in their different perceptions of the meaning of causes, individuality, and definitions of disease. In chapter 3, problems of medical education observed by medical teachers are described, together with their remedies. But because the remedies represent changes that do not deviate from existing thought, better solutions might be found in a different way of thinking. Accordingly, a basis for a new logic of disease is outlined. Its components include individuality, remote as well as proximate causes, and a definition of disease that derives from the principles of evolution and natural selection. Chapters 4 and 5 provide the details of this logic which, in offering a framework of ideas for genetic medicine, require some changes in conventional medical thought.

2

Inborn Errors and Chemical Individuality

It might be claimed that what used to be spoken of as a diathesis is nothing else but chemical individuality. But to our chemical individualities are due our chemical *merits* as well as our chemical shortcomings; and it is more nearly true to say that the factors which confer upon us our predispositions to and immunities from the various mishaps which are spoken of as diseases, are inherent in our very chemical structure; and even in the molecular groupings which confer upon us our individualities, and which went to the making of the chromosomes from which we sprang.

—Archibald E. Garrod, *Inborn Factors in Disease*

That reader of Shakespeare who complained that the plays were flawed by an unrestrained reliance on clichês has a counterpart in medicine who will groan when confronted by yet another reference to Archibald Garrod and his inborn errors. But Garrod's "clichês" represent no less profound insights into the variety of human disease than those of Shakespeare into the diversity of human behavior. Shakespeare's lines are so familiar because they express with such economy those crises and turning points of life that claim our interest because they are universal and representative of us all, while Garrod's propositions, no less universal, claim our interest because they are representative of individuals.

Garrod's observations lay almost unnoticed for many years, but in the 1950s, inborn errors, defined as recessive enzyme deficiencies, attracted interest because methods capable of detecting them became available. Since then the description of new deficiencies has accelerated rapidly. Looking back, it is evident that the definition has expanded, too, revealing the complexity and universality of the idea.

The history of this flowering of a concept central in medical thinking is readily observed in the several editions of *The Metabolic and Molecular Bases of Inherited Disease (MMBID)* (1,2). The first appeared in 1960, with the inborn error as its theme. The editors advanced their intention to present "the pertinent clinical, biochemical, and genetic information concerning those metabolic anomalies which have been grouped under Garrod's engaging term, 'the inborn errors of metabolism'" (3). They also recognized that the existing list of inborn errors was exhaustive in neither number nor quality, and this sensitivity to undiscovered disease was extended in later editions to a definition of the inborn error enlarged beyond recessive enzyme deficiencies. Each edition included not only new disorders inherited in all Mendelian modes but also diseases previously excluded because they did not fit the prevailing restricted definition of an inborn error. For example, the second edition included defects of serum proteins and clotting, and in the fourth the immune system made its appearance. By the sixth edition, 374 disorders were listed, embracing defects in an all-inclusive list of proteins, cell types, and organs, and the definition of the inborn error had been extended to cancer and developmental defects due to chromosomal anomalies. In the current, seventh edition, there are 469 inborn errors, an increase of nearly 30 percent.

Given this pace of discovery and description of new disorders, the editors may be wondering if they have come face to face with what Garrod foresaw as early as 1909: "Among the complex metabolic processes of which the human body is the seat there is room for an almost countless variety of such sports" (4). He also observed that many of these might be missed because they had not "advertised their presence in some conspicuous way." But modern technology is designed expressly to discover those advertisements, no matter how subtle, so the editors of *MMBID* have given notice that their book will embrace any disease as soon as some glimmering of its biochemical-genetic attributes is perceived. And, the hundreds of chapters now included are devoted to molecular descriptions of mutant genes, the proteins in which the mutant effects reside, and the impact of each upon its homeostatic system and, ultimately, the whole organism.

Obviously this expanded definition embraces not only the monogenic inborn error but also those disorders called multifactorial, which constitute the chief bane of humankind. It imposes no barrier to the inclusion of, say, prostatic hypertrophy and varicose veins, which in the general consensus are hardly perceived as due to inborn errors. In fact, although varicose veins are often familial, I know of no extensive genetic analysis, but family studies have shown both hypertrophy and cancer of the prostate to be associated with at least one gene of dominant effect (5,6). Since it is a reflex in the 1990s to proceed to a molecular exploration once a gene is suggested by genetic analysis, who can doubt that the eighth edition of *MMBID* will list these disorders together with the mutants at each relevant locus? Surely we are witnessing a change in medical thought no less profound than that which occurred when morbid anatomy gave way to biochemical interpretations of pathogenesis. It is a change in the canon.

Medical Thinking

GARROD'S THINKING

The development of Garrod's thinking has been perceptively recounted by Bearn in *Archibald Garrod and the Individuality of Man* (7). The biographer shows how the idea of the inborn error crystallized in Garrod's mind while he studied patients with alkaptonuria (7,8). In such patients the inborn error lay in their inability to degrade the benzene ring of homogentisic acid for want of the enzyme assigned to that step in the pathway. This idea led Garrod to infer that alkaptonuria was only one of what must be a nearly limitless list of variations that account in the aggregate for a chemical individuality that identifies each human being no less definitively than the more obvious physical properties by which each of is known. Few of the variants that Garrod knew in his lifetime were diseases defined by disability or threat to life. Indeed, had he perceived all inborn errors as diseases, the extension to chemical individuality might have had less appeal. That is, had he had to define inborn errors as we have done, in the context of overwhelming, often lethal diseases, it is palpably less likely that he would have seen such catastrophes as simply one end of an uninterrupted distribution of the variation that characterizes the species.

Bearn also directs our attention to Garrod's recognition of the evolutionary implications of his ideas. The diversity in the composition of proteins that differentiates one species from others suggested to Garrod that such variation did not stop at species borders but continued into chemical individuality so that it was not interspecies diversity but chemical individuality that formed the substrate for natural selection and evolution.

Late in his life Garrod summarized his thoughts in a second book, *Inborn Factors in Disease* (9). In this book he relegated the rare inborn errors to a lesser role as opposed to more frequent disorders for which he used "diathesis," a word that had been discredited, he said, because the idea was lacking in substance. Redefined as "susceptibility based on chemical individuality," the concept became infused with meaning. Such individuality must be a vital ingredient in the cause of any disease, since "in every case of every malady there are two sets of factors at work in the formation of the morbid picture, namely, internal or constitutional factors inherent in the sufferer and usually inherited from his forebears, and external ones which fire the train." He thought that these internal inherited factors were generally latent and "apt to be revealed sooner or later by the effects produced by external influences which are innocuous to the average man." Indeed, "for some individuals, those trifling traumata which go to make up the wear and tear of daily life are apparently the provoking cause of grave disorders." Many of these thoughts are drawn together in the last paragraph of *Inborn Factors*, which was quoted at the beginning of this chapter.

We cannot know what Garrod meant by the "molecular groupings which confer" mentioned in that paragraph. Certainly he didn't mean the DNA. In fact, he never had any particular interest in genetics (7). Nor could he have meant amino acid sequence in proteins since the recognition that such sequences confer specificity came only after 1940 (10). But it is clear that he saw that people differ in susceptibility to disease as a result of hereditary chemical variation, itself grist for the mill of natural selection and evolution. Obviously, Garrod could not have imagined how today we can give genetic and molecular body to the concept of diathesis, and should a historian quarrel with a too-modern interpretation of an idea that is really an adumbration of a concept of disease just now taking shape, such a critic might at least agree that Garrod provided a substrate for the development of modern ideas, a structural foundation, a mode of thought that is, in any case, more important than whether or not he was interested in or knew anything about genes.

So the enlarging conception of the inborn error as it is taking shape in *MMBID* is something Garrod anticipated and would have been delighted to observe. And it is the basis for the reorientation of our thinking about disease. Unlike Garrod we do know about the DNA that specifies the proteins that both constitute and regulate the unit steps of the homeostatic systems that characterize our species, and we know a little about how their variation confers biochemical uniqueness on each human being. And, in principle, we know how to use that knowledge to explain the origins of disease. Such an expanded definition of the inborn error tells us that all diseases arise out of some condition of incongruence between a chemical constitution and those environmental factors that "fire the train."

The expansion in Garrod's mind of the idea of the inborn error, originally defined as a recessive enzyme deficiency, to a chemical individuality that differentiates human beings and takes the form in some of a diathesis or vulnerability to disease, all stemming from the imperatives of evolution, represents a transcending logic that makes sense of what must otherwise seem random. So to pursue Garrod's thinking to the end, we must seek a logic of disease compatible with outcomes of evolution as the principle from which all else flows.

GARROD AND OSLER: A CONTRAST

Archibald Garrod succeeded William Osler as Regius Professor of Medicine at Oxford. There is a prophetic symbolism in this. Osler, or the Oslerian ideal—it is not easy to separate the man from the myth—dominated medicine in his time as few have done before or since (11). And in large degree the ideal persists to this day (12,13). Disease is accepted simply as a fact of life and it is the doctor's duty to deal with it. Osler's book *The Principles and Practice of Medicine* begins on page 1 with the diagnosis and treatment of typhoid fever

(14). There is no preliminary discussion of the nature of disease, of who is likely to be sick, who escapes, or why anyone should ever be sick at all. The function of a medical school, Osler says, is "to instruct men about disease, what it is, what are its manifestations, how it may be prevented, and how it may be cured" (15). As for medical education, "the student begins with the patient, continues with the patient, and ends his studies with the patient, using books and lectures as tools, as means to an end" (16). Osler put his considerable weight behind the idea of bedside teaching, of student participation in hospital care. Indeed, he said, "It is a safe rule to have no teaching without a patient for a text, and the best teaching is taught by the patient himself" (17). Such experiences with hospitalized patients formed the embryonic doctor's conception of disease as a puzzle to be solved.

To solve the conundrum the clinician was expected to use all five senses, a profound knowledge of pathology, and a broad experience of disease to arrive at a diagnosis that accurately reflected the pathological process that produced the signs and symptoms. That is, in Osler's time, diagnosis was based on morbid anatomy and, then as now, knowledge of pathogenesis was needed to formulate any more than symptomatic treatment.

We adhere to the Oslerian ideal today, and if morbid anatomy, the Clinical Pathological Conference, and finely honed senses have given way to biochemical and molecular diagnosis aided by visual techniques that peer into remote recesses of the body, we still adapt our treatments to what we can learn about pathogenesis. And although we often fall short, we are still exhorted to pay at least as much attention to the needs, fears, and comfort of the patient as to the products of technological devices. In the Oslerian vein we ask, "What disease does the patient have and how do I treat it?" The emphasis is on the disease and how its effects are to be reversed. The patient, who is perceived as representative of the class of people with the disease at hand, might be anybody. The same question, phrased in the Garrodian context, might be "What disease does this particular human being have? Why does he have it at this time in his life? In what way does he differ from the others among whom he lives? What can I do to restore this person's unique orientation to the environment?" Like Garrod, Osler perceived disease as "chemicophysical," but unlike Garrod, he never advanced the idea of biological individuality among patients.

Although both physicians no doubt wore striped trousers and a black coat when seeing patients in consultation, their ideas were poles apart. The difference between them is this: Osler, the activist, saw in a patient a broken machine and was at pains to tell the world how to fix it; Garrod, a contemplative man, saw the patient not as a broken machine but as a less well adapted product of evolution and the disease as a consequence of a unique individual's encounter with an environment for which he was uniquely unfit. Why this difference? Osler accepted the age-old maxim that viewed the body as a machine, but the inborn-ness of alkaptonuria started Garrod on a trail of original thought. To his mind there could not be only one, or even a few, inborn chemical qualities; there had to be many, and if many, they constituted a chemical individuality each of which represents a unique test of natural selection, an experiment in evolution. Osler's knowledge of evolution is not in question, but his silence on the subject suggests that he gave it minor emphasis, whereas Garrod perceived it as a starting point in education.

Osler taught us how to practice medicine; Garrod, how to think about it. Osler conjured with facts; Garrod, with ideas. Oslerian thinking is organized around treatment and management. It is a practical approach in which the student is perceived as an apprentice. It is pretty much what we do in residency training. Garrodian thinking, in contrast, is about concepts: what diseases are and why they exist. In the expansion of the idea of the inborn error, in accepting susceptibility as a consequence of chemical individuality, and in recognizing that both concepts flow from evolutionary necessity, we are witnessing a transition from an Oslerian medicine to ideas that represent a natural elaboration of Garrod's thoughts. No one would deny that Osler was the hero of the medicine of the twentieth century. It is likely that Garrod will be the icon of the twenty-first.

3

The Transition from Oslerian
to Garrodian Medicine

In the 1980's, medical education has been under attack by many critics, including prominent university and foundation leaders, The Association of American Medical Colleges, the federal government, and the general public—not to mention the self-criticism of medical school officials themselves. What is striking is how little the complaints about medical education heard today have changed from those made by medical educators and informed citizens since the turn of the century.

—K. M. Ludmerer, *Learning to Heal:*
The Development of American Medical Education

Ludmerer is here asserting the continuing triumph of the Oslerian ideal. There have always been flaws evident in medical education and practice, but no change in the canon has been suggested. Have things changed since Ludmerer's book was published in 1985? In a summary of 24 reports published between 1910 and 1993, Christakis confirms Ludmerer's observation by emphasizing the similarity of proposed reforms intended to bolster and reaffirm ideas rather than to change them (1).

The previous chapter outlined some of the contrasts in the thinking of Garrod and Osler, the two Regius professors. The question to be taken up now is whether those contrasts give us guidance for responses to calls for reform in medical education. Some may say that we have already attained a Garrodian state of mind, that the rich lore of human biology and genetics is sufficient to inform a logic of disease. No doubt we are on our way to that goal, most notably perhaps in our grasp of the implications of inborn errors, but in our growing understanding of more complex diseases, too. The discovery of chemical individuality in atherosclerosis, high blood pressure, and diabetes, for example, shows how our gaze is shifting from types to the individual. The variety of the risk factors, both genetic and of experience, tells us that each affected person suffers a singular version of each of these diseases. But examination of medical textbooks suggests that we still have a long way to go. While it is true that genetics—that branch of biology that embraces the idea of individuality—has become a medical watchword, there is every reason to believe that human genetics has been adapted to existing medical thinking, rather than having been allowed to change it.

In what follows, the basis for present medical thinking is compared with an alternative. A contrast is most informative when polarities are brought out, but reality is likely to reside somewhere in between. The best of all worlds is attained in the doctor who cleaves to the Oslerian ideal in his practice and the Garrodian in his thinking.

Prevalent Medical Thought

Human society is based on ideas. They inform and shape all our actions, and are often deeply embedded in and interlaced with our identity and self-esteem. They lie there unarticulated and unexamined, and when threatened by a contrary idea, however rational, they are likely to be fiercely defended. Medical education is based on such firmly rooted ideas, which are seldom examined with the thought of any sweeping change. But as Christakas showed, when it is accepted that changes are necessary, it is to the details of existing education and practice that attention is directed, when it might be that what is needed is some fundamentally new idea (1). And if the new idea meets the need, education is likely to be compelled in logic to follow. Discoveries in human biology and, particularly, in genetics urge just such a search for new ideas.

It should be noted that there are differences between medical thinking and medical practice. The former embraces the ideas that guide and constrain medicine. These are given up reluctantly, sometimes being retained even after events have overtaken them. Medical practice, in contrast, changes readily according to the compelling dictates of new data. And that is appropriate. Changes in the thinking that forms the basis for practice should be slow and carefully negotiated.

The Body as a Machine

The prevailing metaphor of medicine is that of the body as a machine that the doctor is called upon to fix when it breaks; the doctor's role is that of an engineer who uses technology in the service of practical utility (2–6). This metaphor is apposite in summarizing today's events, however complex they may seem. Biology is composed of hierarchical levels, each shaped by the one below. Molecular biology is the bottom most and thereby illuminates everything above. Examined in this way, the body *is* a machine, and molecular biology and genetics are showing us its most fundamental components. We are being given glimpses of how the machine is assembled and integrated and of how its automatic controls keep it together and capable of life.

Because the engineer is expected to fix the disabled machine, the governing criterion of this view of medicine is cure. Of course, reality requires that amelioration be accepted, if only until details of the breakage that point to the actual cure are discovered. And there is faith in the capacity of science to find a cure. This optimism has been expressed by Lewis Thomas, who said, "I cannot imagine any category of human disease that we are precluded by nature from thinking our way around. . . . Disease comes as a result of biological mistakes . . . the mechanisms of disease are quite open to intelligent intervention and reversal whenever we learn more about how they operate" (7). Medicine has been defined by Seldin in just such a context as "a narrow discipline. Its goals are the relief of pain, the prevention of disability, and the postponement of death by the application of the theoretical knowledge incorporated in medical science" (8). The basic sciences, he said, furnish a theoretical framework for clinical medicine, consisting of physiological homeostasis with its powers of communication and regulation. So medicine uses biology to provide insights that lead to the discovery and explanation of pathogenesis, the better to invent an appropriate treatment. Herein lie the triumphs of medicine: cell and molecular biology show where and how disease has distorted homeostasis.

This is where Thomas's "thinking around" is going on, and the rate at which information is accumulating ensures that no one can encompass more than some limited fragment of the whole. For example, Osler carried *The Principles and Practice of Medicine* through eight editions by himself. Now in its twenty-second edition, the book has five editors and 159 contributors (9). This pattern is the rule now, whatever the book's subject or however narrow the specialty. So when observed from some Olympian height, there is an inescapable sense that here at last, in all this concerted effort, the promise of continuous and open-ended progress is being fulfilled, and that if there is an end to it, it will only be after all the questions have been answered. If we know the sequence of base pairs in the entire human genome, shall we not be well on our way to the millennium (10)?

SIGNS OF UNEASE

This engineering mentality dominates medical thought, and through its influence on the classification of diseases it has shaped medical institutions. For example, specialization has followed the classification of diseases by organ system, etiology, age, and sex, with consequent influence on the organization of departments and divisions in medical schools and hospitals, and with obvious reflection on medical teaching, training, and care. It is a system that worked to public advantage, but, given the rapidity of recent change, it can surprise no one that there are signs of strain. Thoughts identifying this strain have appeared in many books, reviews, and papers over the past twenty years, publications that represent a comprehensive analysis of medical education and practice (11–27). They report the thinking of medical academicians, historians, sociologists, and other observers; some are the proceedings and recommendations of meetings at which the diverse views of scientists, physicians, ethicists, and administrators were forged into assessments of prevailing conditions and counsel for the future. One of these perceived "a continuing and accelerating erosion in the education of physicians," while another muses on "the prevailing biomedical model based on Cartesian dualism and the monoetiological, or seventeenth century, approach to understanding the origins of disease" (14,17). All express misgivings about (a) medical education, (b) the doctor-patient relationship and the public interest, (c) the fragmentation of the medical enterprise, and (d) an apparent inability easily to accommodate prevention.

Some Questions

The Facts

The questions that emerge from the deliberations of these individuals and bodies are of three kinds. First, what is it about medical teaching that disappoints, even disillusions, students? Is it the mountain of facts generated by modern biology? These facts, in all their baroque detail, are said to be too great a burden for any mind to bear, and it is apparent that the massive accumulation of information has engendered centrifugal forces that have fragmented the medical enterprise into many self-contained subdisciplines without at the same time providing a countervailing logic to hold them all together. Biology was supposed to provide the "theoretical framework for clinical medicine" (8), but apparently does so imperfectly. Gunderman tells us that students themselves perceive a need for a "mental framework" for understanding health and disease (28). Is this a consequence of incompatibility in teaching aims? Do the teachers of the preclinical years not bring out the coherence of the facts and their relevance to medicine?

Human Identity

Second, the reports ask, by what means can we bring the benefits of science to bear on disease without omitting the identity and human qualities of patients? It seems that emphasis on facts has drawn the doctor's attention toward disease processes and away from the biological and social individuality of the patient. This detachment has been remarked by many. For example, Cassell suggested that we have come to think that technology will do the doctor's work (29). In making a diagnosis, technology is presumed to replace the doctor's subjective judgment and to take the uncertainty out of the process. But in doing so, both doctor and patient are diminished; the former becomes in some degree a passive conduit for information provided by technology, while the latter is reduced to little more than those elements of physiology that have been subjected to the scrutiny of diagnostic machinery. The individuality of the encounter is neglected on both sides, and the civility of a meeting of two human beings is omitted. Also missing are those concerns for the patient's social and spiritual well-being Walsh McDermott called "samaritan functions" (30). Reiser also holds these views, pointing out that the technology of diagnosis causes a primary physician to see his patient "indirectly through a screen of machines and specialists," estranging him from both his patient and his own judgment (11). Again, the doctor-patient relationship is the victim; the current of identity that animates a human relationship is deflected.

This fading out of the presence of the patient and the humanity of the medical encounter is nowhere better exhibited than in the history of grand rounds. Beginning as a demonstration of the virtuosity of the professor as clinician and doctor, grand rounds were conducted on the wards, where the professor and an entourage of residents and students moved from bed to bed to speak to, examine, and encourage several patients. The patients saw themselves as interesting to important doctors who addressed them by name and who heard and answered their questions. But in time the exercise was moved to a lecture hall where, although patients were still present, the encounter was limited, the better to discuss the disorder represented. Next, the actual patient was dispensed with and the "rounds" became a review of one person's problem which, in his physical absence, became more and more abstract. Finally, the patient disappeared altogether and the details of a disease that could affect anyone became the subject of a formal lecture accompanied by slides. In this evolution, the decline of individuality is the inverse of the rise of typological thinking: all patients who share the same disease could be discussed as one.

The technology of the doctor-patient encounter is best employed in our hospitals, which are expressly intended as places for diagnosis and treatment of complex disease. With their focus almost entirely on serious disease, hospitals now have little to do with the outside world. Rosenberg likened the hospital to a department of defense: both are "captives of high technology and worst case justifications. In both instances the gradient of technical feasibility becomes a moral imperative" (31). So, is the hospital the best place to teach medical students? Is it the best place to recapture the initiative for the physician, especially the nonspecialist, to promote a rational integration of science with patients' personal needs?

A Social Context

A third set of questions arising from the reports explores the seeming difficulty of accommodating the origins of disease in social conditions observable in both families and communities. Indeed, it was often remarked that the hospital is an unlikely place to practice preventive medicine, or to teach any aspect of primary care.

No one supposed that questions of the social origins of disease were new; they have been asked before, particularly by adherents of social medicine, a movement that began earlier in the twentieth century but never attained much momentum. In their view, disease was so much a consequence of social conditions as to require that individual doctors be responsible for assessing the impact of society on individual patients, while the whole profession would strive to promote changes in the social, economic, and political climate to favor the health of all (32).

Efforts to establish social medicine in the medical curriculum in this country in the 1930s and '40s were ineffective (33). In the next decades new technology together with penetrating biochemical and molecular insights into pathogenesis were more attractive than social concerns to medical students keen to participate in something new and promising. The idea of preventive medicine just wasn't competitive, especially since apart from abolishing poverty and improving housing, nutrition, and education—none of which was much influenced by medicine—there were few preventives in sight for the diseases students saw in teaching hospitals. Even so, the impetus begun by social medicine emerged again in the 1960s and '70s. In medical schools it took the form of creation of departments of family and community medicine, renewed stress on teaching primary care and preventive medicine in the community, and an emphasis on patient individuality.

An example of how these features of medical care could be integrated with conventional modes was advanced by Engel (34,35). It is his view that a description of disease is incomplete as long as the psychological and cultural dimensions are neglected. The "ripples" of effects originating in molecular abnormality are subject to modification as they extend upward through a hierarchy of increasingly complex levels to account for the signs and symptoms of disease in a particular person. Accordingly, the kind of understanding needed for management of each patient can be attained only in a vertical analysis in which the specific modifications of those ripples are explained as properties of systems, each of which is a component of a more complex system above it until at the top is found the patient with his own account of what ails him and how it affects his relationships with his family and community. This model supplies several features not often explicitly expressed: (a) the individuality of a patient is central to diagnosis and treatment; (b) individual expression is explained by an analysis in which the influence of each level on others is emphasized; and (c) the samaritan functions are integral to management because the patient's psychological and cultural attributes are seen to be involved in pathogenesis.

A FOURTH QUESTION MIGHT HAVE BEEN ASKED but was not—namely, to what degree has the conduct of medicine been influenced by social trends outside medicine? Doctors are first of all people, susceptible to the qualities of the cultural environment. For example, the upheaval among the young in the 1960s affected medical schools no less than other elements in universities. The students of that time are now middle aged and have set their mark on medicine. Has that mark been shaped, however subtly, by the sometimes violent events of that time? Further, there have been changes in public attitude—a decline in civility, a heightened distrust, a degree of self-centeredness, a readiness to appeal to law—that are clearly reflected in today's doctor-patient relationship. Nor have physicians escaped the prevailing emphasis on financial gain. No doubt sociologists are examining these issues, but recognition of the influences of these and other social trends by the movers and shakers of medicine is far more likely to lead to solutions (if there are any) than will a cold-eyed examination from outside, no matter how perceptive and penetrating it might be.

REMEDIES

The past ten or fifteen years have seen many efforts to meet the reported shortcomings in medical education. The introductory years of medical school have been modified in several ways. In one, grasp of the required information has been improved by reducing its amount, employing fewer lectures, and promoting self-teaching (36). Further, biology and medicine have become more integrated, particularly at the several schools that have turned to problem-based learning (37). For students in the upper years, some schools stress the virtues of communicating (38). Evidently observing one's own ineptitude on a videotape provokes the recognition that communicating with a patient is an art that must be learned. Other innovations have included reorganization of faculty-student relationships (36), teaching in the community (including in practice settings), and courses in medical ethics that have been incorporated into the curriculum of nearly every school. Some have also instituted courses in "the humanities," in which views of disease in novels are observed. There are also courses on "the physician in society," which examine the penetration of medicine into society.

Several conceptual changes have also been offered. Gunderman proposed a better integration of the reductionist facts with the clinical characteristics of the sick patient (28). Reiser suggested ways for patients to work more efficiently with physicians (38). Freymann and Woodward urged inclusion of public health in the curriculum as something integral to medicine, rather than extraneous (39,40). White and Connelly described the need for a new emphasis on relationships between medical schools and their communities (41), while others saw a need to establish, or to reestablish, better ties with parent universities (42) and to reaffirm the tacit contract between medicine and the public (18,19). Finally, there were suggestions that the times called for a return to the general practice of medicine (43,44).

It is an impressive effort that has been rewarding, but whether and how well these changes have succeeded in establishing a new infrastructure of medical thinking is not clear. The question is, are the changes directed to the core of the problem? It is assumed that we have got somewhat off track, that what we do now, were it done better and in some ways differently, would be ideal. And so the remedies are intended to strengthen and diversify the system as it stands. But there has been little question of whether what we do so successfully may be itself the problem, or even that we might be blinded by success to deficiencies in the formula that led to such achievements. One such deficiency might be an imbalance in the integration of biology and medicine.

The Integration of Medicine and Biology

We say that medical schools and university hospitals are integral components of the parent university. Such a vision of partnership became the fashion after the Flexner report in 1910, but Ebert sees this union as a myth, a pro forma relationship; the medical schools are isolated from the rest of the university by their size and command of public funds (45). There are also philosophical differences. The actual connection and potential point of integration of university and medicine is the preclinical faculty of the latter, who teach medical students but whose interests are not in medicine or even in human biology. Furthermore, they are outnumbered and outweighed by the clinical faculty who, in contrast, are deeply engaged in the double business of providing medical service to patients and of teaching students. Many of the clinical faculty are trained in the basic science necessary for their research, and perhaps it is the duty of these medical scientists to do the integrating of biology and medicine. But since the focus of clinical scientists is on pathogenesis, it is natural that it is a selective biology that they teach. There may be, then, something of an intellectual gap between the abstractions of biology and their practical application to individuals in the clinic. If the students see learning the facts of molecular biology, biochemistry, and physiology simply as a chore, could it be because those facts are not perceived to be embraced in biology's own framework of phylogeny and development, all traceable to natural selection and evolution? And if that is so, might the lack of a grasp of human biological identity and individuality contribute to the much-lamented lack of concern for patients as individuals, unique in genotype, development, and experience?

Perhaps we do not ask these questions because we fail to see a second deficiency, also disguised by success. It is possible that the metaphor of the machine—however honorable its pedigree, however much it seems to go straight to the heart of the matter, and however much it appeals to the typically American dream of an engineering solution to any predicament—is actually wanting in the face of these self-same facts. It is as if the germ of change is not in the metaphor; it is not fertile, not generative of new ideas. No principles flow from it. It is at once unconstrained and constraining. There is nothing inherent in the metaphor to suggest any limit, either in the variety of disease or in treatment. We know that we are unlikely to find treatments leading to the regeneration of amputated limbs or ways that the homeostasis of an old man can be reversed to become that of a youth. But we know these things as a result of observations of molecular and cellular processes; they are not predicted by the logic of the notion that the body is a machine. Nor is there any coherence in the metaphor to hold medicine together. The only property all diseases have in common is a break in the machine. At the same time, the machine mentality is an intellectual straitjacket, neither seeking nor concerned with the social causes of the breaks that need fixing. The spirit of prevention is not in it, nor has it anything to say about the impact of disease upon the lives and feelings of those who experience it, or about their variation and individuality.

It is not that the metaphor is not based on principles. The rules of biological homeostasis are implied, and it is in the complicated network of homeostasis that the breakages occur. But there is nothing in the metaphor that allows us to infer where the human machine came from, how all the machines are related, or how they all fit into the economy of the rest of the biological and social world. And the machine model omits the arrow of time; it is essentially ahistorical. Its history is only that of the illness at hand. It does allow that a machine may wear out, but there is no allusion in it to the phylogenetic past nor necessarily to the ontogenetic experience of the sick person.

We need such information if we are to understand the reasons breakages occur at all, how or why they take the forms they do, why they affect one individual rather than another, when in the lifetime, and whether and how either the multifarious breakages themselves or the diverse individuals who experience them fit into any grand and unifying biological scheme. We need to know these things to be able to continue to perceive medicine as a single discipline, integrated and made coherent by a set of unifying ideas, rather than as a congeries of disciplines that focus each independently on its own diseases. It is also possible that in the answers to these seemingly peripheral questions of where and how and why we will find biological constraints that limit what can be done to fix the damage or that move the most appropriate disposition from treatment to prevention. So it may be that what is needed is a new outlook in which the reasons why disease occurs, the forms it takes, and the people who are affected can be seen to be a consequence of how human beings have evolved. And herein lies the path to a genuine integration into the university.

An Alternative

Whatever alternatives there may be must above all reconcile medical thinking to the troubles cited above. In so doing they cannot dispense with the gratifyingly successful concept of the body as a machine but must instead complement, enhance, and express it as a biological idea with a logic so cogent as to carry all before it.

The alternative developed in this book begins with the idea that although it is entirely reasonable and even desirable to think of the body as a machine, the human machine has qualities lacking in those created by a human mind and hand. For example, the human body was never designed; it was, if anything, refined. Design implies purpose. A machine is designed to do something in some context, and both purpose and context are taken into account in the design. Further, such designed machines may have complex mechanisms for maintenance and control, even allowing them to adapt to variable conditions. Flaws can be corrected in a new design, and different versions of the machine can be created to accommodate new tasks and purposes. But once a design is set, all its units are very nearly identical, and the plan a repairman has before him is as accurate for one unit as another.

The human machine, however, was not designed. It evolved in a selective process in which species come into being unit by unit. Each unit is a unique open system that uses its phylogenetically derived wisdom to develop in an ontogenetic process in which homeostatic mechanisms are constructed and integrated to make use of, adapt to, and shape and be shaped by their surroundings. Each unit is also capable of participating in reproducing new singular units to be submitted, in their turn, to the selective process. No mechanical device develops according to internally coded information, and no such machine reproduces itself. Human machines, like mechanical devices, have flaws and can be abused or overwhelmed by their environment. While these flaws may represent disaster for individuals, they originate in the necessity of the species for variation, the wherewithal to meet new and unforeseeable conditions. So, unlike any manmade machine, the means whereby species thrive in unforeseen conditions lie within the living machines themselves. This means that the alternative to conventional medical thinking proposed here is characterized by principles based on and emanating from natural selection and evolution. These principles explain aspects of disease not accommodated in prevailing thought and respond to the questions posed by troubled observers of the medical scene, including those concerned with reconciling reductionist facts with the feelings and concerns of individual patients.

The idea of an appeal to evolution in thinking about disease is not new. Garrod spoke and wrote of it freely and cited the writings of others (46,47). Although Garrod enlivened the idea, it was seen by others as banal, too obvious to develop further, and so it receded into the shadows. Nor is evolution given much attention in modern medicine; the word does not appear in the indexes of the most widely read textbooks of medicine, surgery, pediatrics, or obstetrics. But why should it? Evolution is of no interest in the coronary care unit or even in coming to a diagnosis. But in forming our thoughts about the biology of human development, homeostasis, and disease, we cannot avoid it.

Evolution is the touchstone of biological thought; nothing in biology makes sense apart from evolution. So the logic of disease must be developed in an evolutionary context, and the possibility of doing so is vastly better now than it was in Garrod's day. Now we know the molecular details of the evolution of gene families and of the conservation of DNA sequences in genes. Now we can demonstrate such conservation between organisms as disparate as drosophila, or even *E. coli,* and Homo sapiens, and show the effects of mutants in all. Now embryology and ontogeny, until recently a black box, are comprehensible in molecular terms, and much of the apparatus of cellular structure and function has been revealed. Now it is possible to comprehend a molecular evolution and to think of medical issues in that context, the better to answer questions of where we came from and how we are related to one another and to other forms of life, as well as why anyone suffers disease, what forms diseases take, and who among us is likely to experience a particular disease at which time in ontogeny and in what form.

The Concept of the Machine and the Alternative

How do the machine concept of disease and that of the alternative compare? The former is narrow; the alternative, broadly based on evolution and natural selection. The machine idea begins with the molecular details at the bottom of the biological hierarchy and works its explanatory way upward to details of pathogenesis and symptoms but does not depend upon the individuality of the patient. The alternative begins at the top of the hierarchy and works its way down to the molecular level; that is, it begins with an individuality that includes expressions of variation of both genes and experiences. Both concepts can be applied simultaneously in the diagnosis and treatment of a patient. The machine approach tells us that disease has its origin in adaptive failure of unit steps of homeostasis. The alternative points to the origin of those unit steps in the patient's unique inheritance, as well as in an equally singular ontogenetic career pursued in a setting of particular experiences. This necessitates as intensive a study of the patient's social and cultural characteristics as of the biological, promoting a degree of intimacy with the patient not found in the machine concept.

Human variation is such that each case of a disease is unique, and if we are to understand its origins, we must explore social variation no less than biological, and if we do, we test the hypothesis that fulfillment of the samaritan functions is directly proportional to the attention given the uniqueness of individual patients. I do not contend here that the necessity to see in such detail the patient's condition in history, in the present, and in an uncertain future must inevitably elicit sensitivity where none exists. Doctors are no less variable than patients, and some will always be content to recite a list of present and potential vulnerabilities arising from both genes and experiences, leaving the patient to figure out what to do with the information. Others, however, will see such details as an invitation to explore and exemplify the art of medicine. If the concept of disease that informs a doctor's actions omits the necessity to attend to any but the most central details, then the doctor-patient relationship is left to sensitivities unrelated to the medical mission. But if that concept includes, as a first principle, the individuality of each patient, then the intimacy engendered in dealing with the details of that individuality as they affect the patient in both the present and the future may enhance the civility and concern expressed in the encounter. It is also possible—even probable—that when the duty of the primary physician is seen to include so extensive an exploration of history and genetic propensity, the doctors who take up such work will be suited by temperament to do it.

This alternative may be uncongenial to some, at least to the degree that it is at variance with conventional thought. So if it is to be taken seriously, it may require new ways of looking at familiar things—perhaps even a new intellectual infrastructure that gives new weight to individuality, evaluates causes differently, and offers definitions of disease responsive to critics' concerns regarding the coherence of ever-increasing information, the patient as a person, and the social responsibilities of medicine. The following two chapters examine some of these issues.

4

Individuality and Causes

Population thinkers stress the uniqueness of everything in the organic world. What is important for them is the individual, not the type. They emphasize that every individual in sexual reproducing species is uniquely different from all others. . . . There is no typical individual and mean values are abstractions. Much of what in the past has been designated in biology as classes, are populations consisting of unique individuals.
　　　　—Ernst Mayr, *The Growth of Biological Thought*

Ernst Mayr is an evolutionary biologist who participated in the "modern synthesis" of the 1930s and '40s that emerged as neo-Darwinism. One of his interests is the evolution and variation of birds, and his observations of the variety within populations of these and other living organisms led him to conclude that it is individuality that is the chief characteristic within populations rather than any criterion of sameness. He called this concept "population thinking" as opposed to "typological thinking." But population thinking, however necessary for the accomplishment of medical aims, does not come easily to human beings, who seem to prefer similarities to differences (1). And yet, individuality is a constant in life. Nowhere is human variation so brazenly, so clamorously exemplified as at an airport. There, although everyone is recognizably human, of one sex or the other, and bent on travel, meeting someone, or working at the airport, each projects an individuality expressed in unique assemblies of qualities, including height, ponderosity, gait, color (both natural and applied), bodily and facial expression, handedness, and choice of dress and ornamentation that varies from uniform to bizarre, from plain to gaudy, from that which expresses some public function to that which screams for attention to its blatant otherness. No doubt about it—it is chaos. But it is a constrained chaos; amid all the exuberance of expression there are no monsters, no satyrs, no centaurs or mermaids. Nor are there any attached clusters; each is a separate individual. And, however hard to believe, there are limits to all these variations. Individuality has its limits.

Each of us expresses two kinds of individuality. First, we are each an indivisible unit of classes—gender, ethnic group, nationality, political party, occupation, and the like. The distinction here is that of the class, not of the persons of which the class is composed. At the same time, each of us is in a class of our own in which we express a unique endowment and unique experiences, and thereby impart variety to the many biological, behavioral, or cultural classes to which we belong. This means that each class is characterized by a range of expressions of classness, and although empirical observation reveals that consensus is common, outliers are infrequent and may even be considered as classes themselves. Teenagers assort themselves in such a range of expressions. Outliers are called "geeks" or "nerds," but what is "cool" is central tendency for them, if not for their parents. Theirs is the central tendency of rebellion, a mild or even amusing rebellion but nonetheless cleaving to a central tendency of rigid ideology. So the first kind of individuality is distinguished by the types or categories into which human beings can be sorted and the second by the ranges of the qualities expressed by the unique individuals composing each of the categories, and these differences inform our thinking.

When we think typologically, we think in types and categories, we draw up lists of qualities that express the essence of the class and differentiate it from others, and to characterize that essence we calculate statistical parameters, means, and dispersions. In medicine, these maneuvers lead to the description of a "classical case" composed of the qualities that typify the model against which to compare the properties of candidates for diagnosis. Individual variations are accepted provided they do not violate the essence of the diagnostic entity. Thus, it is the class, typified by the mean, that is paramount; the mean is perceived to express the essence of the class, and in medicine it is likely to determine the direction of management for all.

In contrast, in population thinking individual expression is paramount, and the emphasis is on heterogeneity, not homogeneity. The statistical parameters that characterize the whole population are perceived as abstract representations of the degree and range of the variability expressed by the individuals aggregated in the class by virtue of some common features. Here the class itself is an abstraction; it has no essence and stands only as a tentative and convenient symbol of the degrees of similarity exhibited by the individuals it embraces. It was Darwin who first drew the attention of biologists away from the ideal to the actual variation among individuals, noting that type had no reality and that the only reality was the individual, heritable variation (2).

Epidemiological studies are designed to characterize populations, to extract their essence, and to use the information to propose risk factors that point to preventive measures to be observed by all. But before long, new qualities, often genetic, emerge that distinguish elements within the whole for whom the original preventive may be either unnecessary or inadequate. The population was all along composed of variable individuals. Thus, epidemiology and genetics are complementary disciplines. The former describes and quantifies the qualities in populations that appear to be related to outcomes. Genetics, in contrast, perceives no essence but describes the qualities of the individuals that compose the population. The epidemiologist says, "This represents a risk factor," to which the geneticist replies, "Yes, but risky for whom?" Of course, it may be risky for the whole of the species, but more often the degree is variable depending upon the endowment, development, and particular experiences of the individual.

The concept of the body as a machine implies typological thinking; machines, even when hand made, are built undeviatingly to a blueprint, so all are identical or nearly so. But the Garrodian concept of chemical individuality implies population thinking that embraces individual particularity; each unique human open system accommodates uniquely to a unique pattern of environments and experiences. As Garrod put it, "Each is an individual and not merely a member of the human race" (3). The medicine of today tilts toward the typological. Indeed, it is ironic that a profession so devoted to the care of individuals should care so little about individuality. Perhaps it is inevitable. We live in a multicultural society that adheres rigidly to types. Such separation can lead to what it is intended to prevent: the polarity of opinion around stereotypes of sex, race, and the like.

Medicine is no exception, having assorted itself into so many specialties and subspecialties, each with its own essence. In medicine, the typological mentality is supported by aggregation of physicians into HMOs, wherein a fine-tuned variety in managing patients is not exactly welcomed. Indeed, what could represent typological thinking more completely than the agent of the HMO who makes sight-unseen decisions according to a standard?

Other typological simplifications are genetic disease, handicap, and disability. Monogenic disorders are designated "genetic" disorders as opposed to "environmental" diseases, of which infections are chief. But we know of many forms of monogenic immunodeficiencies—no less inborn errors than phenylketonuria (PKU)—that fulfill the name of disease only when they accompany the infections to which their victims are vulnerable. So they are not either genetic diseases or infections; they are both. The severe immunodeficiencies are likely to be only one end of a distribution of immune competence that ranges from more than sufficient to totally deficient (4). So typological thinking is limiting even where it seems most pertinent.

As for handicap, there is the egregious example of the XYY chromosome constitution. Because this clearly abnormal karyotype was discovered among men in a Scottish prison, the press leaped upon the Y as "the violence chromosome." As it turns out, the XYY karyotype is associated in some of its possessors with mild mental retardation and in some with impulsive behavior, but most fall into normal distributions of attributes. So it was a typological bias that led the press to include all people with this karyotype with other forms of handicap, which causes the typological thinker to perceive them as set apart. It is the special burden of handicapped people to be seen by some as "different" and so to be segregated in society despite the more numerous ways they resemble those called "normal." As they so often protest, they are "a part of the main" who need help to surmount their disadvantage, and who with it or despite it, wish to fulfill the role of citizen (5). But they may be victims of the tyranny of classification, a mentality that stresses handicap without recognizing compensating qualities that can reduce or surmount it. This is a point made again and again by the disabled, who emphasize the undoubted talents and attainments of so many of their own.

All human beings comprehended within labels are individuals, too. There are all degrees of disability, and all degrees of adaptation to it. Such individuality is always observed in the genetic analysis of disease. Whether the principal cause of, say, an inborn error is a mutant at one locus or at several loci, as in some diseases of complex origin, genetic heterogeneity is the rule. The more detailed the analysis, the more loci shown to be involved in cause, the more nearly do we approximate uniqueness in the clinical expression of each individual said to have the "same" disease, the same handicap, or the same disability. And the more nearly do we account for the genetic variety that led, through the uniqueness of development and the particularity of experience, to the exuberant diversity of humanity observed at the airport.

CAUSES

The nature of causes has provided philosophers with many an hour of puzzled thought (6,7). The problems, as perceived by epidemiologists, are those of establishing (a) association between a presumed cause and its effect; (b) their relationship in time; and (c) direction—that is, outcome must be shown to be a consequence of cause. When compared to geneticists, epidemiologists are always at a disadvantage. For the geneticist, the segregation of a phenotype establishes association, direction, and time all at once, so today the central preoccupation in genetics is establishing the biochemical and physiological connection between gene and segregating phenotype. But this analysis, which clarifies proximate cause to the last nucleotide substitution in the DNA, omits the causes of causes, those forces that lead to or away from conditions that favor or prevent the advent of proximate cause. For clarification on the relationships among causes, we turn again to Ernst Mayr.

Two Currents of Biological Thought

Mayr distinguished two principal currents of biological thought by the kinds of questions they raise (2,8). One, which traditionally includes medicine, is functional biology, concerned with the structure and function of elements from molecules to organisms. The questions a functional biologist asks are preceded by *how:* How do organs work? How do cells communicate? How do molecules interact? Functional studies focus on the type; variability is not of interest. For example, biochemists and molecular biologists are interested in species-specific mechanisms, while medical investigators concentrate on the details of pathogenesis; both probe deeply, but narrowly. Natural history, the second current, is the realm of the evolutionary biologist who asks questions preceded by *why:* Why is a species the way it is, particularly in its adaptations and in its variation?

These two currents of thought coincide at the level of the genetic program. Functional biologists' questions have to do with everything that happens as a consequence of decoding the DNA. Evolutionary biologists are interested in the history of the DNA, in mutation, gene duplication, chromosome organization, sex determination, segregation, selection, and the dynamics of the gene pool. The former are interested in proximate causes, the latter in ultimate causes—ultimate because they represent the wherewithal for evolution.

But genetic causes are not all. Obviously an open system is in and of the environment and experiences it throughout life. So proximate and remote causes must also reside in a no-less evolving social and cultural environment: proximate in experiences of the moment, remote in the cultural tradition and social organization that make experiences possible. So if we wish to explain disease, both kinds of causes are germane—the proximate to account for the origin of pathogenesis and the remote to account for the origins of the agents of disease, what forms diseases can take, how vulnerability is attained, and the specificity of the encounter with disease.

Causes of Disease

When we speak of the cause of a disease—whether a mutant gene, a toxic substance, or both together—we mean that which sets in motion the physiological processes we call pathogenesis. Any of these causes recognize aspects of homeostasis with which they are "incongruent," precipitating either struggles to compensate or the breakdown that leads to disease. The word *pathogenesis* embraces all the various pathways whereby different individuals attain the phenotype of disease. The specificity of the "case" is conferred by remote causes that characterize a particular person as being in the wrong place at the wrong time and lacking the capacity to resist the pathogenic effects of proximate causes that led to the singular pathogenesis of a person who brought to the encounter a unique genotype, ontogeny, and experience of life. Does all this uniqueness make any difference? There are those who would say, "Not much—pathogenesis dictates treatment." And so it does. But it is the person, not the pathogenesis, that is the object of the treatment, and it is the person no less than the pathogenesis that bears the singular stamp.

An example may be useful. Consider a male hemophiliac child injured in a collision of automobiles, one driven by a drunk driver. The child was taken to a hospital where he was transfused with HIV-positive blood, which led to AIDS and, in time, death due to infection. The mutant that specified the deficiency of factor VIII is the cause of hemophilia; the trauma caused by the collision precipitated a transfusion, which led to AIDS caused by HIV, which made the child prey to the organisms that caused his death. All are proximate causes.

But there are remote causes, too. The evolutionary necessity for mutational variation to submit to selective test is one remote cause. The enormous size of the factor VIII gene, which encompasses 186,000 base pairs and 26 exons and has more than 150 identified mutations, is another. And even though the reproductive fitness of untreated hemophiliacs is near zero, the size of the gene and the number of different sites for mutations that make a difference account for an incidence of hemophilia as high as 1 in 10,000. A third remote cause is the mutagen that induced the mutation, whether drug, radiation, or failure of the repair mechanism that should have removed the defect, itself, perhaps, a consequence of a genetic variant. A fourth is the location of the gene in the X chromosome that ensured that the sequence of events occurred in a male, and a fifth is a consequence of the randomness of segregation that endowed this particular male child with the defective gene—after all, he might have got his mother's other X, or his mother might have inherited her mother's normal X. The child's disease made itself known in neonatal life, so a sixth remote cause is its origin in a defect of so vital a function as blood coagulation. Seventh is the qualities of the HIV, with its lethal effects on the immune system. Eighth is the transgression of rules for speed and direction that make possible orderly traffic on congested highways. Ninth is the antisocial behavior of the drunk driver, itself possibly influenced by a predisposing endowment to alcoholism, as well as by whatever experiences work over such a susceptibility. And a tenth remote cause lies in the motivations of those who give or sell blood.

The proximate causes listed are well known to everyone; the tragedy of AIDS and its transmission to hemophiliacs, among others, has become a feature of our lives. But the recitation of only the proximate causes makes an incomplete story that lacks specificity as to who precisely was involved. It provides no indication as to why things happened as they did, and no connecting links to the biological and social communities in which the events occurred. It is the remote causes that provide that specificity and those connections, making a real event out of a set of abstractions. In this example, there had to be not only a concatenation of proximate causes, but those proximate causes had to be made specific by the causes listed as remote. It had to be that specific, male child, that particular mutant derived from that child's mother, that blood derived from a donor drawn from the relatively small population of HIV-positive people, a pool made even smaller by testing for the virus in donors. And the accident had its specificities, too, in the split-second timing of occurrence, the conditions of the highway, and the temperament of the drunk driver as well as the lenient laws that fail to rein in repeat offenders. Had the child been an unaffected male sib, by chance the recipient of an alternative X chromosome, or a female sib possessed of the same mutant as her affected brother, there might have been no need for a transfusion and no AIDS. So it is in exposing and understanding the remote causes that we see why human beings get sick at all, who among us is vulnerable to what, and when in a lifetime we are likely to experience the vulnerability. We are all shaped by the evolution of our species to accommodate to some experiences and not to others, and we are each the beneficiary and the victim of our special aliquot of that biological history.

But let us be practical. When this hemophiliac child arrived at the hospital, all that mattered was that he had suffered an accident; he was bleeding and in shock. How the accident occurred was of little moment; what had to be done was to expand his extracellular volume, raise his blood pressure, and stop the bleeding. As part of the volume expansion, blood would be used for obvious reasons, so matched blood was the first priority. That is, the pathogenesis, the consequences of proximate causes, had to be reversed immediately; the procedures for doing so are the same for everyone, regardless of the origin of the injury or the identity of the victim. It is, then, proximate causes that are at the center of acute medical care, and remote causes are just that—remote. And since so much medical care is acute and episodic, much medicine is transacted as if remote causes did not exist. But since it is they that, in promoting the more immediate factor, confer the stamp of individuality on the case and make plain the patient's connection to family, community, and species, it cannot be in the patient's interest—or in that of the family—to overlook them. Nor can any medical education worthy of the name be propagated in their absence. Omit remote causes and what is left is not education but training.

The disparity between the two approaches to medical education is obvious. The engineering mentality is drawn only to the immediate reasons for illness, to pathogenesis and to what needs fixing, and in the sense that such treatment fulfills the stated (and limited) aims of medicine, it is successful. But a deeper understanding of a disease in the context of a specific individual and family can be attained only by taking into account those factors that make the proximate causes specific. And it is this specificity, the recognition of how each unique patient came to experience a unique version of the disease, that compels attention to prevention so easily neglected when individuality is ignored.

It is now evident why individuality and causes appear together in this chapter. They are intimately intertwined—indeed, are in some ways one. If individuality is expressed in the specificity of the alleles that constitute the genotype and in the trajectory of development determined by the congruence of the products of those alleles with experiences of the environment, then the potential for disease lies in incongruities between a homeostasis bearing the stamp of phylogeny, ontogeny, and experience and the conditions within which an open system moves. That is, that which confers individuality may be a cause of disease.

Chapter 2, in which the views of the eminent professors were compared, advanced the idea that the inborn error, now perceived as a variation in a unit step of homeostasis, is a central feature of medical thought, while this chapter promotes the idea that individuality is an expression of the integration of such unit steps. Then chapter 3 proposed that a logic of disease might originate in the qualities of natural selection and evolution. That is, the objects of selection, whether positive or negative, are the phenotypes that originate in the variation of unit steps of homeostasis. So the genes that specify the variants of those unit steps are one proximate cause of disease, while the experiences with which the variant steps are incongruent are a second. And finally, all of the forces that conspire to bring together the genes, the development, and the experiences of each particular open system constitute remote causes. So to the variation in the unit step of homeostasis that constitutes the basic element in the structure of the logic of disease, we now add individuality and causes. The next chapter reveals how these elements relate to descriptions of disease.

5

Definitions of Disease

When a man is ill, that is, when he feels dis-ease, he has experiences
which are partly his own, partly open to others. This is his individual sickness which in exactly this particular form will never repeat itself in others
or even in himself. But the sick man, his family and neighbors, the physician (if there is one), all will try to understand what is happening to him.
—Owsei Temkin, "The Scientific Approach to Disease:
Specific Entity and Individual Sickness" (1)

Temkin's paragraph highlights several features of the concept of disease. Some expressions of one person's illness are individual, some
are shared with others; the concept is both singular and general. Also, disease
engages the thought of the sick person, the physician, family, friends, and
other social agencies. Everyone defines disease according to particular knowledge and past experience, giving it many meanings: physiological, emotional,
social. Merely the use of the word *disease* raises the question of its nature. One
might suppose, therefore, that conceptual definitions of disease would be
given prominence in medical education and thinking, but, on the contrary,
medical textbooks seldom include such definitions. Conceptualization of disease is usually left to a student's own enterprise and experience, or to informal discussion about health and illness or what it means to be sick. Physicians'
own definitions, if they think about it at all, may be refined by personal encounters with sick patients or occasionally by their own experiences as patients; probably the latter lead to more definite opinions about it than anything else.

Our language is indicative of our thoughts on the subject. We say a person
"comes down with" a disease, "has" it or is "felled" by it, as if it were something that came from somewhere to do us no good. Or we suffer an "attack"
of something against which our immune "defenses" are aroused. Even the
word *patient* conjures up a vision of an enduring victim. But the textbooks are
silent as to why we choose such language to describe these events.

Obviously there are conceptual puzzles here, grist for philosophers' mills, so why do doctors take disease for granted or act as if it needed no elaboration? First, let us be clear: it is *disease* that eludes definition, not *diseases*. The latter are defined exhaustively in the textbooks in terms of (a) subjective reports including pain, discomfort, and disability; (b) departures from some ideal state or statistical norm; (c) abnormalities in structure and function of organ systems; (d) sets of specific signs and symptoms; and (e) specific outcomes. These expressions characterizing groups of patients are given a name, and the pathogenesis is examined for leads to the design of management. Abstract definitions of disease have been derived from such observations, but such exercises are little noticed in the lore of medicine (1–20).

Second, physicians for all their science are strongly empirical. Where, they may say, is the virtue of tedious haggling over something self-evident? A definition must above all be useful. Where is the value to doctors of a definition that leads to no particular action? In any case, today everyone knows that a disease is defined in reductionist terms that emerge from a molecular analysis of a disturbed homeostasis.

Third, definitions of disease may be tautological; disease is a lack of health and health is a lack of disease. This lack of specificity is apparent in the World Health Organization's representation of health as "a state of complete physical, mental, and social well being," a conclusion that only adds to the ambiguity. Is a person out of social synchrony necessarily diseased? The WHO definition is perhaps an expression of what has been called the "medicalization" of society, in which the idea of illness is expanded to include such behavioral deviance as abuse in families, shoplifting, compulsive gambling, or even unhappiness. Such sociological distinctions have been stretched so far that we must all be diseased in one way or another (21). And some doctors contribute to the ambiguity by engaging in such medically marginal activities as plastic surgery for obesity and aging countenances. These actions are defensible on the grounds, say, that a too-distinctive nose can impair social adjustment and ravage self-esteem. But does it constitute disease?

Fourth, and perhaps most important of all, little academic attention is given to definitions of disease because it is the patients who define it in reporting how they feel, how their complaints began and developed, where they hurt, and how their distress has affected their lives. Thus, as long as medical care is offered only when a patient appeals for help, we can make do with tacit definitions of disease, something that in our bones we feel we know. Surrounded daily by patients who proclaim their illness and more often than not have some visible, palpable, or measurable abnormality, the doctor perceives no value in an abstract characterization of something faced daily in reality.

But there are consequences to knowing something in one's bones. Knowledge stored at some unanalyzable level is unlikely to be examined for validity;

change is likely to be resisted. It must also lead to intolerance of alternatives and to isolation from contrary opinions. For example, there are plenty of philosophical and sociological analyses of the nature of disease as a social phenomenon, and sociologists have examined doctors at work, but none of this literature figures prominently in the medical curriculum (1–20). Tacit, unexamined certainty may also account for the much-lamented failure of doctors to listen to patients' stories of how they are affected, not by the specific disease they have, but by disease itself. So, perhaps we should listen more carefully to the voices of philosophers, historians, sociologists, and patients, and so imagine that disease has dimensions that go beyond molecules and homeostatic systems to include not only the integrated individuals who are the patients but all the social and cultural contexts of which they are a part. And perhaps then we will perceive and accept the utility of definitions of disease that embrace such variables.

Those who do pay attention to the definition of disease are seldom clinicians or clinical investigators involved with somatic disease; rather, this is the province of sociologists, philosophers, medical historians, and psychiatrists. These observers see such definitions as shaping social responses to medicine (1,2,5,16,20–22). There are also those outside the medical profession who advance "common sense" models in which disease is perceived as a result of breakdown of the body's defenses in people who disregard nature's laws. The consequences are usually described in a mixture of medical and nonmedical language in which vitamins occupy a place of prominence.

One definition offered by clinicians states the following: "In medical discourse the name of a disease refers to the sum of the abnormal phenomena displayed by a group of living organisms in association with a specified common characteristic or set of characteristics by which they differ from the norm for their species in such a way as to place them at a biological disadvantage" (23,24). These doctors prefer to deal with the issue in the context of questions, namely: (a) What does the name of a disease entail? and (b) What is disease? The answer to the latter question is an abstract something that exists as an entity apart from its victims and may have always existed, while the answer to the former, they say, is more realistic and gives prominence to the patient who expresses the signs and symptoms. The first answer defines disease as essentialist, the second as nominalist.

These two points of view have been argued since antiquity. Because they represent constructs that underlie the implicit definitions lurking deep in the minds of clinicians and medical educators, and because they have provided contexts within which so many characterizations of disease have been expressed, they deserve further scrutiny. What follows is influenced by the views, many and diverse, expressed in references 1 through 25.

Two Views of Disease

In the essentialist version of disease, sometimes called ontological, the patient, while not irrelevant, is undifferentiated. It matters not who the patient is, nor from what population drawn; he or she is simply the recipient of this unwelcome entity. Individuality is that of the class. Diseases most easily embraced in this abstraction have unitary proximate causes, and the response to cause and disease in all patients is perceived to be more or less the same, with obvious implications for diagnosis and treatment. It is in this context that we are likely to use language appropriate to an enemy: diseases attack and defenses are mobilized.

The essentialist view is represented in the "classical case." Diagnosis is attained by comparing each patient's manifestations with a list of typical expressions. Treatment, if not automatically dictated by the diagnosis, is reduced to a few alternatives, and a statistical prognosis is based on experience with many such cases. To the thoroughgoing essentialist, disease is defined in terms of a statistical ideal: a patient is one of a class of individuals marked by the qualities of the disease (1,2). The essentialist view is the quintessence of typological thinking. And it is in this vein that the mind is encouraged to embrace the idea of a disease-free society. If there is nothing in biology we cannot "think our way around," why can we not go forward until all diseases are curable?

The second position has it that disease is represented as simply the response of individuals to experiences for which adaptive mechanisms are inadequate. An extreme expression of this "nominalist" or "physiological" view is that there are no diseases, only sick people (1,2). That is, diseases derive their characteristics from the nature of human beings, so that similarities in clinical expression originate in our common humanity and differences in the variations that make each of us unique. Here the causes are not necessarily harmful in themselves but become so in the presence of "some limitation in the inventory of adaptive resources" (6). Such limitations, expressed in variations of unit steps in integrated homeostatic systems, may extend to the whole species or, in rare conditions, to very few individuals. Here dispersion holds reality rather than the abstract mean, and treatment and prognosis are determined by the special qualities of each case. Here individuality is that of the patient who, even while representing the essentialist disease class, also represents his or her own self.

It is, above all, population thinking that characterizes the mentality of the nominalist view, a mentality that is far less congenial to the idea of a disease-free society than is the essentialist. Even while prevention will reduce the incidence and prevalence of disease, the quality and extent of human variability is likely to foil attempts to circumvent it. Perhaps disease is like Mount Everest. It is often said that the mountain has been "conquered," but the reality is that the few who dare to climb it have become familiar with it and know its quirks, so an increasing number reach its crest. But the mountain is still unfathomable; it still takes lives and will always do so.

As to causes of nominalist disease, the proximate stem from the remote that almost necessarily conjure up thoughts of prevention. For example, if a congenital anomaly is shown to be associated with a specific drug, it follows naturally that pregnant women should avoid that drug. But a further necessity is also invoked: there should be some regulation of the manufacturer of the drug, who, in an entirely legitimate enterprise, distributed a medication that proved to be injurious to some pregnant women and their offspring. This viewpoint prevailed when the sale of thalidomide was discontinued but continues to be defied by the tobacco industry.

These are polar positions. Medicine, nominalist until the early nineteenth century, became essentialist when it became possible to associate physical signs and symptoms with morbid anatomy, and even more so with the discovery of bacteria. Now it has begun to move back toward the nominalist position, but slowly. It is easy to see why. The appeal of the essentialist position is strong. It forms the basis of the body-as-machine mentality, and its strength lies in its perception of the unity and homogeneity of entities. It is the disease that captures the attention of the doctor who asks the Oslerian question, "What disease does this person have and how do I treat it?" And since the differences among patients consist of variations on a single theme, one treatment should suffice for all. Obviously there are modulations—for age and sex, for example—and a certain amount of fiddling in individual management is inevitable, but the beauty of it is that once the diagnosis is in hand one proceeds to treatment by the book. Further, since it is proximate causes that account for pathogenesis, medicine can be perceived as a "narrow discipline" (26); attention to conditions in nature or in social organization that enhance or reduce exposure to causes are the province of other agencies.

But in the strength of the essentialist position lie its weaknesses: there is a serious risk of overlooking clinical and biological heterogeneity, and the emphasis on the disease is likely to be at the expense of the patient whose special properties and private concerns may escape the doctor's notice. The approach is also sterile; it is like asking only where and how the machine is broken without wondering why it broke.

The appeal of the nominalist position lies in its attention to human biological, developmental, social, and behavioral individuality and in its assumption that the disease at hand represents some incongruity between these expressions of self. Individuality here is that of each person's unique genes, development, and experiences, and the immediate, precipitating causes of disease are perceived as deriving from the convergence of biological and cultural currents that are channeled into families by inheritance of both genes and mores. Here it is the Garrodian questions that are pertinent: How and why is this particular human being ill, what treatment is appropriate for so peculiar a constitution, and what differentiates this patient from others in the population whence he or she is drawn? The weakness of the essentialist position is the strength of that of the nominalist, which is alert to how individuality has influenced clinical expression with its implications for heterogeneity and specificity of management and prognosis. Further, because the focus of the nominalist is fixed above all on the patient's particularities, the probability of attention to the samaritan functions is much enhanced.

There is another strength. Because it defines disease as quantitative variation rather than separate entity, the nominalist view accommodates easily the shifting, indefinable point at which health becomes disease or disease health, as well as the broad margin at which there is disagreement as to whether such disabling conditions as, say, alcoholism or panic attacks are to be called diseases at all. When it is the individual that is emphasized, not the entity, the name employed to describe the condition is of little moment. In contrast, the essentialist tradition requires us to say that a person has a disease or does not. If this proves difficult, essentialists resort to the designation "subclinical" or "social deviation," which does nothing to help the either-or quality of the definition.

What is the weakness of the nominalist position? Again, its weakness lies in its strength: because it emphasizes the individual, it reduces the concept of disease from something grand and embracing to merely sick individuals. But to be practical, if we do not classify we will be nowhere at all, and if we avoid trying to group cases for treatment, we will be in worse financial straits than we are.

Conclusion

The contrasts between these views of disease are easily summarized. One, which I call Oslerian, is essentialist and is approached typologically. It emphasizes likeness between cases, means as opposed to dispersions, and proximate causes—especially abnormalities in the molecular composition of homeostatic systems. It conceives the body as a machine to be fixed by a doctor when it breaks, and omits the necessity for a social framework within which to define disease. The other view, which I call Garrodian, sees disease as a consequence of some incongruence between a patient's individuality and the conditions of living. This nominalist position is approached in a populational turn of mind, emphasizes individual variation in the biological constitution of the patient, and while not neglecting proximate causes, it seeks their origin in remote causes deriving from biological and cultural history—which is to say that disease in individuals is a byproduct of the necessity to preserve the species. Here the role of physicians is to use their grasp of individuality to find ways to skirt the proximate causes and to make prevention the primary aim of medicine.

Today, the prevailing concept lies somewhere between these extremes. Our growing understanding of the extent of human molecular and genetic diversity in health and disease is moving us toward the nominalist position. This view, in which disease is perceived as a consequence of incongruence of the molecular properties of some homeostatic device and the environment is more firmly based in variation and individuality than that of the body as a machine. So it should be possible to work within it to employ biological rules to compose a logic of incongruence that may do for disease what the rules of congruence do for normal biology. And since congruence is an evolutionary concept, so must be incongruence.

The concept of disease as an outcome of incongruence is the antithesis of that of the broken machine. It is more tolerant of prevention than that of the engineer and it exposes a curious irony. The more precise the definition of the molecular detail of the incongruent state, the more compelling the need to discover that with which it is incongruent. This need is satisfied in those monogenic disorders in which the variant step is incongruent with an integrated homeostasis within the cell. But for disorders in which the variant step of homeostasis is incongruent with some unknown aspect of development or experiences of the outside, it is the developmental and social conditions within which the disease occurs that must be defined. So the irony is that the more we pursue the reductionist agenda the more we are thrust back to the social framework; the ultimate in reductionism is but a prelude to integration.

Finally, in this chapter one new element has been added to the structure of the logic of disease: its definition as a consequence of incongruence between one or more unit steps of homeostasis and conditions of the environment. In the two chapters of the next section I review the circumstances under which this concept might be accepted in both medicine and biology.

II
A Logic of Disease

What exactly is meant by a "logic" of disease? *Webster's Third International Dictionary* defines *logic* as "a statement of the formal principles of a branch of knowledge," and as "interrelationships or connections or sequences of facts and events seen by rational analysis as inevitable, necessary, or predictable." So the question here is, are there principles of disease that flow by means of predictable connections and sequences from the facts of evolution and natural selection? Are there regularities in the nature, frequency, and characteristics of diseases that can be shown to be consequences of the human genetic and cultural condition? And does the whole range of diseases have some common properties that stem from the human substrate they all share? If so, such a logic could be useful to the medical teacher in providing principles on which to construct a framework for the facts (1). For the practitioner it would draw attention to the origins of each patient's disease in the qualities of that particular person's endowment, development, and experiences. The idea of such a logic of disease is well within the Garrodian canon—indeed, *Inborn Factors* is just such an argument—and altogether foreign to that of Osler.

A critic might protest that human physiology and the pathogenesis of disease are far too complex to allow the elaboration of such a logic: living organisms encompass too much randomness, they are not simple linear systems, their moment-to-moment behavior depends upon their own state. But even in chaotic systems such as the weather, where conditions may change hourly, long range predictions of climate are usually fulfilled. It is the rules of "climate," rather than "weather," that constitute the logic of disease proposed in this book. A critic might also say that any such logic must defy composition: the facts are too many and too diverse, the diseases too varied, the homeostasis too complex to be embraced in a set of principles. If such principles are truly comprehensive, they must be banal; if they are not, then no logic will be apparent. But in the preface to the first edition of *Molecular Biology of the Cell,* a book that comprehends much of what is known about the structure and function of cells, the authors say, "There is a paradox in the growth of scientific knowledge. As information accumulates in ever more intimidating quantities, disconnected facts and impenetrable mysteries give way to rational explanations and simplicity emerges from chaos" (2). If simplicity emerges from chaos in the biology of normal cells, why not in that of cells caught up in the processes of disease?

The first principle of this logic is that it flows from the biology of Homo sapiens, itself traceable to natural selection and evolution. Disease is a byproduct of the necessity for a store of variation to preserve species in the face of variable conditions. Mutation, expressed in differences in the proteins that act as unit steps in homeostasis, supplies that variation. It is through these unit steps that the influence of both genetic and environmental variations is expressed. They are the interface between nature and nurture and constitute the capacity of the individual open system to adapt. Now, since mutation is random, some of the variation in unit steps is sure to be disadaptive, expressed in ways that are incongruent with fulfillment of the missions of the systems of which those steps are a part. Such variable unit steps, together with components of the environment with which they are incongruent, constitute proximate causes of disease whose remote causes are (a) genetic events such as mutation that account for the variant steps of homeostasis, together with recombination, segregation, drift, and other forces that account for the distribution of their products; and (b) the cultural and social history of the experiences with which the variant unit steps are incongruent.

But disease occurs in individuals, those classified both as representative of the species and according to individual phylogenetic and ontogenetic histories. Accordingly, while diseases can be classified in the essentialist vein, individuality defies such assortment by virtue of the variety of both the biology and the experiences of the individuals so classified. That is, although practical necessity requires that we classify, each individual has his or her own disease. Clearly this logic exceeds the scope of the body-as-machine model, but in the form of the broken unit step of homeostasis, it includes it and thereby represents a synthesis of medical and genetic thought.

Such a synthesis is fertile in predictions about disease in relation to age at onset, severity, frequency, sex differences, organ system, symptomatology, and the like. But the logic can evolve only when the ideas of biology and medicine become so interlaced as to attain almost the identity of a new discipline. This evolution is occurring now in the resolution of contrasts between the aims of biology as expressed in genetics, molecular biology, and cell biology on the one hand and medicine on the other. Some of these contrasts and convergences are reviewed in chapter 6, while chapter 7 outlines the synthesis itself.

A Logic of Disease

6

Biology and Medicine

Contrasts and Convergences

M edical education has been criticized for failing to integrate biology and medicine in the preclinical curriculum. But the critics are vague about what they mean by integration and how to attain it, and silent as to why there is not already a satisfactory integration. This may be because biology and medicine are such different disciplines that the adherents of neither think in ways suitable for the attainment of the other's goals. Inevitably the comparisons that follow force each discipline into a typological mold, but they are drawn in a spirit of population thinking, recognizing that (a) the two disciplines have long perceived their affinity, (b) there is increasing confluence of thought, and (c) there are biologists who grasp the motivations of the medical mind, as well as physicians who are comfortable in both spheres.

RELATIONSHIPS BETWEEN BIOLOGY AND MEDICINE

Medicine is a much older discipline than biology, but through much of its history, empiricism ruled the doctor's behavior. Now that biology is changing medicine, how might the relationship between the two be most profitably expressed?

One way is to acknowledge that there is nothing in medical science that is not explained by biology. Indeed, while there is much in biology that is not germane to medical aims, medical science is best represented as a special case of biology. Nevertheless, medicine, while today acknowledging its duty to biology more than ever before, is still inclined to define that duty parochially. Some investigators, many students, and most practitioners still overlook aspects of biology that answer the why questions—why disease, why this individual, why at this time of life, why this family, and why this ethnic group. We have come routinely to perceive common experiences as risk factors, but it is not yet routine to ask, "Risky for whom?" That is, in medicine, biology is preempted; it is not yet truly integrated. Medical thinking is clothed in biology but is not altogether informed by it. More than forty-five years ago I was outraged to hear a famous mouse geneticist (a mere mouse geneticist, as I thought him then) proclaim medicine as a branch of genetics; lèse majestê if ever I had heard it. Now I see the wisdom of his view. He was saying that medicine is a special case of biology. If that is so, then, in common with other aspects of biology, the answers to all of the questions we have about disease must ultimately be traceable to natural selection and evolution.

Goals

The biologist's goal is to illuminate some aspect of how living things work, how nature is ordered and organized to preserve and perpetuate life. Such aspects are sometimes formulated as "problems of biology." Exhibit 1 shows the table of contents of a book by J. H. Maynard Smith that carries that title (1). Each chapter includes subsidiary problems differentiated by objective and method of study into two broad categories: (a) the molecular detail of structure, function, and reproduction of cells, organs, and organisms; and (b) the study of the origins and reproduction of populations and species. However unrelated these objectives seem, work in both bears on the comprehensive question of what ensures the continuity of life, to which questions of the continuity of species and of individuals are secondary. So, although the biologist may focus sharply upon some restricted issue—say, oxidative phosphorylation in mitochondria or the identification of new species in Brazilian rain forests—whatever is found will be easily traceable to some aspect of evolution. The work is evidence of a preoccupation with both the proximate causes that describe how things work and the remote causes that reveal their origins.

Now compare Exhibit 1 with Exhibit 2, the table of contents from David Weatherall's *Science and the Quiet Art* (2). It, too, could be called a "problems" book—*Problems in Medicine*. Both books, written by distinguished representatives of their field, belong to series intended to examine where we are now and where we are going, but the tables of contents show how different are the goals in the two fields. Maynard Smith's looks at the elements of congruence, Weatherall's at those of incongruence. The former is an account of an unending search for generalizable truths, the latter for truths that serve practical ends. And in sections V and VI Weatherall reveals how medicine faces a constraint that biology escapes: that of fulfilling the direct social obligations that have required the investigation. The biologist's problems are of choice, those of the medical investigator, of necessity.

Thus, the agenda of medical educators, investigators, and practitioners differs from that of biologists. The former study how things don't work, how things went wrong. They tend not to seek encompassing generalizations. For example, when biologists ask how selection and other mechanisms work to attain evolutionary ends, they express no interest in that which is of consuming interest to the physician. They do not ask what effect these processes have had

EXHIBIT 1

Table of Contents, *Problems of Biology* by J. H. Maynard Smith

EXHIBIT 2

Table of Contents, Science and *the Quiet Art* by David Weatherall

on specific individuals, especially those subject to what biologists describe, without irony, as "purifying selection." But such individuals are precisely the focus of medical interest. Physicians are compelled by necessity to find out which biological process has failed in each individual, how it failed, and what can be done to repair it or to compensate for the damage. Here the generalizations extend not to all diseases, but only to other individuals with the same complaint. It can be no surprise, then, that medical education and research are concentrated on proximate causes, according their remote origins only a mild interest or omitting them altogether.

But the incursion of genetics into medicine has had a notable effect. For example, such concepts as heterozygote advantage, exemplified in variants of hemoglobin and glucose-6-phosphate dehydrogenase, are known to medical students, and the idea of founder effect crops up in medical conversations. These ideas arise wherever medical people are puzzled by the relatively high frequency of genes that appear to have no redeeming feature. Further, genes contributing to common multifactorial disease may be even more frequent, invoking the idea of genetic polymorphism, heterogeneity, and genetic vulnerability. These concepts represent the direct imposition on medical lore of the thinking of Fisher, Wright, and Haldane, and they have been accepted without reference to their provenance—which is perhaps the fate of most ideas. But without provenance there is the risk that these will take their place among all the other unrelated facts that the student is asked to remember. Ideas of founder effect, polymorphism, and even gene frequency, if defined outside the context of population genetics, lack coherence. It may not be necessary to develop the ideas historically—although the story has many features of human drama, including competition, contention, and above all, startling surprises—but enough of that story must be told to apprise the student of the relationship of disease to the ebb and flow of the gene pool. It is here that the aims of the population geneticist and the physician are made one.

Individuality

Although as citizens biologists and physicians might share a variety of social and political views, their respective goals determine quite different standpoints from which to look at life. For example, biological thought takes for granted the enormous apparent waste of life—the profligacy of seeds (including human sperm), losses in prairie and forest fires as well as among hatching turtles making their way to the sea. But, in fact, it is not waste at all; it is insurance against extinction. Biologists also accept the amorality of wild life, in which one species is maintained at the expense of another, although seldom to the extinction of either. To the biologist, life proceeds at a stately pace, and the scientist is observer, analyst, and interpreter of the intricate associations whereby the earth's organisms attain a homeostatic organization. It is a balance maintained by virtue of the adaptive variability expressed in the lives of the trillions of living individuals, whether microorganisms, insects, plants, or human beings. To the biologist, each of these numberless individuals is a vehicle for the transmission of genes and a means for generation of the variability required to maintain the species. In this view, individuals represent the variegated materials from which an indifferent nature creates the fabric of species; that is, individuality is valued for its contribution to the homeostasis of the population. Only ethologists, including those intrepid observers of families and herds of elephants, lions, gorillas, baboons, hyenas, coyotes, bears, and the like, are drawn to study the characteristics of the particular individuals that form the populations they study. They observe the behavior of each animal, both apart and in relation to one another, and they reveal their humanity in the choice of names they give the objects of their observation.

In sharp contrast, medical thinking includes action, a readiness to interfere with nature wherever a threat to even a single human life is perceived. To the physician, each human being is an individual with an option to pursue life, liberty, and happiness, and it is the business of medicine to correct encumbrances to those pursuits. In fact, as an adjunct to social amelioration, medicine has helped to nullify Malthusian constraints on the proliferation of populations by treatment of individuals suffering traditional scourges. In this treatment, individuals are traditionally distinguished as "cases" of the disease. Differences among cases are perceived as variations on a common theme, and individuals are distinguished only according to how they relate to the classical case.

But molecular genetics is modifying this view to include individual uniqueness in disease. Now we are more likely to perceive the variation not only in relation to the classical case, but as individual expression based on genetic and developmental particularity. Here is a genuine example of integration of biology and medicine. Here biologists' interest in individuals as exemplary of whatever property they may be studying and as variants necessary for the preservation of species has, at the level of the DNA and its products, merged with the medical need for knowledge to individualize diagnosis and management. Here the work of both reductionist and population biologist is put to use in the solution of the individuality of disease, and in the resolution of a curious paradox: the interest of the biologist in the contribution of individuality to adaptation and evolution ignored the identity of each individual, while medicine, however focused on individuals as cases of disease, too often overlooked their individuality. Today we have the wherewithal to allow both biologist and physician to focus on both at once.

Families

A central feature of biology is the union of two gametes to engender a zygote, providing continuity with the past and a precursor to a new and unique individual. In the course of forming the gametes, new mutations are introduced, recombination shuffles the genes to form new combinations, and segregation occurs. Fertilization then supplies another source of variation in the form of new combinations of parental chromosomes. How these ends are attained has occupied the thoughts and energies of many functional biologists, and the molecular details of the structures involved and how they work are now understood to an astonishing degree. In this work, families, whether in the abstract or the specific, are of only the most marginal interest. In contrast, population biology deals with family formation as the means whereby the variants of gametogenesis assembled at fertilization are exposed to selection. So, mating systems, genetic and protein polymorphism, reproductive fitness, ethnicity, and migration form the wherewithal for the work of population geneticists and demographers. But here, too, the family is an abstraction, even when the data are derived from real exemplars.

In medicine, however, the physician's attention is focused traditionally on actual individuals in relation to specific complaints—that is, machines break down one at a time. But obstetricians, pediatricians, and family practitioners constitute themselves as specialists in problems wherein the family is the unit. To them, the relevant biology is functional, but genetics has brought into medicine questions about consanguinity, ethnicity, and family history of illnesses (including the distribution of affected members) as evidence of the participation of variant genes in the cause. Here it is obvious that no assessment of mode of inheritance of disease can be made outside the context of the family. Further, for some purposes, whole families are the basis for linkage work that leads to the detection and description of genes of medical moment. Indeed, questions of family are becoming staples of all doctor-patient relationships, regardless of specialty. They represent the recognition of remote causes that underlie the proximate, and they emphasize the significance of such causes in thinking about prevention of disease.

Uncertainty

While uncertainty and ambiguity bedevil the lives of biologists, they do not handicap their work. Lack of knowledge suggests work to be done, and uncertainty is readily sublimated in hypothesis. If there is no adequate hypothesis, no "handle" on the problem, the biologist is encouraged not to take it up at all, or to await the means to make the study possible. Indeed, Medawar called science "the art of the soluble" (3). Some scientists are distinguished by their timing, their sensitivity to the accessibility of a problem. In any case, the biologist plans his studies, and while competition may promote work at odd hours, it goes according to plan, changing only when results suggest a change.

The physician, in contrast, must tolerate, even embrace, uncertainty and ambiguity. Patients are sick at inconvenient times and appeal to the doctor for relief, expecting action even when the basis for making decisions is inadequate. Sometimes the decision has to be to do nothing, to await developments. Such exigency makes research of some kind necessary, even when the problem is not well defined. It is this need to expand and refine the bases for making decisions

A Logic of Disease

that distinguishes the clinician's research from that of the biologist. The distinction is not that of basic as opposed to applied research, but lies in the original aim of the work. The biologist describes and explains congruence. The clinical investigation may be explanatory, too—this time of incongruence—but the original intent is to reduce or eliminate the uncertainty and ambiguity of decisions that may have to be made in the absence of complete understanding.

It might be added that today, there is some rapprochement of investigators in which congruence and incongruence are studied by the same methods and, increasingly, by the same people. After all, at the molecular level, the difference between outcomes of interest to biologist and clinical investigator might be as little as the substitution of a single nucleotide.

Time

A salient difference between biology and medicine lies in the significance of time. When Max Delbrück, a physicist, began to think about biology, he was startled to realize that everything in it is "time bound" (4). The organism "is not a particular expression of an ideal organism, but one thread in an infinite web of all living forms, all interrelated and all interdependent. . . . It is but a link in an evolutionary chain of changing forms, none of which has any permanent validity." This is in contrast to physics, where "the material and phenomena . . . are the same here and now as they were at all times and as they are on the most distant stars." In other words, every individual representative of every species has a relationship through time to every other; each shares the history of the DNA.

Each such individual has also the history of its own development, its own lifetime. Biologists perceive ontogeny as a prelude to phylogeny; the development of each individual represents a test of the robustness and viability of the species. Indeed, time is built right into living organisms since they all express temporal rhythms varying in periodicity from moments to lifetimes. We are, for example, more likely to experience strokes and heart attacks in the morning because of rhythms expressed in platelets. Similar views are found in Jacob's *The Logic of Life:* "Every living being is inevitably the result of a history that includes not only the sequence of events in which its ancestors participated, but also the succession of transformations by which that organism has been gradually fashioned" (5). So time is not something to be taken for granted or ignored; it is at the heart of the logic of disease.

In traditional medical thinking, however, species and the history of the DNA are of marginal interest. The physician's attention is held by what must be done now. In biology as in Ecclesiastes, "To every thing there is a season, and a time to every purpose under the heaven, a time to be born and a time to die." Not so in medicine, where if imminent birth will be harmful, the time to be born is changed, and a primary aim is to defer death as long as possible. To these ends medicine is practiced cross-sectionally: obstetrics, pediatrics, adolescent medicine, internal medicine, and geriatrics all represent compartments wherein the nature of the work is determined by the age at onset of disease. Such a narrow focus is likely to minimize the physician's appreciation of the unity and continuity of a lifetime that proceeds from zygote to dissolution, as well as to obscure the historical quality of development in which the attributes of today carry the stamp of the past.

But our thinking is changing in two ways. First is in the recognition of the predictive powers of genetics that can influence reproductive decisions for individuals found to harbor undesirable mutants and allow estimates of recurrence rates for familial diseases. This, in turn, is affecting the compartmentalization of medicine. Divisions and departments of genetics cross age boundaries to reveal patients as people with pasts that began in the lives of their ancestors and futures that will be colored by genes inherited from those predecessors. Here the biologist's idea of time is imposed on the pragmatism of medicine.

Second, we now recognize that predispositions to diseases of late onset reside not only in the genes but in experiences of early life. Once, the natural history of a disease included only the time from some overt onset to its end. Now such a history may be traced to conditions of susceptibility that, depending on both genetic conditions and contingent experiences, may develop from onset of subtle expressions in utero through a steady progression of pathogenesis to overt manifestation. It is as if people grow into their diseases. Atherosclerosis and hypertension are examples.

Progress

Biologists and physicians alike partake of prevalent ideas. One such idea is progress, a prominent concept of our century. It is our belief that civilization moves in a forward direction toward some goal (6,7). It is undeniable that there has been a steady, even accelerating, progress in the accumulation of information and insight about ourselves and the world around us. In this sense, progress is undoubted, but what the goal might be—or even if there is a goal—has not been resolved. Indeed, on this point there is a difference between biology and medicine. Progress in biology lies in penetrating to the core of the secrets of life, even if the search leads to the revelation that life has no purpose, while some in medicine see the final goal as ridding humanity of disease.

Progress in Biology

Until the eighteenth century, all living creatures were perceived as arranged in a grand hierarchy, a "great chain of being" that began with the most microscopic and primitive at the bottom and rose to the angels at the top (7). It was God's arrangement, and because the hierarchy was determined by His ineffa-

A Logic of Disease

ble will, there could be no holes in the chain, nor could any new form of life be envisioned. But with Darwin, a historical dimension was added to the lower-to-higher concept, and there appeared to be a progression in the complexity of life. Species were seen to have proliferated to become the thousands known then—and the millions we presume to exist today. So evolution has brought changes in direction, number, size, and complexity over time. Is that progress?

To the biologist, progress includes two components: direction and value. The directional change is from one state to a better state (8,9). "Better" is described in terms of the amount and chromosomal packaging of DNA, as well as in an expansion of life expressed in (a) the number and kinds of organisms, (b) the number of individuals within each kind, (c) the total bulk of living matter, and (d) the complexity of organisms, including their ability to organize and process information about the environment in order to control it. But although the standard by which better or worse is judged is in some degree subjective, there is no criterion of "best" in the abstract or for all purposes, nor is anything implied about evolution toward any ideal. Indeed, the ideal in biology, if there is one, is not perfection but imperfection—embodied, for example, in a sufficient heterozygosity to allow adaptation to changed circumstances. A perfect homozygosity is a prescription for extinction. So, biologists recognize that however progress is defined, the process might be interrupted if the environment were to change, and then other adaptations, other organisms, might be perceived as higher or better. Progress in biology is contingent. After all, millions of once well-adapted species are now extinct.

The Medical Idea of Progress

Medicine participates in the idea of an inevitable and continuous progress in our understanding of the pathogenesis of disease so that the way to management will be revealed. Cure is often mentioned in this connection. No one questions the extraordinary accumulation of knowledge of human biology or the remarkable advances in technology that have made it possible. The virtues of such undoubted medical feats are incontestable, but are they precursors of an era of perfect health or a world free of disease?

The decline in rates of mortality for many diseases is undeniable; in the developed world the average lifetime has been expanded and morbidity has been displaced toward old age, resulting in the "rectangularization" of the mortality curve (10). This progress is in part a consequence of modern medicine but perhaps even more of such social changes as improved housing, diet and hygiene, and public education. The decline in premature death from heart attack, for example, must surely be in some degree due to the efforts of the American Heart Association to promote the benefits of a healthy diet and exercise.

These successes have stimulated thoughts of eliminating individual diseases—the example of smallpox is often cited—and finally of doing away with disease altogether. That would indeed be progress, but is it possible? Some who have been willing to speculate put their faith in technological development and in Lewis Thomas's "thinking our way around." Some—including Thomas, though perhaps with tongue in cheek—have suggested that the rectangularization of the mortality curve might be pushed to the limit of the innate human plan, so that we should each go to pieces all at once like the Deacon's wonderful one-hoss shay in Oliver Wendell Holmes's poem (10–12).

For their part, biologists are unlikely to be able to imagine such a world. As long as species continue to generate new mutations and new combinations of old genes in their quest for adaptive variation, and as long as microorganisms participate in the mutational and recombinational dance, freedom from disease will remain a dream. And there are obstacles beyond the biological. As long as we continue to devise and invent new conditions of living, and to manufacture substances that neglect or overwhelm human endowment, we shall continue to have disease in vulnerable individuals. Human diversity opposes the end of disease.

No doubt few physicians foresee the elimination of disease, but the contrast in thinking outlined here is a consequence of the appeal of biologists to evolution, in which progress is always spelled with a lowercase *p,* and that of the physician to the metaphor of the machine which accommodates easily to the principle that anything that breaks can be fixed—all that is needed is more knowledge.

CONCLUSION

The characteristics of the thought of these two disciplines derive from the principles upon which each is based. Those of biology are variation, natural selection, and evolution; that of medicine is the body as a machine. When the two are perceived as confluent it is because the thinking has become more nearly biological; the common ground is to be found in what flows from the dominant idea of evolution. But when they are perceived as in strong contrast, the differences are those that distinguish the medicine of Garrod from that of Osler. The lesson is plain. A logic of disease can be constructed only when medical thinking is informed by biology, when it is based on what flows from evolution. The next chapter presents a formal synthesis of the ideas of medicine and biology as it is represented by genetics.

7

A Synthesis

It is perhaps unnecessary to state the obvious conclusion that if one is to understand the metabolism of the organism . . . in the most complete way possible, genes must be taken into account. . . . . The biochemist cannot understand what goes on chemically in the organism without considering genes any more than a geneticist can fully appreciate the gene without taking into account what it is and what it does. It is a most unfortunate consequence of . . . the inflexible organization of our institutions of higher learning that investigators tend to be forced into laboratories with such labels as "biochemistry" or "genetics." The gene does not recognize the distinction—we should at least minimize it.

—G. W. Beadle, "The Genetic Control of Biochemical Reactions" (1)

The necessity to come to grips with molecular aspects of all our problems has dissolved the barriers that worried Beadle; cloning and manipulation of genes is to be found in the departments on the clinical side of the street no less than on that of the basic sciences. So genetics and molecular biology have been the means whereby clinical and basic medical research have been unified. The gap between biochemistry and genetics has been more than minimized—it has been obliterated.

THE EVOLUTIONARY SYNTHESIS

Genetics was also an instrument of the unification of biology, a consequence of a dramatic exchange of ideas among geneticists, paleobiologists, and systematists during the 1930s to '50s (2–4). The geneticists, accustomed to populations in which the only contrast was between wild type and mutant, began to accept the evolutionist's view that natural populations are composed of individuals so variable as to make the wild type–mutant contrast almost meaningless—that is, typological thinking gave way to population thinking. In contrast, the evolutionary biologists saw that although the object of natural selection is always the phenotype, not the genes, phenotypic differences nearly always reflect genetic variation. There was a merger in which both sides agreed that the meaning of proximate causes is never completely clear except in the context of remote causes. Both sides perceived their meeting ground to be the phenotype.

The catalysts in this rearrangement of thinking were population geneticists, who perceived evolution as an outcome of changes in gene frequency particularly by natural selection, and evolutionary biologists, who saw that although shifts in gene frequency alone were an insufficient explanation of evolution, neither paleontology nor taxonomy could go much farther without accepting the genetic origin of phenotypes. Both perceived above all the continuity of the new position: micro-evolution is at the root of and continuous with macro-evolution. It was this continuity that constituted the unifying principle. Geneticists, hitherto preoccupied with the physical basis of heredity and with definitions of the gene, assumed new responsibilities for explaining evolution, while evolutionists accepted the fluctuations of gene frequencies as underlying explanations of evolution. Other biologists, including botanists and zoologists, followed suit, and before long the unifying influence of what was soon called the "evolutionary synthesis," or neo-Darwinism, was reflected in universities by the consolidation of evolutionary biology, genetics, botany, and zoology into departments that bore the simple name "biology." Each group carried on with specialized research and teaching but all in the context of a single discipline unified by the principles of natural selection and evolution.

A Synthesis of Medical and Biological Thought

Another synthesis is in progress today with genetics as the integrating principle. In the last chapter I contrasted the goals of biologists and physicians and showed where differing points of view were shifting toward accommodation. This shift represents the beginning of a synthesis of medical and genetic thinking. What does *synthesis* mean in this context? It is the antithesis of analysis which, in medicine, means the reduction of proximate causes and pathogenesis to their molecular identity. Synthetic thinking characterizes the humanities, while in science and medicine analysis predominates (5). But since "synthesis provides a framework of interpretation and analysis of particulars that helps propel thought and feeling to important truths" (5), the idea of such a union should be examined.

This fusion of genetic and medical thinking is in two parts. In the first, genetic variation, population thinking and recognition of remote causes add a significant dimension to the already well established reductionist analysis of disease and pathogenesis. In the second, genetics, as defined in the first, informs medical thinking about diagnosis, treatment, and the relationship of medicine to patients, the family, and society.

A Logic of Disease

Holton has elaborated a system for evaluating the potential for synthesis (5). These principles are (a) the elements to be fused should be both inclusive and historically valid; (b) the synthesis should be embraced within some single principle; (c) the union should lead to predictions beyond those suggested by the separate elements; (d) the elements should cohere in fashioning a new viewpoint; and (e) the impact of the synthesis should reach beyond that of any of the components to influence the culture wherein it occurs.

Does this synthesis of medical and genetic thinking qualify? The elements to be fused appear in Table 1, which contrasts characteristics of the engineering or machine attitudes to disease with the alternative that, when combined with the machine mentality, should constitute a basis for a genetic medicine. Thus, the comparison is in no way invidious; the alternative is not intended to replace the machine approach but, by adding new dimensions, to liberate it. The table lists six elements of thought about disease and seven outcomes, or directions the thinking takes in leading to application. How do these elements qualify according to Holton's principles?

1. *Historical Validity and Inclusiveness.* The components of both ideas and outcomes represent historically affirmed staples of thinking about medicine and genetics. All are accredited by long usage; in none is there incompatibility. As to inclusiveness, no elements have yet been found to imperil the synthesis.

2. *A First Principle.* There is an enveloping idea that, while not implied by the machine model, easily embraces the product of the synthesis. The causes

Table 1 **Elements of the Synthesis**

	The Body as Machine	The Alternative
	IDEAS	
Causes	proximate	remote
Thinking	typological-reductionist	population
Individuality	as member of class	as class of one's own
Focus	genotypes	phenotypes
Time	ahistorical	historical
Evolution	irrelevant	basis
	OUTCOMES	
Variation	discrete	continuous
Experimental approach	analytical	synthetic
Relation to environment	genes versus experience	genes with experience
Application	specialism	general, family
Management	therapeutic	preventive
Education versus training	training	education
Coherence	dispersing	unifying
Icon	Osler	Garrod

and characteristics of disease are a consequence of incongruities between individual endowment as expressed in ontogeny and the conditions of homeostasis of open systems abroad in the environment. Each is a new test of selection and grist for the mill of evolution.

3. *Cohesion of the Systems.* It might be supposed that coherence would be defied by the power of reductionism, which lies in its lack of limits. Like the hydra that generates two heads for every one lopped off, the answer to each question evokes new ones. But coherence of the elements within the synthesis at hand is easily demonstrated. When each of the thought processes listed in the alternative column is added to that expressed in the body-as-machine column, the scope of potential thought and action is enlarged. Individuality is introduced, thinking is populational, the focus is on phenotypes that are a consequence of genetically specified unit steps of homeostasis adapting to experiences in ontogeny to produce a continuity of variation and disease. Remote causes are introduced to deal with the "why" questions. In raising these we are questioning the goals of conventional medicine and even probing the limits of our ability to "think our way around." Asking questions and groping for answers characterize education very well, distinguishing it from training as nothing else can.

4. *Prediction.* Contemplation of the machine model leads to no particular predictions, beyond some likelihood that any machine will break and that some parts are more breakable than others. But genetics is the most predictive of sciences, not only of modes of inheritance but also of likelihood of disease depending upon genotype. Indeed, it goes farther to predict that (a) given what is known about mutation, any unit step of homeostasis is likely to be a site for genetic aberration; (b) symptoms, severity, and age at onset will depend upon type of mutant and the degree of its selective disadvantage; (c) by virtue of the numbers and types of allelic variants in the gene pool, each member of any species is genetically unique, a uniqueness no less likely to be expressed in disease than in health; and (d) depending upon mating systems, migration, isolation, and the like, each population is likely to differ in representation of the alleles of its gene pool, distinguishing each by specificity of disease and number of cases. Thus does the synthesis make predictable how, why, when, and under what conditions the machine breaks down.

5. *Cultural Reach.* The machine model is quite indifferent to the environment beyond recognizing that the breakdown is often a consequence of particular experiences. It does not necessarily prompt the doctor to inquire minutely into the quality, quantity, or other aspect of precipitating events, or necessarily to feel or express responsibility for a society that tolerates or promotes an experience injurious to some of its members. But when this model is clothed in the alternative to constitute a synthetic viewpoint, individuals are distinguished as to the phenotypic effects of experiences representative of their

culture, and the discovery of such a genetic vulnerability predicts some probability, great or small, of a disease when the patient is exposed to a provocative agent. Such knowledge of propensity is likely to lead physicians to discover in their patients specificities of both susceptibility and experience and to become their advocate in promoting social change where hazard exists. Indeed, a principal impact of the synthesis may be in according to prevention the cachet hitherto reserved for treatment.

In the union of medical and genetic thinking, nothing appears to be incompatible with the provisos proposed by Holton. We may therefore confidently expect genetics ultimately to permeate medical thinking and education. This process of slow but accelerating spread differs somewhat from that of the evolutionary synthesis, which was hastened by active dialogue among the participants (2,3). Genetics made its first overture to medicine about fifty years ago with the founding of the American Society of Human Genetics. In outlining the origins of the society and the publication of its journal, H. J. Muller, its first president, observed that "an unfortunate compartmentalization has for many years hindered persons in medicine and in the other specifically human disciplines from attaining the necessary knowledge of genetics, and *mutatis mutandis,* has hindered geneticists from mastering the necessary human subjects." He hoped, therefore, that the new society and journal would work to "avoid that dilettantism which has in the past characterized so many attempts to study human genetics" (6). In the interval, a strong medical-genetics enterprise has sprung up, and now we are on the threshold of a genetic medicine. Muller would have been delighted.

There is a further difference between the evolutionary and the medical-genetic syntheses. In the former, genetics promoted the reductionist view and evolutionary biology imposed coherence by relating the genes to integrated phenotypes. In the latter, it is the other way around. Here medicine promotes the molecular approach, while genetics, in the form of a populational and evolutionary perspective, curbs and integrates a runaway reductionism.

In contrast to these differences, there is an aspect in which the evolutionary synthesis and the logic of disease are in perfect accord: the point of union of both is the phenotype. In the former it was accepted that it was phenotypes, not genes, that were the object of selection, but it was also clear that genes specified the phenotypes. Similarly, in the latter, the machine approach ends with the description of the unit step(s) of homeostasis involved in the pathogenesis of a disease, while the genetic approach carries on the description to the specificity of the single case.

Thus, in the synthetic logic we have the best of both worlds. The molecular analysis accounts at once for the unity of life and its diversity. The unity is mediated by molecular biology and biochemistry through which we comprehend our homeostasis. The diversity is exemplified in the individuality of integrated functions, in the patient, in the disease, and in the cultural frameworks that furnish agents of provocation, as well as in the social networks whence patients come and which support them in their illness. It is a merger of Oslerian and Garrodian thinking.

Uses of the Synthesis

In the outline of the synthesis, evolution fulfilled the requirement of a first principle and in Table 1 it is listed as the basis for the alternative way of thinking, so it must be through evolution that the argument for a logic of disease and a genetic medicine can be developed. But what is evolution? The subject remains as lively and contentious as ever. But for medicine, the arena is greatly reduced; the questions are more nearly answerable. We are not primarily concerned with whether, or how, natural selection is responsible for the complexity and integration of human homeostasis but with how it deals with variation in that homeostasis, especially that which interferes with homeostatic adaptation. So for the purposes of this book, we might say that evolution is defined by the processes biological organisms undergo to attain the morphological, physiological, and genetic characteristics that identify species. It proceeds by descent with such modification as may be useful in attaining adaptive flexibility in unstable environments that are partly of the species' own making. The modifications are a result of the proliferation, whether by selection or chance, of genetic variation that facilitates the broad range of congruence required for the reproduction and development of individuals and for the continuity of life both between and within species. The success or failure of such variants in fulfilling these missions is likely to be reflected in their frequencies in subsequent generations.

Words and phrases in this definition most pertinent to the logic of disease are species identity, adaptive flexibility and development, descent with modification, reproduction, frequency, and range of congruence and continuity of life. These key words and phrases can be elaborated into propositions that embody the elements of the logic and the structure of genetic medicine, and it is to developing and integrating these elements that Parts III through VI are devoted.

This is the book's key chapter. Everything before it led up to it and all that follows is elaboration. It may be that the reader's sense of continuity will be reinforced by occasional reference to its concluding paragraphs and to Table 1.

III
Species Identity

Species identity was one of the phrases employed in defining evolution and as constituting an element in the structure of the logic that underlies genetic medicine. What do the words mean?

Species begin in isolated populations that evolve to lose the capacity to reproduce with those whence they originated. Other qualities distinguish them, too, even while retaining resemblances, both physical and molecular, with predecessors. Among these are ways of dealing with the environment, whether in exploiting it or adapting to it. Such qualities are both promoted and constrained by genes that specify proteins that integrate to form a homeostasic apparatus peculiar to the species, and while the structure and flexibility of such an apparatus may be adaptive for experiences imposed upon and chosen by that species, it may be limiting for others. Which is to say, it is a wise species that knows its own environment. The single chapter in this section reveals some conditions in which human ingenuity has exceeded human homeostatic adaptation.

8

Lessons from Phylogeny

Whatever is, is right.
—Alexander Pope, *An Essay on Man*

We need not subscribe to the eighteenth-century ideology that informed Pope's essay to see that this line has some use as a metaphor for the relationship between a species and its environment. We might assume that if a quality exists, it has stood the test of selection and might have served a useful function at some time and in some place. It need not be the best possible adaptation—evolution is a process of tinkering—but whatever is selected could represent, or have represented, some advantage.

ADAPTATION

The search for such useful functions is the essence of what evolutionary biologists call "the adaptationist program." It is defined by Williams in this way:

> Adherents of this program, when confronted with a biological phenomenon, try to envision it as an aspect of an adaptation. An adaptation is some sort of biological machinery or process shaped by natural selection to help solve one or more problems faced by the organism. The phenomenon may be interpreted as a necessary component of the imagined machinery, or as an unavoidable cost of the machinery or as some incidental manifestations of its operation (1).

Williams and Nesse called our attention to the necessity to add explanations based on evolutionary biology to the proximate causes of disease (1,2). There is, however, some controversy about the adaptationist program. Some suggest that its advocates rely too heavily on natural selection and are too ready to invoke plausibility as evidence thereof (3). That is, selection is not the only reason for whatever is; other causes may prevail. For example, changes in the gene pool may be due to migration or founder effect, and there is evidence that most human protein polymorphism arises without selection. Further, although organisms unquestionably adapt to their surroundings, they also redesign the environment to suit themselves (4). So if an animal seems ideally suited to its conditions, it may be for reasons of its own. Human culture is perhaps the most extreme example. It is also true that selection cannot act on each quality separately. Physiological and morphological development are so complex and so constrained that some qualities that seem to be adaptive may have been carried along without selection because of their tight integration with others that were under intense selective scrutiny (3). Further, this kind of constraint must extend beyond individuals to phylogeny. An example is the upright posture of Homo sapiens: perhaps we are not ideally suited to stand erect because so much of the architectural design we have inherited from the dim past is unsuited for it. So, although much of whatever we are may have been attained by natural selection, some qualities may be attributable to evolution by other means.

But for genetic medicine, whatever is, is a context in which disease may occur. Whatever is, whether adaptive or not, represents the distribution of existing states, the normal against which to measure the abnormal and to describe potential incongruities, defined by the range and fluid conditions of human culture. Conventional medical thinking does not include concern about the evolutionary origins of potential incongruities. Medicine concentrates on violations of the norm that are expressed in dysfunction, discomfort, and disability, and their meaning in phylogeny is seldom questioned. But we cannot understand those variations fully until we have asked in what way they are a consequence of evolution. Several ways come to mind: (a) mutation ensures that whatever is can go wrong and will do so within whatever constraints evolution may have imposed; (b) the kinds of disease that can occur are constrained by the specific paths taken by evolution; (c) diseases are a result of limitations of a genetically, and so phylogenetically, conditioned homeostasis in the face of experiences for which it is unprepared; and (d) it is even possible that disease may be at its worst where adaptation is best, where it has been conserved across species and is tolerant of environments but in individual cases is brought down by mutation.

We don't know the answers to questions of evolution's role in disease. There is no tradition in medicine for asking or answering them. But for medical thinking informed by genetics, questions of phylogenetic significance are natural, even obligatory. This chapter provides examples to illustrate three such questions: (a) shared genetic heritage may mean that intolerance to particular experiences will cross species barriers; (b) species differences will be expressed in species-specific incongruence; and (c) since cultural evolution is so much faster than biological, a species' repertory of adaptations is likely, in time and in particular instances, to be exceeded. The first example describes a popular human experience, not shared by other species, that has proven harmful to many individuals. In the second, a species-specific adaptation exerts, to human detriment, an unanticipated constraint, and in the third, what in Paleolithic times presumably represented ranges of adaptation are now perceived to be ranges of vulnerability. The conditions under scrutiny are run-of-the-mill disorders, seldom perceived in any evolutionary context. But it is that context that unites them, that gives coherence to the idea of disease.

The Use of Tobacco

Plants and animals are not widely known to seek or tolerate an atmosphere of smoke; it seems that only Homo sapiens purposely dilutes inspired oxygen with carbon monoxide and any number of other substances, mutagenic, carcinogenic, and otherwise toxic. At some time in the twentieth century, a biologically informed society might have made these observations and taken warning, rather than waiting to be convinced by the weight of empirical evidence. But we are more alert now; the example of tobacco has been generalized. Today no substance capable of the range and extent of damage plainly caused by tobacco could possibly be widely advertised and legitimately sold— except tobacco, and even that is seriously threatened. So if in the past a wide-awake Darwinist had observed that inhalation of smoke is unnatural throughout the animal kingdom, the possibility of its being harmful to man might have been carefully examined. But, as it happened, the hazard of smoking became apparent in Britain only when it was observed to be strongly associated with an otherwise unaccountable rise in the incidence of bronchogenic cancer, and in the United States only when a surgeon observed the frequency of heavy smokers among his patients with lung cancer (5,6). The observations were entirely empirical; no one had tested the hypothesis that smoking might be damaging. Evidence of the relationship of smoking and chronic obstructive pulmonary disease and heart attack came only after suspicion of the malign effects of smoking had been aroused.

Today we know that smoking is associated with cancer of several organs in addition to the lung, chronic pulmonary infections, atherosclerosis, and heart attack, reproductive hazards, and, indeed, abnormality of nearly every organ system. It is an imposing list and new associations continue to be found. Every year the *Index Medicus* includes upward of a thousand papers recounting these hazards and their consequences. Such a list is a stern commentary on the perception of the body as a machine to be fixed when it breaks, and a powerful recommendation for prevention. One wonders how and when it will end. Not soon, given the long incubation periods that attach to some of these disorders. The collective impact on mortality has been appraised by Peto et al., who concluded that about 80 percent of deaths of individuals between thirty-five and sixty-nine years of age in thirty-one "developed" countries during the 1980s were attributable to smoking (7). So smoking is now a principal contributor to early mortality. Medical educators might do well to teach the virtues of nature's examples.

Breastfeeding

No one would deny that human milk is the "natural" food for newly born human babies; evolution has seen to that (8). Breastfeeding leads to temporary amenorrhea in the mother and a natural spacing of pregnancies of around two years (9). Without this natural contraception, more frequent childbearing may promote disease and mortality for all infants embraced within the narrowed interval (9,10). But for many reasons—some of necessity, some trivial—infants may be fed nonhuman milk.

We act as if birth represents a discrete discontinuity from intrauterine life. Indeed, we date our lives and count our age from the moment of birth, and we celebrate the event annually. But these are cultural observances that have little to do with biology, because birth is in fact a far less abrupt change than it seems: it is more like doing the same business under new conditions. At birth the infant becomes autonomous with respect to physiology and development but must still conform to the trajectory set in utero and supported by the maternal environment. Some of the infant's physiological equipment needs time to adapt to the new environment, and it is human milk that has been designed by nature to supply the antibodies, nutrients, and other substances the infant lacks. In a sense, the breast has assumed the homeostatic role of the cast-off placenta.

Cow's milk is the most popular substitute, but is it appropriate? Apparently not (11). For example, the development of the human neonate is well behind that of a newborn calf, so we may question whether cow's milk, which is adapted to the needs of calves, is attuned to the dynamics of early postnatal human development. That it is not is suggested by the discovery that average attainments on tests of cognitive development of premature infants fed cow's milk were found to be significantly less than those of their breastfed coevals (12). Further, a comparison of learning-disabled children with controls showed that significantly fewer of the former were breast fed (13), and scores in language attainment tests of fifteen-year-old children were significantly higher among those who had been breast fed (14). If acuity of visual evoked potential (VEP) is in any way a surrogate for those cognitive functions, some insight into their deficiency is obtained in the results of a study in which deficient maturation of VEP acuity observed in babies fed cow's milk was corrected by the addition to their diet of long-chain polyunsaturated fatty acids normally abundant in breast milk but wanting in that of the cow (15).

There are other protective effects of human as opposed to cow's milk, though the reasons for them are not always clear. Protection against diabetes may be attained by avoiding cow's milk proteins (16), while the evolutionary origin of protection against diarrhea is demonstrated by the discovery in hu-

Species Identity

man milk of a glycolipid receptor analogue that binds to *Shiga* toxin, thereby depriving the toxin of a means to adhere to its target receptors (17). Another example of protection against microorganisms is a mucin in human milk that specifically binds rotaviruses (18), and still another is the enhancement of response to *Hemophilus influenzae* vaccine in breastfed babies (19). Other antimicrobial agents in human milk are secretory IgA, maternal IgG and IgM, lactoferrin, fibronectin, lysozyme, and elements of the complement cascade.

So, human milk is best for human babies. No data exist to attest to the dangers of human milk when fed to calves, but we have every reason to suppose them to exist. For example, proteins in human milk that protect against microorganisms that threaten human babies may leave undaunted those that are inimical to calves. Oddly enough, the evolutionary significance of human milk has been remarked for years, but until recently medical thinking managed to ignore it, so we have been given all sorts of milk substitutes—some facsimiles, some representing "improvements"—but human milk is a cardinal example of Pope's axiom, or possibly of that of the later, less elegant poet, who said, "If it ain't broke, don't fix it."

The Stone Age and Modern Times

Human cultural evolution has raced so far ahead of its biological counterpart that human beings are ill equipped genetically to adapt to environments that change almost every day. And gene-environment incongruence is an incitement to disease. Eaton and his colleagues summarized the evidence for a state of "dissonance" between life in the developed world and that of ten thousand years ago (20). Before that time there was no agriculture and human beings lived precariously as hunter-gatherers. The disparity between a life of exposure to nature and that of today is such that, unless the genetic evolution of our species has been more rapid than we think, we are now traveling on something like the genome of the Stone Age, a genome that in some respects is unsuitable for some of the habits, customs, and experiences that prevail in our society. If this is true, disease may be a consequence, and high blood pressure, atherosclerosis, diabetes, obesity, and diverticulitis might have such an origin.

Evidence bearing on this hypothesis derives from two sources: (a) similarities between human genes and those of related primates suggest that the former are much the same as they were in prehistoric times, and (b) the few remaining tribes living under conditions resembling those of the Stone Age, although afflicted with microbial and parasitic diseases, are spared some of the diseases we observe so frequently today.

Genetic Likeness

The human proteins that we know resemble closely those of other primates, especially the chimpanzee (21). Amino acid sequences are startlingly—

some might say humiliatingly—similar, so alike that the differences between humans and other primate species are thought to be a consequence of developmental and regulatory genes. The divergence of hominids from other primates occurred several million years ago, so this stability of amino acid sequences in proteins illuminates the very marked disparity between cultural and genetic evolution. That is, many of the diseases we experience today must be a consequence of our cultural evolution rather than of significant change in our gene pool.

Observation of Tribal Societies

Several tribal societies have been investigated but none so thoroughly as the Xavante and the Yanomama in Brazil and Venezuela, observed by Neel (22). Although Neel is emphatic in differentiating these societies from those of the Stone Age—for example, some of the food of the modern populations is cultivated—they are so similar as to provide useful insights into life in those times. The idea of Neel's study was to define the population structures within which the evolutionary forces that account for the characteristics of the human species might have operated before the modern era. The qualities studied were mating patterns, differential fertility, survival, the genetic composition of the population, and health.

Assessment of the latter indicated that it was of a high degree. The diet was remarkably varied. Although most of the calories derived from plantain, the daily fare also included cassava and meat, mostly from small animals and birds but also from frogs, lizards, and insect larvae. Obviously, refined carbohydrates were unheard of. As to physical condition, vision was on the average better than U.S. standards, dental caries and malocclusion were seldom observed, and obesity, diabetes, and hypertension were rare. Infant mortality was lower than might be imagined, perhaps because of spacing of babies and prolonged breastfeeding. Serum cholesterol was very low by our standard, as was blood pressure, which reached the neighborhood of 110/65 at adolescence and rose no further, however long the life. And the near absence of sodium in the urine indicated a low-salt diet that may well have had some bearing on the lack of hypertension. Infections, especially malaria and hepatitis, were frequent; the survival curve, when compared to that of the United States, revealed a much reduced life expectancy, due principally to death by infection or trauma.

These observations constitute a definition of "a norm for humans that has obtained for millions of years, departures from which may create new evolutionary pressures even as old pressures diminish" (22). That is, this is the way people were before industrial progress brought material abundance and relief from infections as well as from other selective pressures. Both sources of evidence point in the same direction: when compared to what we believe the hu-

Species Identity

man condition to have been thousands of years ago, our genetic strengths and vulnerabilities have not changed very much. Only the way we live has changed.

CONCLUSION

"*Non nocere primum,*" says the Hippocratic oath. Although this warning is presumed to apply to doctors who treat individual patients, it is no less applicable to societies that set norms for individual and community behavior. Today this admonition rules the judgments of federal and state authorities about what is acceptable for public use and is represented in the elaborate designs of clinical trials. So we acknowledge dangers discovered by empirical observation, and in general we face them constructively, sometimes despite organized resistance. Probably the empirical way was the only way. It is only recently that we have begun to appreciate the complexity of the human organism, to realize how precisely integrated it is and how likely are efforts to "fix" one part of it to interfere with that integration.

Forty years ago alterations to cow's milk intended to make it "simulate" human milk led to serious disease. In one of these "adjustments," phosphoric acid was added to cow's milk, a maneuver that changed the calcium:phosphorus ratio from 2:1 to 1:1. Result: tetany of the newborn, a sometimes fatal disorder (23). A second treatment omitted folic acid. Result: macrocytic anemia (24). A third was deficient in vitamin B6. Result: convulsions (25,26). These adjustments were a consequence of ignorance. While it was recognized that breast milk was best, the efforts to make cow's milk resemble it were misguided because so little was known about the actual composition of either.

The ignorance is still being dispelled, and chief among the agents of this new understanding is the recognition of our phylogenetic kinship with all life, a kinship expressed not only in metabolic and molecular similarity or even identity, but in ecological relationships that are disturbed at our peril. Perhaps in our expanding grasp of the complexity of disease, we are discovering the lesson evolution teaches so plainly: the integration of physiological systems constrains further evolution to fit precisely with what already exists. This suggests that we can understand disease only insofar as we can see (a) how each individual component of each homeostatic device relates to others, (b) how these relationships are integrated into hierarchies of emergent qualities not predicted by the unit step or even the homeostatic device of which it is a part, and (c) that treatments are likely to succeed only when their impact can be restricted to restoring the homeostatic step or steps that have gone awry. So a first principle for medical education might be this: contemplation of the human condition, which is so nearly exclusively turned inward, ought equally to be turned outward to see ourselves as bound to the life around us in relationships that it is in our interest to observe and take warning.

It might be argued that the environment and our place in phylogeny are the province of ecology, paleontology, and anthropology, or at least of environmental medicine and public health. It could be argued, too, that since it is toward patient care that nearly all students will move and since such disciplines as ecology are little applied in practice, they have no particular relevance to medical education. But if medical education is to transcend medical training, the ultimate destinies of the students are not at the beginning of much concern. It is the ideas that integrate medicine that must occupy students' minds, not their own future outcomes. Indeed, decisions on future outcomes ought, perhaps, to be strongly influenced by those ideas.

IV
Adaptive Flexibility:
Homeostasis and Development

Joshua Lederberg has said that "the principal perspectives of human biology are the evolutionary, the developmental, and the ecological" (1). Lederberg's observation informs this introduction and the next five chapters, in which the homeostasis of the steady state is shown to be compounded of those of the genes, development, and environments, including cultures.

The most obvious evidence of the interactions of these homeostatic devices is the lifelong stability of our individuality. In ordinary social commerce, human individuality is not in question; we have little difficulty in identifying one another, whether by physical appearance or by behavioral characteristics. Further, we each cultivate a social front compounded in part of these physical traits, which we set off by a choice of hair style, clothes, or other such trappings, and in part of our manner, forms of speech, and qualities of character, responses which, in the course of becoming ingrained, are increasingly sharply delineated and refined, becoming ever more individualistic, more defining of self.

The constancy of this distinctiveness is maintained despite the quality, intensity, and duration of our experiences, the intimacy of our relationship to the environment, and the flow of time. We are all open systems moving freely in an environment that we inhale and exhale, ingest and egest, accrete and excrete, which we see, hear, feel, smell, and taste, to which we adhere by gravity and within which we cohere in families, communities, and societies. We are never at an equilibrium but in a steady state in which the concentration of cellular components is more or less constant, the rate of income equals that of output, and the rate of formation equals that of degradation, entropy is at a minimum, and efficiency is at a maximum. In addition, we shed and replace the cells of many of our organs so that although throughout life we are ourselves only and no one else, it is through many incarnations that we have maintained identity and stability. How?

The individuality of human beings is a reflection of the individuality of homeostasis, a straightforward concept that is deeply embedded in medical thought. It is usually defined as the steady state, an outcome in which an open system is given access to and protection from the external environment. Recent usage includes in the definition the mechanisms by which the steady state is attained and that sustain constancy and continuity under ordinary conditions as well as in the face of experiences that, unless opposed, could be injurious.

As it is generally expressed, the idea of physiological homeostasis is strongly typological: although it is the steady state of the individual that must be maintained, the ways in which different people might attain that stability are seldom distinguished. But a typological understanding cannot account for the ability of each particular human being to retain unique identity in the face of a the variety of experiences of a lifetime or the constant turnover of cells. Archibald Garrod's understanding of homeostasis was of necessity rudimentary, but he perceived that any such uniqueness would have to be based on what he called "chemical individuality." Today these two currents, the typological scheme and the idea of individuality, flow together, and we know both the molecular details of homeostasis and how it can vary as a consequence of molecular individuality arising from genetic variation. We also know that it is the uniqueness of our genetic program that ensures our identity throughout development and aging as well as in the face of experiences that test our capacities to adapt.

So, human physiological homeostasis is dependent upon genes, and the individuality of homeostasis is dependent upon the particular genome of each human being. But physiological homeostasis has a further basis, emphasized particularly by C. H. Waddington (2). That same genome that accounts for physiological individuality also constrains the developmental trajectories taken throughout life, trajectories that are influenced by how the outcomes of the genetic plan are shaped by forces of the environment (2). Physiological homeostasis is therefore an outcome of the forces that shape the gene pool and account for individual aliquots thereof and of the genes and ecological conditions that determine development and preserve identity throughout life.

There is still another component. Homeostatic systems are the means by which organisms adapt to the environment. But the environment is not static. It, too, has order, context, rules, and forces that shape it. There is a homeostasis of the environment that changes through time, and physiological, developmental, and genetic homeostasis are intelligible only in relation to that of the environment.

Physiological homeostasis, then, is dependent upon a homeostasis of the genes, a homeostasis of development, and a homeostasis of cultures. And it was Waddington's observation that since the adaptive state of the moment is a product of both the history of the lifetime and that of the species, the properties of both species and individual organisms can be understood only in the context of all three of these time scales (2). By extension, if we wish to understand congruence and incongruence, homeostasis and disease, it will be in the context of those same three time frames.

Cultural and political history can also be represented in the context of similar time frames, a concept characteristic of the French *Annales* historians (3,4). History begins with an almost timeless background phase composed of the physical environment and including the geographical, climatological, and evolutionary cycles within which human history works itself out. Here the analogy is to Lederberg's evolutionary perspective and Waddington's phylogenetic time scale. Second is a history of more easily calculable time, which embraces the rise and fall of empires, cultures, and economic systems, in analogy to the developmental perspective of Lederberg and time scale of Waddington. Finally, there is a more immediate history of events in which individuals occupy the stage. This is analogous to the ecological perspective and the time scale of the moment. So there is in history a basic substratum, an ontogeny of cultures, and a record of immediate events in which individuality can be discerned. Each of these historical levels embraces, enables, shapes, and constrains the next. The ontogeny of societies and economic systems is plainly characterized, promoted, and constrained by climatic cycles, the availability of natural resources, and the whole of the biological environment, while local and immediate events are dictated and conditioned by the cultural state of the moment, in which the acts of individuals can be seen to exert an influence. But it must be clear that while the most local and immediate history has its own circumscribed validity, more complete explanations must reach back into the other time frames.

An example of the aptness of these three historical views and their interactions is given in the homeostasis of immunity, specifically the formation of antibody. Phylogeny is represented in a timeless history of assembly through selection of several hundred genes pertaining to antibody formation. In development and the intermediate historical range, these genes are shuffled to equip each individual with a set of lymphocytes, each of which is capable of producing a single unique antibody (5). There is also a winnowing process in the thymus that eliminates any that could produce an antibody reacting to self. And lastly, the ecological perspective, the time scale of the moment, and the immediate history of events are all fulfilled in a clonal expansion of particular B lymphocytes in response to antigen, a process in which specificity is further refined by somatic mutation. Thus, evolution, ontogeny, and experiences of the moment have conspired together to create a responsive mechanism, increasing at each step the individuality of the process. It appears that it is impossible to understand such a mechanism outside the context of the three time frames.

Today in medicine we express a strong tendency to analyze both health and disease only in the moment-to-moment time scale, in the realm of homeostatic resiliency, of proximate causes, and of the breakages that need fixing. But if we are to include individuality in our thinking and to understand how remote causes influence individual proximate causes, we have to take into account the origins of the biological constitution of each person as well as how over a lifetime he or she came to a particular expression of disease. Indeed, medicine is nothing if not a historical pursuit. Although somatic mutations occur and play a salient role in cancer, for example, genes that participate in most diseases are inherited, and some may have been in the gene pool for many generations. Obviously they are there at conception, and even though onset of disease may occur late in life, the products of those genes may have been adaptively limiting for a long time. So it is up to the physician to inquire into inheritance and development as well as into the position of the moment. Such an archeological quest will be rewarded by signs and traces, whether historical, physical, or of the laboratory, that give evidence of how far back into the patient's life the incongruent state reaches. This intermediate phase of the history of disease is too little emphasized in medical education.

In the next several chapters I examine the integration and interdependence of the several forms of homeostasis. It will be seen that the mechanisms of physiological homeostasis are mediated by molecules that carry within them information that distinguishes both species and individuals. If we would understand the meaning to a particular individual of the disease that affects him or her, we must see that disease first in the larger context of the person's role as a member of the species. Thus, we proceed from the typological to the individual.

Adaptive Flexibility

9

Physiological Homeostasis

The Homeostasis of the Moment

Textbooks of physiology, biochemistry, and molecular biology may not even mention the word *homeostasis,* let alone define it so clearly as to cause a student to see it as a guiding concept. When the word is defined and employed, it is usually in connection with an isolated system, like salt and water, or glucose, or calcium metabolism. It is not that homeostasis is forgotten—it is at the very heart of both general physiology and our descriptions of pathogenesis—but in this era of specialization it is easy to neglect what the originators of this central concept stressed: the interdependence of all systems and the use of the word *homeostasis* as an expression of the means whereby the steady state of the whole individual is maintained.

ORIGINS OF THE IDEA

A review of moment-to-moment homeostasis, however summary, is most cogent when begun with the views of Claude Bernard, L. J. Henderson, and W. B. Cannon, the physiologists who first conceived and formulated the idea. Although their observations were not informed by modern biochemistry and molecular biology, their concepts have been repeatedly affirmed by the molecular analysis of the physiological systems they described.

Claude Bernard

The idea of an internal mechanism that maintains the constancy of the cellular environment is identified with Claude Bernard (1,2). This notion did not spring fully formed from his mind, but emerged only in his later years. He had first to compare the relationships to the environment of seeds, plants, invertebrates, and poikilothermic vertebrates with those of warm-blooded organisms to appreciate the complexity and necessity of such relationships for mammals (1). In his *Lectures on the Phenomena of Life,* he wrote that "life's expressions are a result of a close and harmonious relationship between the conditions and the constitution of the organism" (2). As complexity increased, more and more of the organism's cells lost contact with the environment, and so had to be provided with mechanisms that could at once give access to the outside and protect against it, a condition whereby the integrity of the cells is respected even while it is subordinated to that of the whole. That is, this constancy, which calls for the autonomy of the cells and organs, exacts in return the integration of all of the organism's elements, including cells, organs, and organ systems, to serve the needs of the whole. The organism is then able to carry on the free and independent life necessary to explore and experiment if it is to enlarge restricted niches or to transcend them.

The integration of these functions of diverse organ systems brought to Bernard's mind the metaphor of a city, a community of individuals who carry on autonomous lives but are always subject to rules that give independence and identity to the whole. Unless the rules of the city are accepted, each individual is possessed of only feeble and inadequate means to combat threats to life or health. By present standards Claude Bernard had little knowledge of what controls the exchanges between the cells and the outside that are mediated by the *milieu intérieur,* but he saw clearly that without such regulation there could be no phylogeny, and that such complexity was a consequence of evolutionary success.

L. J. Henderson

Henderson came to similar conclusions (3,4). Many of his views were formed in studying the maintenance of the pH of the blood, which led him to emphasize the integration of systems, each of which is insufficient for the job but in the aggregate participate in exerting a strong effect. For example, he showed how interrelated are the buffers that maintain the pH of the blood. The $HCO_3–H_2CO_2$ buffer is of itself weak and easily overwhelmed, but when combined with the ability of the lung to regulate CO_2 it becomes a powerful instrument for constancy. So it is the integration of systems—not the systems themselves or their components—that serves and preserves the individual.

Like Bernard, Henderson perceived social analogues. There are similarities between social and physiological regulation; each is complete in itself, but each is also dependent upon the other. Later in his life Henderson became preoccupied with sociology, drawn to the subject partly by its similarities to physiological organization but even more by his interest in the rules whereby the behavior of whole human beings, themselves compounded of interacting physiological elements, is governed. Social interaction seemed to him an extension of physiological organization, which led him, as a physician, to make interesting observations on the doctor-patient relationship. He also influenced the field of sociology (5): Talcott Parsons was a student of Henderson, and due to the latter, the idea of homeostasis, often called *equilibrium,* was taken up in sociology (6).

W. B. Cannon

Cannon embroidered further on these themes. First, he invented the word *homeostasis,* compounded of the Greek roots *homeo,* meaning like (not same), and *stasis,* meaning condition or state. His thoughts are summarized in his book *The Wisdom of the Body,* an especially felicitous title because it suggests an organism capable of choice (7). After all, homeostasis is defined by regulation, itself a consequence of controlled interactions between sensors and effectors that constitute a scheme of self-observation, giving the body a noncognitive wisdom. In his book, Cannon echoed Bernard's thesis that constancy is maintained not by shielding the body from the environment but by regulating physiological processes that made the environment accessible, and he added that the steady state is better maintained by changing the rates of processes than by turning them on and off as a thermostat does. He also expanded the description of the systems involved to include the homeostasis of calcium, the endocrine system, and defenses against infection, and provided a detailed outline of the role of the autonomic nervous system.

Although moment-to-moment constancy was his primary concern, he included changes that take longer, such as the response of the bone marrow to altitude. He also observed that there is an ontogeny of homeostasis: infants and children seem to "grow into" their homeostatic powers, while aging is characterized by a loss of such competences. And finally, he examined the mechanisms of redundancy that provide a wide margin of safety in response to perturbation.

Like the others, Cannon was attracted to the idea of cultural homeostasis (7). Why, he asked, should there not be general principles of stabilization applicable both to biology and to culture? Just as physiological homeostasis provides the individual the autonomy to be and to act without conscious concern for breathing, digesting, metabolizing, and excreting, so do societies organize themselves to fulfill needs common to all, leaving individuals to whatever destinies nature, talent, and inclination lead them.

THAT THIS CONNECTION between physiological and social organization is a natural one is expressed in the words we use to describe the molecular details of communication and "traffic" within and between cells and organs. Cell surface molecules are called "receptors" in analogy to receiving stations; molecules and vesicles are "transported" or "exported," and their "landing" may be facilitated by "docking" proteins. Some proteins need "chaperones" to protect and help them to fold, while signals are "received" at cell surfaces and "transmitted" or "transduced" to promote reactions within. Cells "talk" to one another, specific samples of DNA are called "libraries," and cyclic functions of cells and organs are governed by biological "clocks," while the word *hormone* is derived from a Greek word that means to incite or stir up. It is not that the discoverers of biology's secrets are straining for analogy, it is simply that as products of human culture they use the words of that culture that are appropriate to describe what they see. Had such usage been inappropriate, they would have had to invent new words for new concepts, but the applicability of words in ordinary parlance seems to point to the unity of biology and culture.

Garland Allen suggested that Henderson and Cannon changed the way physiology was studied by emphasizing the importance of the organization and integration of complex interactions analyzed as a whole rather than in their parts (8). While not opposed to reductive analysis, they perceived that it was not enough—that the parts alone could not explain the whole. So it is ironic that not many years later the reductive analysis prevails, and although the idea of homeostasis is integral to our thinking in medicine, it is likely to be used not in relation to the whole, but to such particular functions as signal transduction, DNA transcription, metabolic processes, immune responses, and the like. Nearly every metabolic property is now susceptible to study by the analysis of the appropriate proteins and of the genes that specify and regulate them. It is a triumph of the imperative of the search for structure to explain function.

The irony is that as the details of homeostasis have accumulated, the dreams of its originators—that the idea could be applied to the whole organism—have faded, obscured by the masses of detail. But their time is coming. As a consequence of the Human Genome Project, unanticipated genes are being found whose functions are sometimes deduced by comparing their structures with those of genes that are thoroughly understood. So, by a process that cannot have entered the minds of the progenitors of homeostasis to whom structure always followed function, we now observe structure in search of function, which must lead to integrative biology and the re-enthronement of physiology as queen.

Definitions of Physiological Homeostasis

A Limited Definition

Homeostasis is often defined in the limited sense of preservation of the status quo ante. For example, Murphy and his colleagues have given mathematical rigor to attributes that work to offset perturbing forces, including measurements of the effects of perturbation in terms of such characteristics as (a) excursions about a homing value that represents a state of stability, and which themselves have such properties as delay and lag time; (b) the vigor with which baseline is restored; (c) tolerance or drift around baseline before restoration is required; (d) staggering, a means whereby compensatory mechanisms prevent extravagant overshooting of the baseline; (e) oscillation around baseline; and so on (9). Murphy's model is general; it is applicable to all systems and is useful in research. It is also a cardinal example of the wherewithal with which a student might reason his way through unfamiliar pathophysiology. It is just what the redesigners of curriculum want. It is also a unique effort to link the parameters of homeostasis with the encompassing vision of its discoverers who, although testing their ideas in experiment, went beyond them to outline a grand scheme.

An Expanded Definition

From the beginning, the concept of homeostasis included facilitation of access to, as well as protection from, the environment. And if, in addition, the automatic devices that free the individual for conscious effort and that inform the outcomes of such effort are included, then the word takes on an expanded connotation that embraces all the means whereby an individual, whether bacterium or human being, maintains a steady state in the face of an indifferent world.

And logic does not allow us to stop there. To what end the steady state? Obviously it serves the evolutionary purpose of maintaining individuals to reproduce, so a part of the homeostatic apparatus must be that which promotes that end. And finally, since biological economy requires a period of development, those devices that promote growth, differentiation, and maturation are a part of homeostasis, even while representing a goal that it serves. So the concept is at once narrow and broad: narrow in its definition as the means for maintaining the integrity of the individual being, and broad in comprehending all the machinery required to do so (10).

Integrity of Systems

But the meaning of the word *integrity* as it was used in the preceding sentence suggests something not so narrow after all. It represents the completeness and sufficiency of a system in which everything depends upon everything else. There is no weakest link if adaptation is to be attained. For example, the *milieu intérieur,* that key element in maintenance, must itself be maintained. Concentration of its electrolytes is regulated by ion channels, themselves constructed of gate proteins that have been synthesized in the endoplasmic reticulum (ER), then transported in vesicles to the Golgi apparatus, processed, and exported again in vesicles to the cell surface to take their place in the plasma membrane. And all of these proteins, including those composing the ER, the Golgi, and the vesicles, have had to be specified by mRNA. The mRNA itself is determined by DNA sequences, and both are regulated by still other proteins that direct transcription and translation, neither of which is possible without the many proteins engaged in the synthesis and maintenance of the DNA to begin with. It is like the nursery rhyme "The House That Jack Built," in which each event is both dependent upon the last and essential for the next, as "This is the milkmaid all forlorn that milked the cow with the crooked horn that kicked the dog that chased the cat that worried the rat that ate the malt that lay in the house that Jack built" no one of the events can be deleted without compromising the whole, nor can any be substituted by another since each new event is preceded by the specifying word *this* or *that*. So the word *integrity* in relation to networking of systems means an adaptation, not only to function but to the specificity of each of its elements (11).

All of these physiological processes depend upon recognition and complementarity. Particular amino acid sequences determine particular roles for proteins in structure and function—for example, to assume positions within or on either side of the plasma membrane and there to act as receptors for complementary ligands and as transducers of signals to the nucleus or to other elements within the cell. But, unlike the house that Jack built, there is no beginning nor any end. A fertilized ovum represents a generational transition—an end, a beginning, or a continuity, depending upon how you look at it. Anthropocentrism accords the DNA the purpose of making new people out of old, but a case has been made for the reciprocal notion that a human being is merely a device employed by the DNA to perpetuate itself (12).

Some Characteristics of Physiological Homeostasis

What are the essential characteristics of this integrated mechanism? I cannot rehearse here either the molecular details of its anatomy or the dynamics of its physiology, even though no compelling logic of disease can be formulated in their absence. They constitute the facts that are said to overburden the medical student, and they inform the pathophysiology of disease. They are presented in detail in *Molecular Biology of the Cell* (13), as well as in textbooks of physiology, biochemistry, and metabolism. What is wanted here is a summary of the qualities of moment-to-moment homeostasis that reveals its origins in the genotype and that is compatible with descriptions to come of homeostasis in the other time scales.

Communication

If the homeostatic apparatus preserves a steady state in a fluctuating environment, it must do so by virtue of its capacity to send and respond to signals. The most familiar characterization of physiological homeostasis is that of automatic control through feedback mechanisms, self-regulation by devices that preserve central tendencies in reactions that can speed up or slow down, increase or decrease, intensify or weaken, lengthen or shorten, contract or relax. So physiological homeostasis employs an elaborate scheme of communication to achieve a controlled and coherent intercourse among systems, within individuals, and between individuals and the environment. But communication from what to what and whom to whom?

There are many ways to describe the participants in this system of sending and receiving, but a geneticist might see it as follows. The environment is there to be experienced and is itself under various kinds of controls: physical, biological, social, and so on. How an experience of the environment is interpreted and processed and how its effects are limited is a property of the homeostatic apparatus which is composed of macromolecules, themselves specified and regulated by the genes. That is, the communication is in the first instance between the environment on the one side and the genes on the other, with the anatomic and metabolic apparatus of cells and organs as mediators. So it is not entirely accurate to speak of gene-environment interactions; it is a shorthand notation that can be misleading. Outside influences have always to be interpreted by the gene-determined homeostatic apparatus. This modification of a conventional usage is of the utmost importance to the idea of the inborn error and the logic of disease.

There is a third element in this interaction. It is the qualities of the colloquy between the environment and the genes, which have been shaped by a lifetime of development, maturation, and aging. So the dialogue is carried out in language suitable for all three time scales; the steady state of the moment is attained idiosyncratically by individual homeostatic competences made unique by the particularity of a genotype whose products have adapted to a unique array of events and conditions encountered in the past.

Organization

The descent of the large, complex eukaryotes from prokaryotes is never so obvious as when observing the organization of a mammalian cell. Ordered complexity, self-sufficiency, self-regulation, and diversity characterize both. There are more than two hundred cell types in the human body and a good many more single cell varieties in nature. A prominent difference between pro- and eukaryotes lies in the latter's supracellular organization, which requires differentiation into cell types that gain specialized functions while retaining the elements of self-sufficiency.

A typical cell has properties of a separate organism capable of synthesizing 10,000 to 20,000 proteins, carrying on 1,000 reactions per second, and housing as many as 10^9 protein molecules; each cell has its own homeostasis regulated by signals from within and without (13). Phylogenetic modification is observed in the use of invaginated plasma membrane to serve the needs of the ER, the Golgi apparatus, endosomes, and lysosomes, and to envelop the nucleus. Transcription takes place in the nucleus, translation on the ER, processing of proteins in the caverns of the Golgi, and transport to appropriate destinations is carried out in vesicles, often guided by the proteins of the cytoskeleton. Metabolic processes are facilitated by aggregation of enzymes and substrates on membrane surfaces. The plasma membrane bristles with receptors which, after binding with complementary ligands, send signals through the bilayer to cyclic AMP or protein kinases which, in turn, activate other reactions that often amplify the original signal manyfold. Other receptor-ligand complexes are enclosed in vesicles to be transported to various parts of the cell, after which vesicular proteins are recycled to the surface. It is said that as many as 2,500 such vesicles leave the plasma membrane every second.

The energy that sustains order in this nanoscale community as well as in its macroscale universe is derived from coupled reactions that transfer with high efficiency the wherewithal to fulfill the manifold purposes of both. Energy maintains order; in its absence, endergonic reactions cannot proceed and there is disarray. But there is another source of order that accounts for energy-transferring reactions as well as for everything else: the genes. The genes present a plan which, in specifying the macromolecular design of the cell, determines its role in structure and function. So the genes are the basis for the organization of homeostasis as well as for its continuity.

Complexity and Hierarchy

In differentiating to assume special properties, some eukaryotic cells may lose essential qualities and so must depend upon others to supply what they lack the capacity to make. As the number of differentiated cell types rises, so does complexity, defined by the number of elements in the whole and the irregularity of their arrangement—irregularity as opposed to the regularity of, say, elements in a crystal. But with complexity comes stability, as eager reformers always discover when frustrated by the inertia of massive bureaucracies.

Human beings are comprised of a staggering number of cells—estimates rise to 10^{14}—aggregated into organs and systems according to their differentiation. Each cell, cell type, tissue, organ and organ system has purposes deriving, however indirectly, from the genes, but the purposes of each are interpreted differently depending upon its function in a hierarchy of actions that encompasses the genes at the bottom and the whole individual at the top.

Jacob used the word *integron* to describe the levels of integration in the hierarchy (14). Each integron represents an assembly of elements that fulfills a function not predicted by inspection of the role of each element separately. And each is integrated into a larger set, comprising a new integron to articulate with a set still larger, each acting as a mechanism to engender functions, again not necessarily predictable by reference to the separate elements (10,14). Obviously, each integron transcends previous boundaries to include cells, tissues, organs, and organ systems, ending with the organism as a whole. And each level of the hierarchy of integrons is described in terms of the function of that level and is named according to a description of what it is doing, as "T-cell receptor," or "phenylalanine hydroxylase" if observed at the level of gene product, or "pH of the blood" or "visual processing in the cerebral cortex" when observed at a higher (physiological) level of complexity. Body weight and height and proportionality are more complex qualities that demonstrate relationships limited by the rules of allometry (15). And we may go on to behavioral properties such as appetite and thirst—which, although represented in particular parts of the brain, derive also from actions in other organs that send signals to the brain—or beyond these to aesthetic experiences or even romantic love, which cap all others in being better portrayed by poets than scientists. In the process, the influence of each gene becomes less and less discernible as its product plays its part as only one element of one subset and that subset becomes, in turn, one element of still other subsets. To the degree that this product plays a part in several subsets it is called pleiotropic, and as its effect is less and less discernible, after being exerted through several integrons it is said to have been altered by the products of modifying or epistatic genes. Thus, the more extensive the integration, the dimmer the perception of the effct of the gene, the more pleiotropic and modified it is, and the less rationally can it be called a gene "for" the complex function. Is it any wonder that the drosophilists perceived each gene as contributing to all phenotypes and each phenotype as a product of all genes?

Complexity, then, is compounded of the products of numerous genes; the more complex the function, the more genes that contribute. But the complex phenotype cannot be described simply as a consequence of the additive influences of many genes; the effect of each gene in such a trait is not imposed linearly. Rather, the actions of several are translated into some new function, and the outcomes of these emerge as something else. But the identity, purpose, and function of each gene is in no way altered for being hidden by layers of collaborative phenotypes. At the next mitosis each will be duplicated, and in the germline each will segregate duly; all gene effects mendelize when examined appropriately. Later in the book I describe the contention between the early Mendelists and the biometricians, which could not be resolved until it became clear that continuously distributed characters are no less a product of the actions of individual genes than those that mendelize. The final evidence for the Mendelist view in this now-ancient debate is still being gathered by reductionist investigators who are discovering the elements that compose the phenotypic sets and subsets, tracing them back to their origins in specific genes. We are helped in this when a trait mendelizes because then we know that it bears a relation, however indirect, to a gene at a single locus. The detection of the mendelizing elements of a complex phenotype requires patient detective work passing downward through several phenotypic levels to the gene product and its DNA, or hoping to discover a link with some known element of DNA. But even when a linkage, the locus, and the relevant gene and its product are found, there remains the task, opposite to that described above, of fitting the action of the gene discovered by linkage into the series of integrated functions of which the original phenotype is comprised.

Once it was possible to analyze higher functions—say, the relationships between T cells and the major histocompatibility complex (MHC)—without any reference to the genes; the physiological level was self-contained. But no more. Now the details of the genes themselves must be included, their nucleotide sequences colinear with the sequences of amino acids in their protein products. The aim of molecular genetics is to explain the origins of complex physiological mechanisms and functions in the structure and actions of the genes.

Adaptation

Human beings bear to the environment a relationship that is at once intimate and guarded, amicable and inimical. Each person is enveloped by it, draws sustenance from it, and is, in reference to others, a part of it. Successful living is measured by degrees of adaptation to it, or we might say that an individual's adaptive success is directly proportional to some measure of his sensitivity to the environment.

Sensitivity

What is sensitivity? Is it attunement? Speed and delicacy of response? Nicety of discrimination? It is all these and more. When we say "environment," we usually mean the physical and biological conditions that surround us as opposed to the *milieu intérieur,* although the latter is in no way precluded. These conditions are what they are because of the laws of nature, but what of the laws of society and culture? Certainly to be out of tune with society is always risky— witness the close correlation between SES and disease—but we are more and more aware that to be part of the current can be dangerous, too. In recognition of such perils, what were once nearly universal indulgences have in some quarters and by some people been replaced by an asceticism faintly reminiscent of primitive life. Ice cream, hot dogs, hamburgers, french fries, and indolence have been replaced by salads, fish, skim milk, high fiber cereals, and programmed exercise.

To be out of tune, to be insensitive or inattentive to warnings, to be slow to respond, and to fail to take profit in experience of both biological and cultural settings is to fail in adaptation and to invite disease. This sensitivity, this ability to respond efficiently, precisely, and speedily, is a consequence of the perfection of the integration of metabolic machinery.

Integration

Integration is, then, a second attribute of adaptation. It is essential to be able to generate just the right amount of ATP at just the right time and place, to have efficient DNA repair, to have enzymes and receptors folded appropriately to accommodate substrates and ligands, and to have sufficient dendritic connections and speedy axonal transmission, effective intra- and intercellular communications and transport, and so on. All must be capable of speeding up and slowing down, of turning on and turning off, of supplying not too much and not too little, and always each response, each system, must be in concert with all the others, and within limits. Mechanisms, regulators, and limits—all are built in. They are modifications of nature tracing back to the beginning of life. So it is the genes that specify the macromolecules that function in integrated systems that respond sensitively to perturbations of the environment by sending the signals that activate the transcribing devices that enable the genes to set in motion the wherewithal to maintain, with minimum energy, the steady state.

Rhythmicity

Although much of today's culture is designed to reduce, if not to eliminate, the unpredictable, untoward things happen anyway, and homeostasis is ready for such events. But some of nature is unchanging, eternal, and easily foretold—for example, time passes, the earth rotates, the seasons change. These processes are rhythmical in their fulfillment, so it should be no surprise that our responses vary accordingly. We have mechanisms that can tell time: biological clocks. The anatomical and physiological details of such clocks are being clarified. There are pacemakers that regulate multiple oscillators that characterize different cell types, photoreceptors that communicate with the pacemakers, and receptors for whatever is elaborated by pacemakers and oscillators (16,17).

Most is known about circadian rhythms with their period of approximately twenty-four hours, but there are others. For example, ultradian rhythms have periods of seconds to hours—for example, the heartbeat and the movement of cilia—while infradian rhythms vary from months to years. It has been suggested that circadian rhythms are generated from ultradian, and infradian from circadian (17).

Circadian cycles are ordinarily synchronized with day-night alternatives. But when an individual is exposed to constant light or dark, the rhythms "free run"—that is, they continue to show periodicity but lose synchrony with day and night, running instead on endogenous idiosyncratic time with "days" that are longer or shorter than those of sidereal time. A return to alternating day and night entrains the cycle to synchrony again.

Sleep and activity cycles are known to us all, and jet lag is known to many. But according to Edmunds, "virtually all levels of cellular organization display a circadian time structure, including photosynthesis, DNA replication, cell division, susceptibility to noxious agents, enzymatic activities, concentrations of metabolic products, and so on" (17). Cycles reach their peaks and nadirs according to their own impulses. Body temperature is highest in the afternoon, lowest in the early morning; serum cortisol levels are also lowest in the early hours of the day, at a time when the level of growth hormone is at its highest. And these rhythms are affected by age and development. For example, infants attain a "normal" sleep cycle only after several months, and they achieve a regular cycle of cortisol secretion after two to three years. In general, cycles are longest at puberty and tend to shorten with aging. It has even been suggested that aging may be due to a loss of temporal organization.

Presumably the point of the various periodicities is to schedule physiological functions for some purpose (16). Perhaps an animal's survival in a periodic night-day environment is dependent upon the appropriateness and precision of physiological timing. That is, if certain kinds of challenges are periodic and predictable, there is a selective advantage in a prepared homeostasis.

It is now clear that the clocks' components are proteins engaged, like other proteins, in structural, enzymatic, and regulatory activities, so it should be possible to find the genes that specify them and to account for the rhythms. Mutants that fulfill these expectations have been found in strains of *Neurospora crassa,* in species of drosophila, and in a few other organisms, including mice (17–21). Most act as semidominants, and the effects of mutants at more than one locus are additive. Some are pleiotropic and affect ultradian rhythms as well.

What is the medical significance of these biological clocks? There are several "periodic" diseases—Mediterranean fever and periodic paralysis are examples—and the well attested preponderance of strokes, myocardial infarction, and sudden death in the morning hours coincides with a morning peak in blood pressure and platelet aggregability and a trough in fibrinolytic activity. The blood pressure elevation is associated with circadian rhythms of vascular tone concomitant with daily variation in sympathetic vasoconstrictor activity. So it is in a context of rhythmic undulations of physiologic homeostasis that these catastrophic events happen. That is, circadian variations enhance and reduce the probability of their occurrence, and it is reasonable to suppose that they do so variably according to individual variation in the genes governing these clocks. One set of homeostatic regulators modifies others; the genes specifying the proteins of the biological clocks are epistatic to others that contribute to those aspects of the vascular system that are compromised and so lead to disaster. Other diseases are likely to show similar relationships to variations in rhythms.

CONCLUSION

The molecular details of the means whereby the steady state of the moment is maintained constitute the bulk of the biology appropriated by machine fixers to serve medical purposes. Since treatment is the paramount goal of medicine, the condition of the patient at this moment along with the immediate history of pathogenesis are what is needed to formulate therapeutic tactics. So, one time scale—that of the moment—is preeminent, while those of the lifetime and the biological past are given attention only as they seem to exert some direct impact on the diagnostic or therapeutic process. Such a position, within its own context, makes sense. If one can go directly to a cause that leads to a certain pathogenesis which in turn suggests an effective treatment, why worry about what seems to be irrelevant? Medical treatment is too exigent to be left to the philosophers.

The aridity of this view is exposed in the molecular analysis of the anatomy and function of any moment-to-moment homeostatic device, for no matter how detailed that analysis, it is incomplete without reference to the genes that specify those homeostatic proteins. Here the gene pool insinuates itself to determine the singularity of the genetic background within which the elements of proximate cause wreak their malign purpose. And wherever the gene pool makes an appearance, so does the idea of mutants that vary in both frequency and impact on the phenotypes, not only of the clinical condition that needs immediate attention but also of the pathogenesis that began sometime in the patient's past, perhaps in a form so subtle as to escape notice. That is, in each case we are catapulted into a house that Jack built, wherein the story is incomplete unless all three time scales are given more than a nod.

Failure to consider all the time scales leads to typological accounts of the steady state and its aberrations. Omitting the lifetime and the biological past allows the erection of typological standards of normality with their abstract means and dispersions. But once an appeal is made to the other time scales, it is evident that each person has his own norms that bear a stronger relationship to his own genes and developmental history than to the means for the species. Further, that norm may have varied, and will continue to vary, idiosyncratically over the lifetime. So each person's steady state is unique, and if this is true, treatment of disease, although always in some degree standardized, must vary according to the extent to which individual norms depart from the statistical one. So if 95 percent of the population is embraced within 2 standard deviations, 5 percent, or 1 in 20, is outside it and may need something special (and so may some of those at 1.75 or 1.5 SD). There are also likely to be some who differ altogether—say at the genetic level and so in pathogenesis—even while sheltering within or overlapping the distribution of phenotypic characterization. Clearly, the steady state of the moment cannot be divorced from its origins in development and biological history.

The molecular analysis of moment-to-moment homeostasis defines in modern terms Garrod's idea of chemical individuality. That is, the inborn error, defined by Garrod as a hereditary enzyme deficiency, is only one among many variations that he thought of as comprising a chemical individuality. For Garrod, the inborn errors were only at one extreme in a distribution of chemical variants that distinguished individuals no less than they distinguished species. Today we perceive the inborn error as associated with genes that alter the function of specific unit steps in physiological homeostasis that identify points of vulnerability in the maintenance of the steady state. The evidence for this, accumulating at a pace that at once amazes and stupefies the interested onlooker, suggests that this concept, of inborn error become biochemical individuality expanded to include all gene products, their specificities, their amounts, and their responses to regulation, must be a principal focus of medical thought.

Our treatments are designed to correct, to nullify, or to circumvent the abnormal consequences of the inborn variation. So far, such treatments have been only partially successful. Perhaps this is not surprising given the precision of the works that have gone awry; it is as if we were trying to fix a watch with our hands in boxing gloves. The idea of gene therapy represents a frontal attack; the homeostasis is to be made whole by the addition of "wild type" DNA. The Human Genome Project is expected to stimulate this work, and surely it will do so. But who can doubt that another outcome of the initiative will be to probe the limits of the number and variety of the variants of unit steps of homeostasis that constitute human biochemical individuality? Perhaps this will lead to our beginning to see how biochemical individuality modifies the expression of the inborn errors, how the latter is continuous with the former, and even, in some individuals, how the one becomes the other. That is, we will be given some insights that would be pleasing to the originators of the idea of homeostasis, especially into how the component parts, the unit steps of systems (integrons), are created, how they assemble, associate, and interdigitate, and how they communicate and cooperate with others to form aggregates that are perceived as people or patients.

It was the coherent whole that concerned them and they visualized the whole body as the site of any disease. Here is an excerpt from a paper by Henderson on acidosis:

> There is no one process or phenomenon which is the fundamental or essential one
> . . . each is integral . . . as cause and as effect in a cycle of pathological changes
> whose onset may be at any one of many points and which as a whole . . . constitutes the deranged acid-base metabolism. But this . . . is not the whole of the mat-

ter, for, just as the parts of this cycle engage in the whole of the process of acid-base metabolism, so do they also engage, as parts, in other processes, some of them in the respiration, some in the process of excretion, and so on indefinitely. Thus the condition known as acidosis can only be truly conceived in terms of the organization of the body as a whole (22).

This paragraph encapsulates significant lessons. First, the description of acidosis that includes "each is integral, at once as cause and effect" and "onset may be at any one of many points" may be the first allusion to the unit step of homeostasis as a central theme of disease. Neither Henderson nor Garrod referred to the other's work, but in this paragraph is language that implies compatibility in their thinking.

Another lesson is suggested by Henderson's words. If it is the "body as a whole" that is sick—that is, if the dis-homeostasis of one step or a few steps is reflected in the function of the whole—then it must be the duty of the physician to inquire of the patient just how the whole has been affected, and to take very seriously whatever answer is given.

10

Genetic Homeostasis

The Past

Still, it is indeed true that we inherit an entire province, an entire world. The angle at whose apex we are lodged gapes behind us toward infinity. Seen in this way, the science of genealogy, which is so often placed in the service of human vanity, leads first to humility—by making us conscious of the little that we are amid these multitudes—and then to vertigo.
—Marguerite Yourcenar, *How Many Years: A Memoir*

These observations appear in Mme Yourcenar's memoir, a book that is unusual among autobiographies in being more an account of the lives of her forebears than of her own. She, being French, begins by counting in the male line four great-grandparents in 1850, sixteen great-great-grandparents around the time of the Revolution, and as many as a million forebears in the thirteenth century. Next she derides the idea of a lineage that omits the female line with its no less significant contribution, and then dilates on the folly of tracing one's ancestry only to the "overly splendid figures that dominate the foreground of history," while neglecting the "obscurity and mediocrity" of most of so large a pool. And finally, she observes that if we include our cultural inheritances, "we are the universal heirs of the entire earth." That is, we are what we are by virtue of how we use that which we inherit from the infinity of the biological past as well as from the wealth of cultural history.

Herein lies the reason Mme Yourcenar is so preoccupied with ancestry in her autobiography. She acknowledges the present, yes, but instead of recounting the details of her own life after a perfunctory review of those of her parents, she seeks the origin and evolution of her own character in its continuity with the past. And she perceives that amid the vagaries of that continuity, there is a stability attributable to both heredity and culture. Had she been a biologist she might have alluded to a homeostasis of each.

Genetic Homeostasis

In medical education, evolution is little noticed; textbooks of internal medicine and allied disciplines do not list the word in their indexes. But why should evolution be given attention in medical books? What could be more remote from the exigency of the sick patient? The answer to the first question is that there is no reason, and to the second that nothing could be more distant—when the questions are asked in reference to how and where to fix a broken machine rather than to the origin of its fragility.

But there have been murmurs off stage, as it were. In the late nineteenth century and the early part of the twentieth, disease as natural selection at work was the subject of speculation and of important lectures by well-known medical sages. Evidence favoring the idea was wanting, until Garrod perceived that inborn errors and chemical individuality were substrates for selection. This led to the thoughts embodied in *Inborn Factors of Disease* (1), one chapter of which is entitled "Evolution and Disease." There Garrod says, "in no discussion of the inborn factors of disease can evolution . . . be left out of account." And apropos of natural selection he says, "As to what constitutes fitness to survive, man and nature do not see eye to eye." That is, he saw clearly that human culture had tamed some of the forces of selection even while creating others; if people do not die of predation or starvation, they are likely to succumb to disease.

Since Garrod's day much has been written about human evolution with reference to medicine, perhaps most notably books by Dubos (2–4), Dobzhansky (5,6), Darlington (7), and Neel (8), among others (9). In some of these there are pointed allusions to the origin of disease in evolutionary processes. Now that we know so much about pathogenesis and its proximate causes, now that we know that the homeostatic steps disrupted in disease originate in the unique genotypes of their victims, it is time to seek the origins of the specificities of those genotypes and the remote causes of homeostatic disorder in the forces that promote the evolution of species.

Evolution and Medical Thought

What has evolution to do with medical thought and education? First, we cannot encourage the perception of disease in three time scales if that of biological history is omitted. The forces of evolution shape a gene pool that expresses the species' capacity for adaptation. Unique aliquots are drawn from that pool to begin the singular life histories of individuals whose homeostatic competence is in varying degree congruent with their experiences. Those same forces also account for incongruities in individuals whose heritage includes vulnerabilities that lead to breakages of the machine. So the life history and the immediate state of homeostasis cannot escape the influence of biological history.

Second, what are the forces that give evolution direction and how do they work to preserve and enhance the individual homeostatic powers reviewed in the last section? If life, as opposed to individual lives, has a purpose, it is reproduction. To this end, each species has a gene pool whose stability is maintained by reproduction through which both losses and replenishment are attained. The instruments of this stability are the individuals of the species, who act as filters through which workable combinations of genes pass more readily than those that are not. So there is a genetic homeostasis that serves the purpose of reproducing the species while serving that of individual lives, too, but with the proviso that the preservation of the gene pool comes first. That is, the necessity for replenishment and variation brings in new mutants and new combinations of genes, some inviable, some only conditionally tolerable, some that are compatible with the existing state of adaptation but not necessarily with changes to it, and a few that even enhance the present condition. All of these must be submitted to the test of development and living, so in this necessity to replenish and preserve the stability of the gene pool, we discover at once the origins of the proteins that constitute the unit steps of physiological homeostasis and a source of remote causes of diseases whose proximate causes are the products of mutants.

The means whereby the stability of the gene pool is both conserved and promoted is the province of evolutionary biologists and population geneticists. Genetics is first of all a predictive discipline, so it can be no surprise that genetic theories of natural selection and evolution, specifically those proposed by R. A. Fisher (10), Sewall Wright (11), and J. B. S. Haldane (12), were advanced even before there were data to test them. These theories, first published in the 1930s, were elaborated in a mathematical form that made them general and inclusive of all life. They gave most attention to natural selection, an agency that promotes adaptation to environmental place and circumstance, preserving genes that contribute to physiological stability and eliminating those that threaten it.

It was also agreed, although not without the controversy that seems so often to accompany scientific advance, that randomness plays some part, even in the attainment of the adapted state. Species are constituted of diverse populations that pursue different destinies, reshuffling and evolving gene pools both randomly and in response to different selective experiences. The gene pools of small populations are especially sensitive to random changes, whether due to migration of strangers into them or to overrepresentation of the genes of particular individuals or families. The evolution of a whole species is therefore likely to reflect the evolutionary careers of several or many populations, each marked by local genetic differences but all connected not only by the capacity for successful mating between the members of each, but by certain qualities that characterize the entire species.

In the publications of the pioneers of population genetics, it sometimes seems that the genes and their frequencies are the sole objects of scrutiny, so an unwary reader may conclude that evolution is simply a matter of changes in gene frequency, but nothing could be farther from the truth. Evolution results from the differential choice of phenotypes. It is the integrated individual fish, plant, or human being that survives to reproduce that is the conduit through which genes flow to the next generation. And it is the entire genotype that survives or is lost, unreproduced. For example, a single noxious gene, by imperiling the life of an individual, endangers the survival of that individual's whole genotype, never mind how many good and useful genes it holds. But some genotypes may contain enough modifiers to nullify the potential harm of that noxious gene, or at least to abate its mischief long enough to permit reproduction and so allow it to do its worst in another homeostatic context. So, genes, as they exist in the abstract gene pool, have no selective value. It is only when they are lodged in the variable genotypes of variable individuals that they exert effects based on the competence of their products to function in concert with those of others in their homeostatic systems and in the integrated whole.

It may be easy to demonstrate in a particular environment the selective disadvantage of a gene product that so disrupts physiological homeostasis as to override the influences of other genes or experiences that might exert a modifying effect, but in the same environment to adduce physiological evidence of the selective advantage of a single allele over its congeners is more difficult. The normal condition is attained by integration of the work of many genes. A single gene that exerts an effect that stands out above others in its homeostatic milieu risks definition as abnormal and so is unlikely to represent any advantage.

THE QUALITIES OF THE GENE POOL

It is the individual who is the object of natural selection and drift, in whom the representatives of the gene pool are expressed and by whom an entire set of genes is transmitted to offspring. So, each of us is a unit of evolution, a player in life's game of chance in a way that is promoted or constrained by the particular set of genes we inherit and by how we use their guidance in development and in encounters with our particular environments. Since individual human genotypes are derived from parents and other ancestors as well as, more remotely, from the species and phylogeny represented in Mme Yourcenar's "infinity," some part of each genotype must express constraints appropriate to each of these levels of ancestry. Indeed, we know that there is a good deal of such conservation. Some genes—for example, those that specify heat-shock proteins—vary only slightly in amino acid sequence across the entire range of phylogeny, and we differ very little in the sequences of most proteins from our nearest phylogenetic relative, the chimpanzee (13,14). But we are manifestly not chimpanzees, and each of us is unique in appearance, in behavior, and in how we maintain our homeostatic stability.

Clearly there is a genetic homeostasis that conserves gene pools even while it promotes individual variation. Population geneticists ask, therefore, how much genetic variation is required to account for the phenotypic differences that distinguish each person from all others without altering the characteristics of our humanity. So they attempt to ascertain the constitution of the human gene pool as it appears in the population of human beings living in all sorts of environments and both healthy and otherwise. The proviso of "living" human beings is necessary because while we know of many mutations that are either incompatible with long life or are conducive to early mortality, we do not yet know the frequencies of any genes in the gene pool of the gametes. I say "yet" because, given the high frequency of intrauterine losses of zygotes and embryos, the question will be vigorously pursued when the requisite technology is at hand. Despite the originality and cogency of their theoretical arguments and the rich detail of their mathematical treatments, the early population geneticists had too few data to give real answers to such a question. But lack of data is no bar to speculation, which thirty to forty years ago crystallized into two incompatible positions (15,16).

The Classical-Balance Controversy

Scientific debates are often at first characterized by more heat than light but go on to stimulate investigation that leads to unexpected outcomes—in this instance, some solutions to the puzzle of multifactorial disease. According to Crow, the controversy was precipitated by the diverse interests of Dobzhansky and Muller, the two principal protagonists, each of whom saw the problem through a different lens (15). For one of the contending views, called the "balance" position, Dobzhansky was the champion (17). His interest in explaining evolution led him to propose a high degree of genetic variability in all species, so that more than one allele qualified as "normal" at many, or even most, loci. Although it was agreed that new mutants might be disadaptive, such genes could contribute favorably if they conferred some advantage in heterozygotes not experienced by either homozygote, and before long the familiar HgbA/HgbS heterozygote advantage was advanced in seeming confirmation.

The alternative view, called "classical" in derision by the opposition, was that of Herman Muller, whose preoccupation with the mutagenic effects of radiation caused him to stress the already-adapted state, which he thought had sufficient variation that new mutants would be useless or, more likely, contributory to debility and disease. That is, such genes constituted a genetic "load" to be borne by the individual members of the species, especially in heterozygotes, and expressed as vulnerability or outright disease (18). Further, the load was certain to increase as technological and cultural advances both heightened the mutation rate and relieved selective pressures that in more primitive times had eliminated such genes. These ideas, expressed on both sides at length, cogently and with fervor, could not be tested until the 1960s, when a remarkable degree of genetic variation was discovered in both human beings and drosophila.

Polymorphism

The studies that put an end to this controversy, but engendered another, were undertaken for different reasons. The examination of human variation carried out by Harris was conceived in a mentality conditioned by his work with inborn errors and his interest in Garrod's idea of chemical individuality (19). His question was simply, "How variable is the human genome?" The drosophila work was undertaken by Lewontin, who sought the means to settle the balance-classical argument (20).

Electrophoretic mobility of soluble enzymes was used in both organisms to show that at about 30 percent of loci there were at least two alleles, of which the least frequent was present in 1 percent or more of individuals in the populations studied. This means that each individual is heterozygous at 6 to 10 percent of loci. Such loci were said to be polymorphic because allelic frequencies of 1 percent or more cannot be accounted for by new mutation alone.

Initially it was presumed that natural selection must have favored these polymorphisms, and the data seemed to support the balance theory and heterozygote advantage. But after polymorphism was shown to characterize hundreds of species, it became clear that the numbers and frequencies of polymorphic alleles were too great to be explained by selection alone; the "load" imposed by the mutants was too great (16). The alternative was random drift, migration, founder effect, and the like, so a hypothesis of neutral polymorphism was advanced, principally by Kimura, who had observed that the rate of substitution of amino acid in proteins remained constant through evolutionary time, suggesting randomness rather than selection (21). This theory is made plausible by the observation that allelic differences in enzyme mobility are only occasionally reflected in significant differences in activity.

But the question of whether there is selective advantage in some heterozygotes remains. That is, substantial heterozygosity would reduce species variability, enhancing conformity to the average and reducing the number of anomalous outliers. This question, which has engendered so much controversy, is still unsettled, although studies of some species have demonstrated the reduced variability and enhanced developmental stability anticipated in the hypothesis of heterozygote advantage (16,22). The alternative—that mutants contribute to a genetic load to be paid in illness or death—while clearly not applicable to most of the "neutral" polymorphism, retains some validity in regard to heterozygosity for some mutants associated with recessive disease (23). That is, although Kacser and Burns have demonstrated that heterozygotes for most mutants associated with recessive inborn errors show no deficiency in the flux through an enzyme pathway (24), there are others who do express modified forms of the diseases observed in homozygotes (23).

Polymorphism for structural proteins is thought to be significantly less, but that in the DNA is much more; in introns and nontranscribed DNA, a polymorphic difference is found on the average in 1 of every 200 base pairs. The studies of human and drosophila populations also turned up a good deal of nonpolymorphic variation—that is, alleles with frequencies of less than 1 percent (16,25).

But what does it mean for medicine? First, it is a body blow to essences and typological thinking, a powerful assertion of population thinking, a confirmation of nominalism, and a validation of the observation that everyone has his own disease. In addition, if polymorphism assures the genetic uniqueness of every human being, it also assures the heterogeneity of disease; the more genes engaged in proximate cause, the greater the degree of heterogeneity. No more can we imagine that all people with high blood pressure or atherosclerosis suffer from the same disease. Rather the hypothesis to test is the reverse: all cases are different. The randomness of mutation and the extent of polymorphism predict such differences.

Second, selection must account for some of this polymorphic variation and randomness for more. There are clearly some examples of heterozygote advantage. For example, the MHC loci are extremely polymorphic, with dozens of alleles of such frequency that nearly everyone is multiply heterozygous. Indeed, there appears to be some reproductive disadvantage for matings of homozygotes of the type II alleles. And there is certainly some "genetic load," expressed in disease in people heterozygous for genes that in homozygotes produce more severe symptoms.

The problem lies in how to account for polymorphism locus by locus. For example, do alleles of below polymorphic frequency represent former polymorphisms on their way to extinction or selectively useful genes on their way to becoming polymorphic, even to be established as the predominant allele? Or both? And what is the origin of polymorphic alleles that do not alter function? A compelling case has been made that they attained their frequency by some nonselective means. The question cannot be answered by analysis of amino acid sequence, but it may be possible to use molecular analysis to distinguish the allele that originates randomly from that established by selection (25). The former will resemble its ancestors in intronic and other nucleotide sequences, while the latter need show no such constraint.

Adaptive Flexibility

Third, the polymorphic loci are the embodiment of Garrod's chemical individuality. The human population is divided into as many distinctive camps as there are alleles for each such locus. To this, as an additional source of genetic variation and no less chemical individuality for being less frequent, must be added the nonpolymorphic alleles, but polymorphism alone is sufficient to account for the genetic uniqueness of the entire human population—and then some.

Fourth, not all polymorphic alleles function within normal limits. Under appropriate conditions, some are even associated with disease and so are listed as vulnerabilities or risk factors. For example, neither the vitamin D receptor allele associated with osteoporosis of old age nor the ACE polymorphic allele associated with myocardial damage in heart attacks is likely to be under heavy adverse selection because their complicity with disease is usually evident only after the end of reproduction.

Other polymorphic alleles are harder to fathom. Why are the genes for cystic fibrosis and PKU polymorphic, at least in some populations? Examination of these genes at the molecular level reveals one or two alleles at polymorphic frequencies and dozens or hundreds of rare ones—just the position observed by electrophoresis of enzymes ascertained in all studies of polymorphism without relation to disease. The more frequent alleles usually constitute 60 to 80 percent of those found in patients with the disease, with the remaining 20 to 40 percent being made up of rare genes. How do these alleles, whether alone or in the aggregate, attain polymorphic levels in populations? Perhaps by one of the following:

(a) There may be a founder effect. This, however, explains only one or maybe two common alleles; attributing several alleles to "founder" effects begins to sound more like favorable selection.

(b) There may be some heterozygote advantage, not yet explained or possibly no longer in existence because of changed conditions.

(c) There may be a tight linkage between such undoubtedly pernicious alleles and a much-conserved gene so necessary for normal development that it carries the bad gene along for many generations.

(d) The frequencies may be attained by drift.

It may be that the Human Genome Project will yield the wherewithal, including both the identities of specific genes and the technology, easily and quickly to choose between the above or other explanations. A molecular population genetics will have to await methods to distinguish and count alleles with the facility of simple electrophoresis.

A Gradient of Selective Effect

This discussion of the constitution of the gene pool suggests that, in the race for predominance, all genes are not created equal: some are chosen, some arrive by chance, and some are rejected. Further, there seem to be degrees of stringency in both choice and rejection. Some genes are so effective in their role as to have been essential to the homeostasis of almost the whole of phylogeny, while others are so destructive that they extinguish life. And in between there are permissive loci, accommodating alleles that seem to be about equally competent. These competences are measured against the calls made on the products of the alleles in contributing to the flexibility and stability of physiological homeostasis, contributions that must have varied over millennia of adaptation to changing conditions of the environment. And given the tempo of cultural and technological change in modern societies, today's competence may be tomorrow's inadequacy—or it may be the other way around. But despite such variability, there is a hint of a selective gradient among the components of the gene pool, a concept that is likely to be of interest to medical thinking in linking remote and proximate causes of disease. This gradient will turn up in the book in other contexts.

Conclusion

Freedom and constraint. These are the qualities that provide and preserve the stability of physiological homeostasis: the freedom to function as an independent open system in an indifferent environment within constraints imposed by the original plan; freedom also as a singular individual to maintain stability uniquely.

Both flexibility and constancy of physiological homeostasis are a consequence of the constitution of the gene pool, itself maintained by a homeostasis based on outcomes of reproduction. Genes conducive to reproduction tend to reappear in subsequent generations, while those that are not tend to disappear. The climate for reproduction is set by an environment composed in part of experiences of the external conditions and in part of an internal physiological equanimity, itself an outcome of development. Development is a consequence of the interactions of gene products with experiences through time that constitute a developmental homeostasis that responds to its own freedoms and constraints, while the experiences are representative of the possibilities and limitations characteristic of a social and cultural homeostasis. It was outcomes of such sources of freedom and constraint that Mme Yourcenar seemed to be seeking in writing a memoir that was a local probe of a past that reached to infinity. The next three chapters continue this exploration of sources of variation and stability.

11

Developmental Homeostasis

The Lifetime

My heart leaps up when I behold
A rainbow in the sky:
    So was it when my life began;
So is it now I am a man;
So be it when I shall grow old,
    Or let me die!
The Child is father of the Man;
And I could wish my days to be
Bound each to each by natural piety.
—William Wordsworth, "My heart leaps up when I behold"

The genes that inform and constrain physiological homeostasis do so by specifying and regulating the molecules of which its systems are composed, within the context of whatever cellular and metabolic conditions prevail at the moment. But it happens that such moment-to-moment settings are, and have been, regulated and constrained by the elements that control development. That is, there is a developmental homeostasis that is represented in the longitudinal consequences of innumerable moment-to-moment adjustments. It is a program that provides direction for the promotion, guidance, and modulation of ontogeny, so that the missions of physiological homeostasis are fulfilled in an ever-changing matrix influenced by elements derived from endowment and experience. If the developmental itinerary is represented as a column or tube, this matrix is observed in cross-sectional cuts through it, each slice consisting of the structural and metabolic conditions of the moment. Because those conditions change, each slice is likely to be constituted of somewhat different attributes, different states of organization, all varying in degree according to the distance in time between the slices.

So a coherent assessment of the physical or biochemical qualities of an individual at a given moment must include not only genes and experiences but also elements characterizing the developmental matrix. They constitute the wherewithal for a biological and social biography of the whole species, along with that of each of its individual constituents, a prospectus for the future as well as a record of how that future worked out in the past.

THE PATH TO INDEPENDENCE

Philosophers argue whether or not nature has intention. Biologists agree that there is no design from without, but how to express what seems purposeful? The various parts of organisms seem to have uses that enable the integrated individual to express a purpose—that of reproduction. In *Chance and Necessity,* Monod observes that "all the functional adaptations in living beings, like all the artifacts they produce, fulfill particular projects which may be seen as so many aspects or fragments of a unique primary project, which is the preservation and multiplication of the species" (1). Another way of putting this is that nature imposes three tests upon us all. We must (a) survive long enough to (b) attain fertility, which should lead (c) to successful reproduction. To fail any is to fail nature's intent, but only the first compromises irretrievably an individual life.

Obviously nature's expectations can be fulfilled only by a fully developed organism acting independently, so human biological development may be seen as a path to independence. Although it is useful to think of development in stages, it is, in fact, seamlessly continuous. Birth and puberty, however apparently discrete, are merely transitional phases that lead to fertility and reproduction. Aging is more insidious, more indistinct, and is miscellaneous in its choice of which organ systems fail first. There is some question whether aging is a part of development at all, but if not, it is inalienably coupled with it. Gerontologists speak of a period of maturity between development and aging.

There is another path to independence taken simultaneously with the biological. Tests are imposed by the organization of the environment, which offers the developing open system both advantages and constraints. Ideally, these two ontogenetic paths, one representing fulfillment of biological possibilities and the other acculturation, should reinforce each other. Cultural advantages should enhance the realization of biological potential, while biological advantages should help in exploiting cultural opportunities—and clearly both these things happen. In fact, it is to just the degree that this reciprocity has been attained that human welfare has prospered and the ideals of development have been reached. For example, if increased body size and longevity are representative of attainment of developmental ideals, then modern living has realized a good deal of genetic potential and continues to do so.

But societies, however well intentioned, are not always organized around the welfare of all individuals. Cultural evolution is more rapid than its biological counterpart, so our ontogenetic program, which adapted to environments of long ago, is likely to bring the environment and the developmental program into conflict, with the result of the emergence of vulnerabilities of both species and individual. Such vulnerabilities make themselves known throughout the lifetime, often leaving impressions, depending upon when in ontogeny they rose to overt expression. For example, early onset of disease may be expressed in distortion of physical and mental development, while late onset may hasten or exacerbate aging.

DEVELOPMENT AS A HISTORICAL PROCESS

In the poem that opens this chapter I take Wordsworth to be saying that later life is shaped by earlier experiences and that to retain the aspirations and idealism of youth can help to offset the erosive effects of daily life. Perhaps the poet meant it as a kind of spiritual homeostasis, but for my purpose the poem represents a compelling metaphor that embraces two interacting ideas: the first is the continuity of development, in which the evolution of species is a consequence of variable outcomes of individual ontogenies; the second is that development unfolds in a history of days influenced by endowment and experience, here defined as a path to independence. The metaphor also provides a context within which to expound the idea that all disease results from the means whereby the continuing, and ever provisional, evolution of our species is attained. If we would know why we are subject to being cut down by disease, we should seek answers in the qualities of the contrivances of nature, among which evolution, development, and aging are prominent.

Let us begin with definitions. If the child is father of the man, it is in two ways. First, in accord with species-specific directions, what begins as an embryo becomes an adult, perhaps a centenarian. And second, the child is father of a specific adult by transmitting from the start the information that maintains throughout life his unique identity. That information embodies the "piety" that binds the days each to each, a word that *Webster's* defines as "fidelity to natural obligations." What more natural obligation than to the genetic program that specifies the molecules that carry on the business of life? So, the child is father of a man whose qualities are shaped by experiences of the social and cultural environment, but always within the limits set by the original plan, and our days are bound each to each not only in time, but in the continuous forging of a singular biological and cultural self, a self distinguished from others not only by what is visible but also by how we grow, mature, meet an infection, metabolize a drug, or respond to a work of art. Indeed, it is the particularity of that self that determines whether we get sick and in what way.

Now, how can we use these ideas in thinking about how we change in life? How are our days bound each to each in fidelity to natural obligations? No one needs reminding that we remain our own selves however long we live. If we live long enough, we may become demented and bereft of remembrance, but we remain ourselves for all that. So there is something permanent, a kind of memory that binds our days each to each, a memory that transcends remembering.

That memory is of two kinds. One is phylogenetic, ensuring that the product of the union of human gametes will be a human being. The other is developmental, endowing that human being with a unique personhood. The first memory makes clear that the development and decline of a human being cannot be a creation of something de novo. If it were, the days would be bound each to each in time only; if no natural obligation were in evidence, the child could not be father of the man since the latter would be shaped by the caprice of circumstance. But if not a creation, is development merely a revelation, an inevitable outcome of a plan? If so, then the man is a faithful product of the plan that engineered the child, and the relationship of the days is foreordained. But the second kind of memory guarantees that they are not, since those days are bound each to each in experience as well as by the DNA. So development is neither a creation nor a revelation; it is both.

The Conservation of Design

How can that be? Remember we are to visualize human development in the context of the three time scales. That is, it is not to be perceived as like arranging a pile of stones into the form of a house. Rather, it is analogous to the manufacture of automobiles, in which the basic elements were anticipated in four-wheeled coaches and carts pulled by horses, and even earlier in primitive conveyances with or without wheels that were pulled by men and women. The automobile improved on all of these, adding an internal combustion engine, placed out of habit in honor of the horse it superseded before the driver, as well as pneumatic tires, gears, brakes of improved design, springs, and more comfortable appointments. Subsequent models added more cylinders, an automatic gear shift, and front wheel drive, novelties that improved the basic design but did not deviate from it, and even later "improvements" consist of such faddish paraphernalia as automatic locks and window openers, stereo radios, telephones, and alarms, ending in a bewildering variety of makes of cars, each offering such an array of "extras" as to allow the consumer individuality of choice. The choice may include them all, or even add such private embellishments as baby shoes or huge dice suspended from the rearview mirror or bumper stickers or even facsimiles of parts of expensive cars, say a grille that resembles that of a Rolls Royce. Alternatively, necessity, or even eccentricity, may take the form of the stripped-down cheap car without extras.

But each "improvement" was added to a plan that stemmed from a previous version of the basic plan that remains inviolate to this day. The options for fundamental change are actually narrow, and although novelty is stressed in advertising, it is always in the context of what has been accepted previously. Although we know that if car designers were given their head, we might have had some truly revolutionary designs, it was the imperative of sales (for which read natural selection) that limited improvements to those that represent only evolutionary change. So the designer of the sleekest Lamborghini is constrained by features of that most plebeian of cars, the Model T Ford. By extension, one might say that the development of the very model of a modern human being represents the integration of innovations into the successful designs of the ancient, prehuman past. The old constrains the direction to be taken by the new, an inhibition that is exerted through conservation of the genetic program.

Genetic Conservation

What does conservation mean? The metaphor of the automobile gives the answer. Nature hangs on to what works. The mechanisms of embryonic development have been conserved throughout phylogeny; gametes unite, blastulas and gastrulas form, the same housekeeping genes turn on, and embryonic genes carry the embryo through processes of cell adhesion, communication, determination, differentiation, migration, and cell death, all processes that at the start are almost indistinguishable across the species. This uniformity is a consequence of genetic conservation of two kinds. One is represented in the formation, by duplication, of families of genes that allow, by mutation, a slow change in the qualities of function so that quite disparate organisms may have the same gene families. A second is observed in conserved sequences of DNA in which similarity, sometimes near identity, of amino acid sequences is preserved in proteins of different species. One example already cited is the family of heat shock molecules that are so conserved that those present in bacteria may be perceived as self by the human immune system (2). Others are mismatch repair genes originally discovered in yeast that, when they appear as mutants in human chromosomes, are involved in colon cancer. There are many others: growth factors and their specific receptors, signaling pathways leading to the activities of transcription factors, and homeotic genes that encode positional information and are conserved not only in the amino acid sequences of the proteins they specify but also in the order of arrangement of the genes along the chromosomes (3). All of these are echoes of the phylogenetic past, retained by some necessity even as the complexity of what we call "higher organisms" is attained by trying out novel solutions within the context of what has already been accredited by selection—what Jacob describes as "nature's tinkering" (4).

What this means is that in some aspects of our developmental and physiological homeostasis we differ very little from organisms we perceive as primitive (e.g., bacteria). In other aspects our genes resemble those of simple, but "higher," organisms—drosophila, for example—and when we come to comparisons with the primates, our phylogenetic brethren, our proteins are said to differ hardly at all (5). So each of us is a sort of mosaic of genes derived from different phases of phylogeny; that is, in the course of evolution, the products of the old have been integrated with the new to emerge as the familiar homeostasis of Homo sapiens. We have a strong inclination to perceive ourselves as nature's aristocrats, but in our genes we are compounded of nature's experiments, some dating back to prokaryotes. Fans of Gilbert and Sullivan's *Mikado* may agree that Pooh-Bah is on to something when, with exquisite hauteur, he proclaims himself to have descended from a primordial protoplasmic globule.

So if we are compounded of the stuff of lesser breeds, how do we differ from other animals, especially from other primates? It is in novelty in developmental timing. The human path to independence lasts longer than that of even our nearest phylogenetic relatives. It is characterized by neoteny, an evolutionary program wherein juvenility is much prolonged and, in comparison to related organisms, retained in adult features (6). For example, not only is the time of growth and maturation of human beings longer than that of, say, the chimpanzee, but as adults we have features that resemble their young. The prolonged growth and maturation has promoted bipedal posture as well as enlargement and increased complexity and plasticity of the brain; the latter persists into adult life, even into old age.

There is, of course, a cost. Prolonged juvenility means prolonged supervision. In comparison to the offspring of even the nearest primate, the human newborn infant is still a fetus, and a far cry from, say, the infant gazelle, who must run competently within minutes or end up as somebody's lunch. And the developing brain is particularly vulnerable to damage and permanent disability from influences which, when applied later in life, leave it intact. So there are diseases of neoteny, but even so, the advantages are obvious. Extended exposure of a gradually maturing nervous system to experiences of a variable environment, together with the mental resiliency to continue to learn at all ages, is a recipe for the adaptive agility that has enabled human beings to live in all latitudes and climates and so to exploit the earth's resources to construct civilizations and to be aesthetically creative. These achievements are a consequence of the nature of learning, a process that is not static, like piling block on block, but historical and integrative. What we learn today has been determined by what we learned yesterday, and tomorrow's learning will be influenced by today's. So the store of learning accumulates and takes the learners into diverse fields of information and behavior. Learning is a metaphor for development, which is also a historical process.

Development Is a Historical Process

All development and maturation are historical; what happens today depends upon yesterday's events, and tomorrow's will depend upon today's (7).

When the first gene turns on to specify a product, it engenders a milieu favorable for the next, and that for still others, and so on. Each step takes place in new cellular conditions that were created in the course of realization of previous steps. Development would be historical whether creative or revelatory, but at its beginning it is predominantly revelatory; there is strong fidelity to the genetic program. It could not be otherwise. Tolerance for variation must be limited at first since it would amount to interference with those most historically preserved elements of design and would result in distortion that became increasingly prominent with further development. So we all begin with much the same developmental trajectory, as if we were an endless parade of twins marching to the monotonous strains of a band with a single tune. But as embryogenesis proceeds and merges into fetal life and fetal life into postnatal, there is more and more latitude for differences in design and rate of growth; there is diversity in experiences of the environment and, progressively, the imposition of a personal stamp on the developing organism. The effects of such experiences are cumulative and, within constraints set by diverse genotypes, lead to variable developmental paths or trajectories—"canalization," Waddington called it (8).

Development is, then, a formative process in which we move through life from the general to the specific, the unspecialized to the particular, and the simple to the complex, all the while defining and refining our distinctions and risking, in old age, becoming caricatures of ourselves. And it is through days bound each to each by actions and reactions of a genetically unique homeostasis with a no less unique set of experiences that such a caricature descends from its progenitive infant.

THE INDIVIDUALITY OF DEVELOPMENT

The path to independence leads but to the grave, but the metaphor of learning suggests that each of us attains that destiny by a unique road. And postnatal development shows it. Although medical students usually refer to infants as "it" in bland indifference even to sex, let alone other qualities, every mother discerns the "character" of her baby, perhaps in utero and certainly at birth. And why not? The infant is already expressing the polymorphic differences with which that baby and no other is endowed. Postnatal development begins immediately to make individuality more obvious. For example, attainment of developmental milestones is increasingly variable with age; nearly all babies sit unaided at or around six months, but walking and talking vary by several months, and even broader limits are observed around the onset of menses, puberty, and the cessation of physical growth. Social development is more variable still. Very young infants respond only to stimuli imposed on them; later, babies learn to evoke responses, and still later to create for themselves an environment in which to react

(9). So by slowing the process of our development into whatever each of us is to become, neoteny provides opportunities for shaping that outcome—some of it by choice and some by the imposition of outside influences—adding thereby to individuality and to the diversity of the species. Neoteny allows us to escape the tyranny of our genes, or at least to temper their rule.

It is illuminating to consider the characteristics of the pilgrimage to independence in a cohort of individuals all born at the same time. If development is historical, it follows that the diversity expressed in the cohort must increase with age. Further, since constraint is constant and history cumulative, individual trajectories must increasingly be shaped by the kind, intensity, and duration of experiences. Later I present evidence bearing on this idea in connection with disease, but a return to the metaphor of the automobile may be useful here. No one would deny intrinsic differences between representatives of, say, the year 2000 models of any one of the many makes of automobile, differences that might well be expressed in durability. There is bound to be variation, however slight, in materials used, quality of workers, conditions within individual factories, and glitches in assembly, all of which will be expressed in how well individual cars perform and for how long, even if all drivers and all conditions of driving were identical, which they manifestly are not. Variations in the latter are expressed in driver temperament and attitude, in concepts of maintenance, conditions of roads, climate, distance, city driving as opposed to rural, and frequency of use. So experiences make a difference, too. Sooner in some cars and later in others, deterioration sets in, first here, then there, ultimately everywhere, until finally, the car disintegrates. And since the material basis for a cohort of these cars all leaving the assembly line the same day remains the same as it was at the start, it is increasingly the varieties of experiences that test the workmanship and quality of each, distinguishing one car from another and differentiating the mode of demise of each. But in human beings this progressive increase in nongenetic variation is not likely to be a smooth progression. Development, although continuous, proceeds by phases, so new genetic sources of individual variation emerge with the onset of each new phase. This means that how the genes and experiences contribute to individuality must vary not only from the start to the finish of a lifetime, but also from the start to the finish of each phase of development.

PARENTAL EFFECTS

There is another source of individuality in development. Although the fetus is shielded from the outside by the uterus and maternal circulation, intrauterine life is marked by parental effects that may leave a lifelong stamp. Examination of some of these follows.

(a) Since all of the cytoplasm of the fertilized ovum is maternal, conditions surrounding the first cell divisions are governed not by the embryo but by the mother.

(b) The presence, in the zygote and in each subsequent cell, of maternal mitochondria may be reflected in development and disease.

(c) Maternal-fetal incompatibilities make of the embryo a potentially incompatible graft. Results of blood group antigen incompatibility are well known, and while polymorphism of the MHC antigens makes inconsonance the rule, paradoxically maternal-paternal compatibility for these proteins reduces fertility (10).

(d) Imprinting of parental genes is reflected in inheritance of disease according to the sex of one or the other parent, the imprinting having created a species of haploidy (11,12). If imprinting is a consequence of the necessity to defend the integrity of membranes and embryo, then such a biological necessity is a remote cause of disorders whose proximate causes are traceable to the haploid effect. And if disorders, why not normal development, too? Might not development be influenced by the unopposed effect of polymorphic alleles?

(e) Variations in the intrauterine environment may have profound effects on development; maternal age and birth rank are examples whose effects may not be apparent until postnatal life. For example, onset of both insulin-dependent diabetes mellitus (IDDM) and schizophrenia is influenced by the age of the mother at the birth of the patient. Further, maternal disease may provoke adverse fetal consequences. Maternal PKU and IDDM are examples.

(f) Parental age at conception may be reflected in new mutations in gametes that can lead to sporadic cases of disease. This effect is more likely to be paternal because of the vastly greater number of cell divisions in the creation of sperm.

(g) Disorders due to external influences on intrauterine life are too well known to rehearse here. Their often profound effects prejudice the lives of their victims, and the differences in consequences depending upon the timing of the insult is further evidence of the historical nature of development.

(h) If neotenous delay means that the newborn human infant is still a fetus when compared to the neonates of other primates, the continuation of an intimate maternal-infant tie is paramount. The virtues of human milk have been remarked. And modern insights into infant development show that substantial advantages accrue to infants whose mothers are verbal and articulate and whose "conversation" is always a little in advance of the infants' development. So what we are later is in variable degree, dependent upon the content of those early days bound each to each by a lively parental investment in our future.

The Foreclosure of Options

I have recounted these aspects of fetal and early infant life one at a time, but in fact every embryo and fetus is subject to some version of each of these variables—and to many others besides, including its own genes. And the course the individual takes must depend both upon the qualities of all these influences and upon how they interact with one another at various times in ontogeny. What happens in embryogenesis is the formation of parts and their coalescence into a unique individual. Each embryonic phase represents another choice, a further canalization, another irretrievable ordination to be supplanted by yet another, each reducing the range of choices for the next. So there is a further progression in development that is a consequence of its historical nature: a progressive reduction in options as choices are made. Canalization, beginning in embryonic life, is expressed in developmental trajectories that take the embryo, its fetus, and all its later products into paths from which there is no return.

To the fertilized ovum all things potential in the genotype are possible, and this total potential state characterizes all cells for a few divisions. But soon there is a positional orientation, and then cells are irreversibly determined and differentiated to fulfill organ-specific purposes; then structures, tissues, and organs are formed from which there is no going back. The integration of cells and organs into a fetus, however remarkable a feat of engineering, has reduced at each step options for development into anything else. That is, of course, just what is wanted. But in addition to qualities that distinguish species, steps of individuation have been taken all along the line so that what emerges at birth is not only a baby, but that special, particular baby that the mother recognizes as her one and only; it is precisely the reduction in options that accounts for individuality.

The history of postnatal life is also one of choices, both biological and social, each of which constrains further options yet a little more. For children, at best, life is a bowl of cherries—all options are open. Young adulthood, at best, is devoted to that sometimes charming, often exasperating, process of "finding oneself," which may take the form of schooling that leads to occupational choices, decisions likely to eliminate most and that may even eliminate all others. For the fortunate, graduate school is likely to impose further limitation. Not that avocations are out of the question, but a professional musician, an architect, a cabinetmaker, or a clergyman—or indeed most of us, having filled our lives with the work that earned our livings—is unlikely to be more than an amateur of anything else.

But these examples represent the best of life. All along the developmental line, some people's choices are foreclosed by lack of educational or economic opportunity, by poverty, and by disease. And some of our choices, even when freely made, may expose the susceptible to disease even while disease is robbing others of the freedom of choice. Still, although our life trajectories send us in diverse directions, it is the supreme gift of neoteny to make those trajectories broad and encompassing, promoting choice and variety within them. Indeed, who can doubt that realized potential falls far short of what is latent?

Aging

Having attained maturity, we lose it—we age. The simplest expression of aging is given in the progression of attitudes toward time: children long for it to pass, youth revels in it, middle age both fears and ignores it, and old age regrets it. "Oh, to be seventy again" was the plaintive sigh of Oliver Wendell Holmes when in his nineties.

The path to biological independence is completed sometime in early adult life; the first two tests have been passed, and the third is, or is not, an option. All systems are at peak performance and seemingly ready to go on forever. But, insidiously and variously, like Carl Sandburg's fog that "comes on little cat feet," aging begins in the third decade, hardly recognized by the individual and for most functions compensated by homeostasis, whose only sign of aging might be a modest delay in return to baseline after perturbation (13). Early expressions are followed by increasing homeostatic disorder; some see aging as an increase in entropy, resulting in a loss of adaptability.

The uniqueness of individual aging is compounded of individual patterns of affected homeostatic systems—indeed, of individual cells (13)—so if it is dust from which we arise and dust to which we return, each aliquot thereof will have traveled a different road. Evidence of this uniqueness is derived from both cross-sectional and longitudinal studies (14). The former reveal increasing variances with age for physiological measurements, while the latter make clear that patterns and rates of aging in different organ systems vary independently, both within and between individuals. That is, few individuals follow the patterns of change predicted by averages of many subjects, and the age of an individual is a poor predictor of performance in tests of physical function. Evidently cleaving to the central tendency is a criterion for passing nature's three tests; afterward we are at liberty to pursue an individual path compounded of not entirely wholesome gene effects and of possibly destructive experiences.

Why do we age and what causes it? If any explanation is favored it is that selection bears most heavily on life before reproduction ends and loses interest, as it were, after that. Williams has suggested that certain genes that are at a selective advantage in youth may be less useful, or even damaging, in later life (15). Others have explained this seeming paradox by proposing that nature wisely invests energy resources in youth and reproduction rather than in the very expensive enzymatic and metabolic equipment required to continue indefinitely to repair the random and cumulative ravages of life's experiences

(16,17). And it is this damage, whether due to oxidants, free radicals, radiation, or other stresses and mutagens, that leads directly, through somatic mutation, to such metabolic aberrations as reduced protein synthesis and degradation, changes in post-translational modification, and failure of DNA repair, all a consequence of damage to the same unit steps of homeostasis that, in diseases of earlier onset, vary in response to mutations in the germ line (18).

So is aging a form of disease, or does it provide a favorable substrate for the agents of disease? The question seems to suggest that there is a process called "aging" that, despite involving the same homeostatic steps, is distinct from disease. According to Rowe and Kahn, aging is "successful" when measurements of physiological functions in older subjects give results in the same range as those for younger people, while in "usual" aging the results of such tests are outside this range, or nearly so (19). This classification calls attention to the heterogeneity of aging, both within individuals, in whom different systems age differently, and between. So successful aging means a physiology more youthful than chronology suggests, while usual aging in one system or all may be perilously close to disease—or at least may represent a heightened susceptibility to threats from experiences that were once well tolerated. So at the very least there must be a point in the usual aging-disease continuum wherein the former becomes the latter or the difference is negligible.

For example, how do we differentiate in this aging-disease continuum the effects of reduced protein turnover due to oxidative damage from the cancers of old age due to somatic mutations that alter proteins that act to constrain the actions of growth factors? Do we call the former aging and the latter disease, even though both are a consequence of alterations in unit steps of homeostasis? Perhaps another way of putting it is that aging promotes homeostatic incongruence that leads to disease, a formula for disease that could apply at any age. So at the least we may say that a debilitated homeostasis, less fit to defy the ravages of usual aging by virtue of its genetic origins and a lifetime of experiences that have themselves contributed to the aging process, succumbs in particular ways to the impact of specific genes and experiences. That is, usual aging contributes to multifactorial disease.

What are the genes that contribute to the specificity of usual aging and to the disease of old age? Gerontology has moved from a backwater to the forefront of science in a remarkably short time (18,20–22). Indeed, it is now possessed of that clutter of molecular information that at once enthralls the molecular geneticists and tries their patience as they struggle to fit new data to old hypotheses or to devise new ones (18,23). Some have turned to nonhuman organisms—yeast, C. elegans, drosophila, and the mouse—where they have found genes associated with prolonged life (24). Those that have been identified appear to specify resistance to the effects of oxidants and other stresses, influences that lead to gene dysregulation, mutation, and reduced protein turnover (18,23). Stresses are applied variously to us all, human beings no less than yeast and drosophila, and we respond according to the capacity for resistance that resides in the products of our genes, expressing thereby our individuality in the qualities of the unit steps of homeostasis in aging no less than in disease (23).

So the problem of aging is the problem of mutifactorial disease; both are a consequence of variation in unit steps of homeostasis. And if the proximate origins of both are the same, how are they different? Perhaps it is a matter of words. During most of usual aging there is little or no dis-ease, and so we do not call it disease. An alternative is to make no distinction and to speak of aging as the most multifactorial of all diseases, a puzzle whose complexity increases in time. But still, in both, the child is father of the man; however late the onset, whether of disease or of the obvious ravages of aging, the stressful experiences have been imposed upon the genetically influenced constitution that has distinguished the person from the start. So our descent into senescence and extinction is no less characteristic of self than is the rest of life, and our individuality is expressed in exaggeration of weaknesses in homeostatic control that have been compensated by the robustness of early and middle life but which become evident in old age as signs of decline.

12

Sociocultural Homeostasis

I saw that fitness is a reciprocal relation, that adaptation in the Darwinian sense must be adaptation to something, and that complexity, stability, and intensity and diversity of metabolism in organisms could not have resulted through adaptation unless there was some sort of pattern in the properties of the environment that, as I now partly know, is both intricate and highly singular.

—L. J. Henderson, Cited in Parascandola (1)

Flexibility and constraint characterize physiological homeostasis, and we know that these properties are imparted by individual genotypes representative of variation in the gene pool. In the physiological sense, these qualities enable an individual open system to explore the environment while retaining its integrated identity. But such an individual is able to do so because the gene pool has been refined through phylogeny to contain genes that make for harmonious intercourse between the physiological homeostasis of the species and the organization of the environment.

This ecological-social-cultural homeostasis was very much an object of interest to all three originators of the physiological concept. Each remarked the similarity between the maintenance of physiological organization and that of human societies. Each was aware that the open system processed the environment to its own profit, even while being protected against it. Henderson conjured most extensively with the idea, arguing that while the environment constrains life to make do with what it offers, what it offers is something congenial for life to exist. So his thinking, expressed in the chapter's epigraph, included the same constraint and flexibility that is characteristic of physiological homeostasis: there is a fitness of the environment within which the fitness of species is worked out.

The literature of genetics is vague about the identity and quality of the environment, usually citing "gene-environment" interactions. In the past, perhaps because both participants in this interaction were nothing but abstractions, they were sometimes described as if there were a competition between nature and nurture, with predominance being given to one or the other. This misapprehension may have been based on a misunderstanding of calculations of heritability, a concept in which fractions of the variance in measurements of traits in populations are assigned to genes or to the environment (2).

GENE-ENVIRONMENT INTERACTION

Apart from substances that interfere directly with replication or transcription, the interaction of the environment with the genes is indirect and mediated by homeostatic devices. The effect is on one or more gene products acting in their appointed roles, roles that are both prescribed and limited by the specificity of the genes. What the genes actually do is provide what the drosophilists called "norms of reaction" within which experience and development have leeway to generate variation. In the logic of disease, this norm of reaction is represented by the developmental matrix (3).

Sometimes the variation is easily traceable to a single gene; more often the impulses of several genes emerge in phenotypes not predicted by the actions of any one of them. For example, a chemical substance alien to normal physiology enters the body and, because of its conformation, is able to bind to a cell surface receptor ordinarily occupied by some other ligand. This perturbs the receptor-ligand system, which signals the necessity for remedial steps; more of the normal ligand is mobilized to compete with and displace the alien substance, more receptors appear, and mechanisms for detoxification go into action. In time the unwanted agent is disposed of or "tolerance" develops and a steady state is resumed. Here detoxification is the phenotype, and variation is not assignable to any one gene, but if the gene that specified the receptor was one of several alleles that vary in their capacity to carry out their mission, the variation in the phenotype evoked by the foreign substance may be such as to segregate and so to be perceived as a genetic trait. And if there is variation in the genes that specify the other proteins upon which the variable receptors reflect, these too may be seen as genetic traits, perhaps as modifiers, or their effects may be called epistatic.

Much reciprocal behavior is encompassed in what in genetic parlance is called "gene-environment interaction," but in reality the interactions are confined to the mechanisms composed of gene products that are charged with the maintenance of congruence or which, if they fail in their purpose, lead to incongruence. Further, we must define the environment as including also stimuli that originate within. For example, in Tay-Sachs disease, deficiency of hexose aminidase A leads to accumulation of unhydrolyzed GM2 gangliosides that physically compress the interior of neurons, leading to their death. Here the environment is represented by the physical properties of neurons that cannot dispose of a normal metabolite. So the environment is best defined as the whole complex of factors within which the business of the maintenance of an individual's life is carried on, including influences emanating from within as well as without.

This is not merely a truism. If we are to have a genuine synthesis of medical and genetic thinking, we must transcend the parochial language of both. What comes to the mind of the geneticist when the idea of gene-environment interaction is introduced is an individual response to a stimulus, strongly influenced by a unique genetic endowment that binds each person to his own developmental past and to that of the species. In contrast, the physiologist, the biochemist, or the student of pathogenesis is more likely to conjure up a vision of the details of the apparatus designed to accommodate the stimulus and so to maintain the status quo, without necessarily acknowledging the variable individuality implicit in the phrase "gene-environmental interaction." The two views are in no way in opposition. They are made for each other.

THE EXTERNAL ENVIRONMENT

The inner environment consists of the organized structure of cells, including the apparatus of physiological homeostasis, and we know that the engines of these qualities, the proteins, originate in the genes, which themselves are subject to organizing principles. But what of the external environment? Of what does it consist? What are its organizing principles, and what governs its structure and function?

There are several external environments. Some were here before life existed. First came the elements of the remote past: water, geology, climate, seasons, and the laws of gravity and thermodynamics. These conditions in which life began will influence the adaptations of open systems until the end of time. From the start, life had to adapt to them and to changes in them, many of which—including, for example, the balance between oxygen and carbon dioxide in the air—are a result of the presence of life.

Some of this environment is immutable, some is indifferent to life; all is indifferent to individual lives, in the sense of not discriminating among those individuals. But that the physical environment has had a powerful influence in human history is the subject of a book written by Simon Schama, called *Landscape and Memory* (4). It shows, in sections titled "Wood," "Water," and "Rock," how human beings not only adapted to these elements of nature but also actively used them in advancing their own designs. In the course of constructing a culture, nature was woven into its texture, becoming "hidden between layers of the commonplace." So, *Landscape and Memory* is "constructed as an excavation below our conventional sight-level to recover the veins of myth and memory that lie beneath the surface." By myth and memory Schama means how in working out their destinies in the contexts of forests and deserts, oceans and rivers, mountains and plains, people adapted to and used these surroundings to create a culture of adaptation. This is what all organisms do, though none so self-centeredly as Homo sapiens. Lewontin, too, reminds us that adaptation is an active process in which the fitness of organisms is enhanced by their competence in creating favorable environments (5). He sees adaptation as an active, constructive process in which organisms create much of their environment. Such a process leads not merely to evolution but to co-evolution, in which organisms evolve in relation to one another.

Other forms of life that constitute an aspect of the external environment were described by Darwin as an "entangled bank wherein plants, birds, insects, and worms coexist in and on a damp earth, different and dependent on each other, and all . . . produced by laws acting around us" (6). The study of ecology reveals the interdependence of all species. Each forms a part of and influences the environment of others, representing a network that some have conceived as a diverse but unified homeostatic system in which, when one part is changed, others react (7,8). How far this "one world" idea can be pushed remains unclear, but that there are interspecies' relationships representing a homeostasis that includes affinities both among species and between species and the environment can hardly be denied (9). Human societies test this homeostasis to its limit, and beyond. In typical human locutions we speak of the "fragile" ecologies of wetlands and forests. In fact, it is not to the fragility of these ecosystems we should allude; they are anything but fragile. Rather, it is the ponderousness of the assault that we should stress. What ecosystem is proof against a bulldozer? It is always some Darwin's bank that the bulldozer destroys.

Competition and cooperation among species have been a part of the adaptive scene since the beginning. Species have evolved accordingly, and the principle of an interlocking, mutually dependent biosphere free to exploit the limitless potential of the DNA but constrained by the properties of the physical environment, by dependency itself, and by random events is an attractive one. So opportunities and constraints confronting individual open systems are dictated by regional versions of the organization of the whole, and local populations evolve in accord with rules both general and regional. At the same time, when species alter their environments for their own reasons, there is an impact on the adaptation of other species and on the organization of the whole.

No species has changed the earth and challenged its homeostasis to such a degree and with such dramatic effect as Homo sapiens. We have imposed our culture and the rules of our societies on the organization of nature with far-reaching consequences for the health of both. That is, both the constantly evolving interrelationships of life on the planet and the organization of human societies and cultures are sources of remote causes of disease. No one can be oblivious to the fluxes in our relationships with parasites, especially microorganisms with their capacity to evolve the most menacing mutants which, in the course of pursuing their "careers," as Garrod put it, they use effectively to our detriment. Some of this threat, including new viruses and the reappearance in drug-resistant guise of organisms such as the tubercle bacillus that were thought to have been contained, , has to do with human habits and choices— for example, the overuse of antibiotics. Thus does human behavior, even that generally perceived as constructive, constitute remote causes of disease. It is both constraining and permissive in determining the repertory of proximate causes.

CULTURAL INHERITANCE

Both the gene pool and our cultural traits evolve. Cultural traits are the ideas, beliefs, and values we live by. They are deeply embedded in the structures of social entities—families, communities, schools, churches, and other groups based on common interests, including cat fanciers and stamp collectors no less than philosophers and manufacturers. Indeed, these traits motivate society. So there are analogies between cultural traits and genes, on the one hand, and between social organization and biological integration, on the other. Culture is to society what genes are to physiology. This analogy between the evolution of biological qualities and the shifts and changes in cultural traits has been given serious attention by several workers, among them L. L. Cavalli-Sforza and M. W. Feldman at Stanford University, R. Boyd and P. J. Richerson at Emory University and the University of California at Davis, respectively, and W. H. Durham at Stanford (10–12). Cavalli-Sforza has also studied the distribution of genes in relation to agriculture (13) and language (14). In that they represent an interface between medicine and the humanities, these books are of great interest for medical education. They are genetic, anthropological, and historical, and they join with those of historians such as W. H. McNeil and A. H. Crosby, who have written of the impact of infections on history.

A principal outcome of the synthesis of genetic and medical thinking is a new emphasis on prevention, which, in turn, means a heightened grasp of the relationships of culture and social organization to human genes and individuality. Some of the thinking of the genetic-anthropological writers is summarized below.

Cultural traits may be perceived as units of transmission capable of mutation. They may be transmitted vertically, like the genes, but also horizontally, as between sibs or coevals, and obliquely, as between aunt and nephew. Other departures from the mendelian-like pattern involve the transmission of ideas or behaviors from one central figure to many pupils or fans, as well as from many to one as happens in the pressure on individuals to accept the conventional wisdom.

Mutation is represented as inventions as well as new ideas and perceptions that all lead to conceptual change. Such mutant ideas have the same kind of influence on transmission and distribution as do genes. Like genes, the cultural units may vary in frequency, and they are subject to selection, proliferating to prevalence or diminishing to extinction. And their frequencies may be changed by migration, as in the adoption of foreign styles, say, or by chance; for example, death may cause a decline in influence of a popular figure and a rise in that of a divergent authority. But unlike biological qualities that change at glacial rates, cultural change may be very rapid, a difference in tempo that is likely to create incongruence and risks for disease.

There is also a cultural form of natural selection—that is, there is a competition of values and for changes in habits. Television, for example, is energetic in persuading us in many directions, not least in changing our habits and behaviors having to do with health. Such a competition is likely to be no less subtle than that which occurs in nature.

There is much interaction between the behaviors determined by culture and the homeostatic qualities promoted by the genes; the former may constitute risk factors for disease. And there is a complex relationship in the evolution, or co-evolution, of both. An apposite example is the persistence of lactase in the intestinal mucosa of some populations (15). This persistence varies directly with latitude and inversely with skin pigmentation and ultraviolet radiation. The hypothesis is that in areas of low ultraviolet radiation, precursors may not be converted to active vitamin D. There is then the threat of rickets which, when untreated, may reduce reproductive fitness. But rickets can be averted by lactose, which promotes the intestinal absorption of Ca^{++}—hence, the persistence of lactase (14). But where the intensity of ultraviolet radiation is high, rickets is not a threat, so lactase is not needed. So cultural and biological traits have evolved together.

A second example is that of the well-known advantage of hemoglobin S in malarial areas. In some parts of Africa, the frequency of the HgbS gene is influenced by diet. The highest frequency is found where yams are cultivated. Yams require sunlight, which means cleared forests and warm, sunlit pools, wherein mosquitoes thrive. Populations that live in forests and eat other food have fewer mosquitoes, less malaria, and less HgbS (11).

So there are intimate relationships between gene frequencies and the way people live. Gene-determined molecules work in cellular environments, themselves influenced by cultural traits that determine social environments. Sometimes these are at cross-purposes and therefore of interest in medicine. The tobacco industry and human health is again an example. The U.S. tobacco enterprise has its own internal homeostasis that includes farmers, manufacturers, wholesalers, retailers, advertisers, marketers, and lobbyists. And it is a part of a larger homeostatic system consisting of community, state, and international trade. The livelihoods of all of the workers named above, as well as taxes and the general economy, all depend on smokers who imperil their health by smoking, and do so in the face of growing social disapprobation. So in this case, physiological homeostasis, subject to injury by smoke, is opposed by a social homeostasis, and we are observing how difficult it is when there is a clash of values to change the prevalent custom, even when that custom is manifestly harmful. Social homeostatic systems are as stubborn and defensive as the physiological version.

There are many other examples of cultural changes that produce ripple effects. Improvements in nutrition and sanitation brought about substantial decline in the incidence of infectious disease long before antibiotics, with profound impact on natural selection and population growth. Selection seemed to be altered, and in detail it was. But today we are observing other kinds of selective pressures, including changes in population density which is responding to education and contraceptives. But here we find another clash of values. People holding unyielding beliefs in a parochial version of the "sanctity" of life resist and block the use of contraceptives by anyone, including those whose views are altogether at variance with theirs. This is an example of cultural selection at work, and the outcome—at least the immediate outcome—is unclear. Another change: Recently in the United States we have seen shifts in dietary habits, stimulated by reports of an association of saturated fat in food with atherosclerosis and heart attack. The impact of these observations has been felt not only in the home, but by the dairy, meat, and other food industries, so that the Food and Drug Administration now requires labeling to indicate the amount of fat and other substances in food sold at retail markets. It is not clear that anyone has suffered. Those who pay attention to such admonitions must be presumed to be better off, while those who do not are in no worse position than they were. As for the affected industries, those that survive in our culture are those that are quickest to make a virtue of necessity. They exemplify Henderson's "fitness of the environment."

CONCLUSION

In this section, gene-environment interactions have been defined as mediated by the devices of physiological homeostasis, themselves composed of protein products of the genes, the unit steps of homeostasis. The environment, therefore, is both internal and external. Species tend to alter their environments to suit their purposes, none more than Homo sapiens. Such alterations are usually systematic, but the human case transcends all others in the creation of cultural influences on health and disease. Human beings are disposed into many kinds of social entities, and the culture represents the expressions of human lives within those bodies. Medical educators often stress the need for an infusion of "humanities" into the medical curriculum. By humanities they mean literature and the arts, expressions of human aspiration and experience they think might enhance students' ability to engage with the emotional and humane aspects of medicine, the samaritan functions. But the humanities are nothing but accounts in diverse media of the cultural condition of the species, so it might be that study of the inheritance and evolution of cultural traits, their influence on social homeostasis and how they interact with their biological counterparts, should fill the need perceived by the educators. This understanding was among the aims of Henry Sigerist and other adherents to the ideals of social medicine (16). In their time there was not the wherewithal to create an effective agenda, but now their hopes are likely to be realized—though in ways they could not have anticipated.

13

Homeostatic Interactions

It is interesting to contemplate an entangled bank, clothed with many plants of many kinds, with birds singing on the bushes, with various insects flitting about, and with worms crawling through the damp earth, and to reflect that these elaborately constructed forms, so different from each other, and dependent on each other in so complex a manner, have all been produced by laws acting around us.

—Charles Darwin

This account of Darwin's bank appeared in part in the last chapter, but it serves as nothing else could as an introduction to the idea of homeostatic interactions. Darwin's observations were, of course, limited to phenotypes, but here he describes the mutual dependence of living organisms that reflects integrations we now know begin with the molecular level.

In the preceding chapters of this section, the idea of homeostasis, first proposed in the setting of moment-to-moment maintenance of physiological integrity, has been extended to phylogeny, to the lifetime as exhibited in development and aging, and to the dynamics of gene pools and the organization and evolution of cultures and societies. These systems embrace biological history, the individual lifetime, and the moment, representing at once the historical contexts of the French *Annaliste* historians, Waddington's three time scales, and the three salient perspectives of biology observed by Lederberg. All must be reckoned simultaneously if the individual is to be understood. That is, it is the unique individual that is the focus and the product of the mutual and reciprocal actions and reactions of these several homeostatic systems.

Certainly they entail reciprocal actions and reactions, but no one of these systems could exist without the others. They are all of a piece. What point is there in genes and genetic individuality except in the context of physiological individuality? And what point in physiological individuality apart from the development of an organism capable of coping independently with an environment consisting in part of other organisms also capable of coping independently with it? The reciprocity is exhibited whenever a significant change is made in any one of the systems. For example, a mutation changes a protein that interferes with a signaling device so that it fails to respond to some condition of the environment, which then must be changed to deal with the alterations in physiology that have impaired the capacity of the affected individual to be independent. These reflections are of marginal interest to the machine mentality, but they are very much to the point in teaching the student. The next question, then, is how our thinking about disease can be made consonant with this integrated way of looking at the past and present of individuals. What have the affinities of the several homeostatic systems to do with genetic medicine?

Health no less than disease is a product of the response to influences of genes and experiences that in turn influence the developmental matrix in which such transformations take place. While there is as much variability in health as there is in disease, the latter disrupts the inner harmony of both patient and family in ways that make overt the variability so little noticed in health. The elements of the logic are listed in Table 2 in a way that comprehends the three time scales in an arrangement that allows the physician to analyze each case according to the array of its constituents—which is to say, to the individuality of the patient, itself an indicator for choices in treatment.

The patient is for genetic and developmental reasons incongruent with some conditions of the environment. In Figure 1 the several factors that interact to produce the disease phenotype surround it, with arrows pointing to it to represent their participation. The phenotype is the pathophysiological state at the time, say, of diagnosis, but it could easily represent any other time in the course of the disease, or even in the state of health. The three contributors each represent their own homeostatic dynamic and time scale. But the position is not actually as simple as that. There are also arrows that point outward from the phenotype, suggesting some reciprocal action of the pathophysiological state on the elements that conspired to produce it in the first place. For example, while all phenotypes reflect the developmental state in which they reveal themselves, they may, in their turn, influence development, with further reflec-

Table 2 **Elements Contributing to the Individuality of Phenotypes**

Genes	Developmental Matrix	Environmental Factors (Experiences)
Major gene	Age	Geography
Modifiers	Sex	Time
	Parental effects	Climate
	Ethnic group	Education
	Cognition	Occupation
	Behavioral attributes	Diet
		Habits
		Socioeconomic status
		Disease

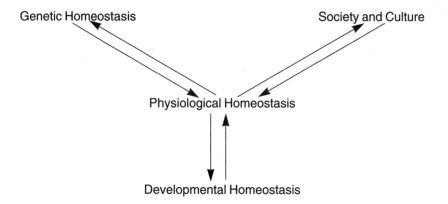

Figure 1 Interactions among genes, experiences, and development are dynamic.

tion on the phenotype. Since time continues relentlessly to pass and ontogenetic imperatives must be met, however badly, increasing distortion of development is the result. Similarly, all phenotypes are in some degree shaped by experience of the environment. When the phenotype is a disease, treatment and management leap to the mind. That is, the outside environment must be altered in some way—whether through medication, hospitalization, or merely changes in habitual routines—with the intention of promoting a return of the phenotype to normal.

This means that the physiological homeostasis, whether inadequate from the start or damaged by some agent or experience, must be supported, even propped up, from without. So doctors, nurses, spouses, parents, and friends become integrated into the homeostatic apparatus of the sick patient. This may suffice; healing may then take place and business as usual may be resumed. But in chronic disease, these props must be permanent, so that the sick individual comes to rely not only upon such residual adjustments of physiological homeostasis as may represent adaptation to new conditions but also upon the availability and quality of social and cultural institutions. These, as we know, vary according to the resources of the sick person as well as the political trends that reflect cyclic changes in prevailing mores. All of this, even when it works, is but a poor substitute for the flexible, resilient instrument nature intended. So, again, there is a dialectic, this time between disease phenotypes and the social institutions created to counter them. The more responsive the dialectical communion, the more likely is the life of the patient to be given meaning and purpose.

Another arrow in Figure 1 represents the contribution of genetic individuality to the disease phenotype. That is plain enough, but what does the reciprocal arrow represent? Obviously, it is the fates of phenotypes that determine the condition of the gene pool; the genes of those phenotypes that interfere with reproduction are deleted by selection, and the frequencies of genes of noxious effect are thereby kept low. So the dialectic here is of a different magnitude: each separate individual affects the composition of the gene pool only infinitesimally. The fates of species hinge not on that of any particular individual, but upon aggregates thereof. But because the aggregates are composed of individuals, an opposing arrow is justified.

All of these reciprocating actions are going on at once, but there are no arrows, say, between development and society or society and the gene pool. Always the influence is exerted upon the phenotype or arises from the phenotype, itself a reflection of homeostatic individuality as expressed in the qualities of the unit steps of homeostasis. So, for a comprehensive view of a disease in an individual, we must reckon with a dialectical relationship in which the disease processes influence variously the conditions that initiated them. Indeed, the dialectical process was going on long before the homeostasis became so disordered as to reach the stage of overt disease. And it is in place in health, too.

An Example

A family I have known for fifty years provides a real-life exemplification of this abstract description (1). This family is afflicted with a chronic disease that has tested its victims' capacity to cope, both physiologically and socially, to the last degree. The disease has influenced every waking moment and every decision of those affected. It is an aspect of their personhood, has informed the banter of their friends and barbed the arrows of their enemies. It has blunted their intellect, constricted their social and cultural options, put them at a disadvantage at school and work, and made them the object of the intervention of a broad array of public agencies. Indeed, they have probed the chinks in the safety net. But this is not the Jukes family. Sibs, aunts, uncles, and cousins who have escaped the blight have succeeded in making satisfactory lives for themselves. For example, while success in school at all levels has eluded the affected, college degrees have been attained by unaffected cousins. The disease is nephrogenic diabetes insipidus, a genetically determined disorder characterized by a failure to concentrate solute in the urine, and it illustrates the interplay between genes, development, and society as nothing else can.

The story began in the summer of 1941 with the admission to the pediatric service of the Johns Hopkins Hospital of a thin, scrawny infant of two months, very dehydrated and weighing no more than at birth. There was a history of vomiting, constipation, and rejection of milk, but an avidity for water. The family history revealed only a normal female sib. Despite his dehydration, the baby produced a dilute urine, so a diagnosis of diabetes insipidus was proposed—but rejected because there was no response to exogenous pitressin. Before much more study could be done, the baby died. Time passed and so did the father. The mother, a vivacious and attractive young woman, soon contracted a second partner and produced three more boys, all affected with the same complaints as their half-brother. In the meantime, Albright had described a model of end organ resistance in the form of pseudohypoparathyroidism, which was applied to this family by Waring et al. (2). Here, too, the end organ was presumed to be insensitive, and the disease was called "pitressin resistant" diabetes insipidus (3). The diagnosis was of little help to the three stricken boys. The eldest was run over by a car at age five; the other two are still alive, both much handicapped by their disease.

The family underwent a second convulsion when the new father decamped, possibly unable to accommodate to the chaos in a household of three constantly restless youngsters who could not sustain interest in anything by day and were up and down all night.

In a long acquaintance with this mother I have never known her to be daunted so I was not surprised to learn of the advent of yet another man in her life. He did not tarry long, but he did participate in the genetic experiment by collaborating in the production of a healthy girl, who has since demonstrated her own lack of taint by producing five children and thirteen grandchildren, all unaffected. The mother, now required to be the breadwinner, exhibited a taste for irony by taking a job as a barmaid. In time she met a fourth man by whom she had four more children: two boys, one of whom is affected, and two girls, one of whom has a less severe version of the disorder. The affected boy, who is markedly retarded, was adopted into another family and has been lost to view. This fourth father, a worker in an abattoir by day and a private detective by night, was a good provider and gave the family a degree of financial stability, even while adding to the burden of affected children. But in time, he too departed.

It must be acknowledged that a certain instability characterized this mother's relationships with men, but her undiminished enthusiasm for a pursuit that others might have perceived as hopeless was revealed in a fifth union, more durable than the rest and untested by more children. It lasted until the man's death a few years ago.

Genetics

This woman engaged in an interesting genetic experiment. Of her ten children by four fathers, five boys and one girl were affected. She, her mother, and two of her three sisters were shown to be carriers by their failure to concentrate urine after a water load and pitressin test, as well as by habitual extravagant consumption of fluid. For example, the mother who rose frequently from her bed in the night in response to the urgent needs of her babies thought it the most normal thing in the world to drink two or three cups of tea at each awakening. She had been doing that all her life anyway. One of the carrier sisters also had affected sons, who were of small stature and mentally retarded. Such evidence favors X linkage, and although no molecular genetic test of this family has been done, in others a gene mapping at Xq28 that specifies the V2 vasopressin receptor has been demonstrated. Other genes that have been implicated, both X linked and autosomal, fulfill the expectation of heterogeneity.

Symptoms

Since urine cannot be concentrated yet solute must be excreted, the dominant symptom is a ferocious and unquenchable thirst and a single-minded concentration on water, a craving that befits the danger of vascular collapse and death after hours, rather than days, of deprivation. In infancy, milk is often rejected, water is preferred to food, and there is an unhealthy standoff: deprivation of water leads to hyperosmolality and dehydration, while lack of any food contributes to failure in growth and development. Frequent infections exacerbate dehydration by causing vomiting, even of water, and failure to thrive and to grow and mature in intellect is the rule. The boys in this family endured innumerable hospitalizations to treat infections and to restore hydration. One of them spent most of his first year in the hospital because of the near impossibility of maintaining both nutrition and hydration.

An Analysis

How do we analyze these patients, their families, and their experiences according to the elements in Table 2 and the dialectical relationships expressed in Figure 1?

Gene-Phenotype

The phenotype consists of a failure to transmit a hormonal signal that promotes renal tubular reabsorption of water, with signs and symptoms in consequence. In our family the mutant is presumed to reside in the X chromosome. Mother and grandmother are both carriers, but we have no knowledge of the mutant's origin. Bode and Crawford reported a similar family in which the disease was traced by hearsay evidence to the eighteenth century (4). Obviously many males were only presumed to be affected, but of twenty-seven males known to have the disease, only two reproduced, indicating a low reproductive fitness. In our family, one affected male had one daughter, hardly up to his mother's or sister's standard. Carrier females, however, are not so handicapped. So an unequal toll is exacted from males who participate in the genetic lottery that is an expression of the need of the species for heritable variation. Here the curse, visited upon sons, is transmitted only by daughters, even unto the seventh generation or more. Will an equitable society ever accord such victims some special concern for bearing such a burden?

Development-Phenotype

This disease is at its worst early in life when the ratio of water need to body size is greatest; it is very difficult for an affected baby to avoid dehydration even while on a normal diet. So the phenotype soon includes retardation in growth and development, which itself further impairs maturation. Later in life the rigors of the disease seem somewhat less, in part because of bladder enlargement. But that, too, has its hazards. One of the males in our family fell into the hands of urologists who, mistaking the cause of the dilated bladder, did a bladder neck resection. A further hazard is the failure of unaware medical personnel to recognize the unnatural extent of their need for water when treating infections or at operation. The eight glasses of water per day said to be good for us all are but a stopgap dose for a patient with this disease, an eye-opener perhaps, after a night of "rest" made up of naps. Wordsworth's lines "The world is too much with us, getting and spending" are appropriately paraphrased as "The world is too much with us, drinking and voiding." There is in both the same compulsive devotion to a single appetite at the cost of that diversity of satisfactions that makes life worth living.

There are treatments in the form of low-solute diets and drugs that inhibit sodium reabsorption, but these failed in our family, more for social reasons than any other. There is no question but that a reduction, say, of one-half of the daily water need and output, enlarges the horizon and increases social opportunities, with positive effects on school, work, and development in general. All this was explained to our patients and to their mother, but the advice was disregarded—indeed, I think it was never grasped.

Thus, the developmental state of very early life affects the phenotype which, in turn, affects development which shapes the phenotype—and so it goes until some sort of uneasy, often perturbed equilibrium is reached. How aging affects the phenotype is unlikely to have had more than an occasional test. The eldest male in our family, the second son of the second father, is now only about fifty years old.

Environment-Phenotype

Certainly no phenotype is impervious to the conditions in which it emerges; indeed, many are provoked by those conditions. Equally, none fails to evoke changes in them. In the case of nephrogenic diabetes insipidus, although experiences of the environment have little to do with whether there is a disease phenotype, they have everything to do with its particular expression: diets that limit solute, or the aforementioned drugs, reduce the rigor of the disease's demands. But above all, the socioeconomic status, the conditions of the home, the parents, the family, the schools, the availability of medical and social support, and the capacity of all to work efficiently together are the factors that determine whether physical and intellectual development can be protected to lead to an independent life. All of these agencies become a part of the homeostasis of the affected child, an extension of the physiological device, and as we know, the cardinal quality of a successful homeostasis is the perfection of its integration. So in this, as in most chronic diseases, we call upon the resiliency of extracorporeal organizations not known for flexible individual responses. Thus, the dialectic is likely to be characterized more by creaks and groans than by effortless efficiency.

Still, like its physiological counterpart, the extracorporeal homeostasis is composed of elements of variable tolerance. For example, a family intelligently concerned and furnished with resources can go some way to avoid or to compensate for bureaucratic indifference. And bureaucracy itself varies according to the humanity of its components. But in our family, with its here-today and gone-tomorrow fathers, its mother reluctant even to discuss abridging her reproductive marathon, and the utter chaos of a home dominated not by the ordinary standard of care and acculturation of robust children, but by a compelling need, night and day, to consume water—even sometimes at the expense of food—and to excrete it, the job is impossible. All of the ordinary activities of childhood and youth—outdoor play, school, the movies, sports—and later the choice of jobs, all are subject to limitations of some degree by this imperious physiological necessity.

SOME GENERALIZATIONS

This family seems an apposite example of a number of generalizations implicit in Figure 1. First, open systems may be incongruent with experiences of their environment in diverse ways, depending upon both genotype and kind, intensity, and duration of experiences. And it is the individuality of ontogeny that gives form to the consequences of the incongruence—that is, to the description of the disease. Second, phenotypes react on and change the elements that determine them and then are themselves changed in a dialectical process. Third, this dialectical discourse, which includes treatment and responses to it, influences homeostasis to effect a cure or to attain an equilibrium, however uneasy and unstable, or to foreclose options with consequent death or irreversible damage. Fourth, ontogeny and aging are historical processes: what we are today depends upon what we were yesterday, and whatever we become tomorrow will be conditioned by what we are today. So, a disease may begin very early in life with consequences that, as in this family, prevail until life ends. Or if it is held in check by a robust homeostasis, a disease may become overt when, slowly, imperceptibly, or all at once, that protective compensation fails, overwhelmed by habitual exposure to something noxious or another disease or enfeebled by inherent frailties present from the start or by aging, the debility shared by all. And this should remind us that medicine is among the most historical of all human missions; the patient's doctor is the repository of his or her history, and the satisfaction taken in the encounter for both parties may depend upon how completely the doctor is in possession of that history (5).

In summary, we might think of our genes as a biological memory that serves to connect each of us with relatives, other human beings, and all of life, present and past. The genes also provide the wherewithal to construct a homeostatic memory that mediates experiences in the context of an ontogenetic memory that preserves individuality through time and change to set on disease a personal stamp. Surely it is the mission of medicine to attend to the individuality of these several memories and to help patients to adjust the qualities of life to the limitations these memories impose.

V
Descent with Modification: Genetic Variation

In the definition of evolution in chapter 7, such concepts as species identity, descent with modification, adaptive flexibility, reproduction, and the like were cited. Both individual and species differences in all of these are a reflection of variation in the genes. In other chapters, too, disease has been defined as a consequence of incongruence of a gene-specified homeostasis with experiences of the environment. So there is reason in pausing to define the gene, not only in its physical and functional details but as a concept.

In fact, it is a capacious and inclusive idea, central to any thought about life—whether in general or of the individual—and as such it is at the forefront of the thinking of genetic medicine. When defined as that which is transmitted through the generations, that which specifies the wherewithal for the homeostasis of both development and adaptive maintenance of organisms, and that which, when changed, becomes the means for the generation of new species and the improvement of old, it can surprise no one that it dominates the opening pages of the book *The Molecular Biology of the Cell* (1).

In other places in this book I emphasize the continuity of congruence with incongruence, of health with disease, so if the concept of the gene is perceived as being of such moment in an account of congruence, ought it not to occupy the forefront of the medical preoccupation with incongruence? Accordingly, Part V is devoted to defining the gene, its variations, and its role as specifier of the proteins of the homeostatic mechanisms that fulfill intentions latent in the genome. As the details of the nature of the gene and its functions have become apparent, the universality of its concept and all its works is increasingly evident in human disease, as in all else. One application to human affairs is in the imposition of the gene product—the unit step of homeostasis—on the classification of disease. Another is in the evolution of vocabulary suitable for a universal discourse that crosses species boundaries.

14

What Is a Gene?

That is, genetics deals with both the problem of heredity and the problem
of variation. It is, in fact, the triumph of genetics that a single theory, down
to the molecular level, explains in one synthesis, both the constancy of inheritance and its variation.
— R. C. Lewontin, *The Genetic Basis of Evolutionary Change*

What is a gene? Since the word figures so prominently in the literature of medicine and biology, as well as in the press and on television, it might be presumed that its meaning is clear. Indeed, some assume that
every schoolchild knows what a gene is. But the word embodies so many ideas
expressed at so many levels that its definition turns out to be elusive; new information that leads to resolution on one level brings ambiguity on another.
And why not? Poets and artists know the stretch of imagination needed to give
expression to concepts that are at once abstract and tangible, that embrace an
essence yet can be measured. For example, the idea of humanity is expressed
in such words as *consciousness, intellect,* and *emotion,* and these definitions
are further elaborated in the dictionary. But still the essence of such concepts
eludes us until we observe them in action and discover their origins. So it is with
the concept of the gene. It is, as Lewontin expresses it, an idea that conveys at
once the unity of all life and the particularity of a single individual. In previous
sections of this book the genes were represented as the architects of physiological and developmental homeostasis, the determiners of both structure and
function of open systems, and, by means of variation in unit steps of homeostasis, the source of human vulnerability and disease. So we have several
answers already for the question "What is a gene?"

This chapter provides a different kind of answer to the question. Here the
evolution of the idea of the gene is traced from a statistical abstraction to a
physical entity characterized in units of DNA. Such a historical elaboration of
the concept discloses the gene's multiple dimensions. That is, although the progression of definitions ends with a molecular description, in practice we continue to use those that have been superseded because medical exigency requires

that we enter the path from phenotype to gene wherever we see an opening. The pursuit of such openings has led us to a generic definition of the gene, but it has also exposed, in panorama, the variety of specificities implicit in the concept. Indeed, as the reductionist definition has been refined, the ramifications of the idea have expanded.

It is not the facts about the gene that are ambiguous; several prominent textbooks agree about the DNA sequences to be included in a modern definition (1–4). Rather, it is in conceptualization that the uncertainty lies, in what elements and functions should be included and in how the defined gene is to fulfill all the roles attributed to it. The history of the physical definition of the gene can be represented in a coherent progression from a hypothetical entity to a circumscribed piece of DNA, but the trajectory of the ideas that generated this progression was anything but coherent. Investigations testing prevalent ideas often ended in results that transcended existing norms and so were rejected for a time or were reluctantly accepted.

Human biology and medicine had only a subsidiary role in the development of gene concepts but are among the chief beneficiaries. For example, the discovery by linkage analysis of genes associated with mendelizing phenotypes, followed by molecular characterization of the mutants and description of their variable expressions, is intended to clarify pathogenesis and, especially when extended to multifactorial diseases, may pay therapeutic dividends.

This chapter takes a developmental path that outlines how each new conceptual definition was attained. It is not a historical account of events but an examination of how the ideas about the gene now in use in medicine came into being.

The Statistical Gene

It is the conventional wisdom that Mendel conceived of "factors" that account for alternative forms of characters that segregate and assort independently. Nothing is said in his paper of the nature of the factors, only that they obey the rules of probability. Recently there has been some "deconstruction" of Mendel's work, some indications that all of what has been attributed to him was not in his mind at the time (5,6). This seems inevitable. Ideas elaborated in one set of circumstances are likely, when adapted to others, to emerge in another form. Olby points out how Correns, one of Mendel's rediscoverers, actually changed Mendel's words, introducing new ideas that were then attributed to Mendel (6). But Mendel never set out to discover genetics; his work was done in the context of the role of hybridization in species and evolution. Still, however and by whomever conceived, the mendelian concepts are so compelling as to have become central themes in the genetics of organisms ranging from bacteriophage to human beings.

An alternative to Mendel is Francis Galton, first cousin to Darwin, whose theory of heredity was based on his observations of human beings. In contrast to Mendel, whose theory of heredity was based on variation, Galton observed how relatives resemble one another according to a statistical pattern (7). Means and dispersions of traits were strongly correlated among relatives, and in parent-child pairs they regressed toward the mean. So Galton's vision of inheritance was entirely statistical, and his theory, which came to be called the "Law of Ancestral Inheritance," accommodated continuous distributions of measured properties in populations, an inheritance compatible with correlations and regression to the mean (8).

The explanatory inadequacies of ancestral inheritance were exposed when mendelism was taken up around 1900, especially by William Bateson (8). The variation that Mendel studied was discontinuous: he showed that traits segregated and assorted independently. Neither of these properties could be explained by ancestral inheritance, which was more compatible with intrafamilial correlation and continuous variation. Ideas of evolution followed. Although Galton himself believed that evolution occurred by discontinuity, his followers, headed by Karl Pearson, subscribed to Darwin's own view that evolution proceeded by small, almost infinitesimal steps leading to continuously graded traits. In contrast, the Mendelists, led by Bateson, visualized evolutionary change much as Galton did—as a process of sudden jumps leading to easily differentiated traits.

This put Galton in the strange position of one to whom both sides of an acrimonious debate appealed for authority. Now mendelism was used as a stick with which to beat the ancestrians, who gave as good as they got in a bitter conflict (8). It was a debate in which each side argued a different subject. Both were right and both were wrong, a position demonstrated first by Yule in 1907 and definitively in 1918 by R. A. Fisher, who concluded that both continuous and discontinuous variation are a consequence of mendelian genes (9). Fisher sent his paper to the *Proceedings of the Royal Society,* where it was rejected by the ancestrians as too mendelian and by the Mendelists as too ancestrian (10). Fisher's was a theoretical resolution that is working itself out today as we use a better knowledge of what genes are and do to discern the mendelizing genes that contribute to heart attacks, diabetes, high blood pressure, and even infections.

In fact, the controversy could not have been settled by the contenders. That is, although both sides referred to "factors" in inheritance, neither distinguished the factors from the traits. Even Johannson, who by 1909 had defined the words *gene* and *genotype,* saw the former as a "kind of accounting or calculating unit," not as a morphological structure (11–13). So the first definition of the gene was altogether statistical.

Echoes of this controversy are with us still. Although mendelian analysis has dominated medical genetics, Galton's correlational approach has exerted a strong influence in population genetics and genetic epidemiology and in the quantitative analysis of complex phenotypes. Out of the controversy there arose two lines of thought in human and medical genetics. One, represented as galtonian, is synthetic and typological; the characteristics of populations, usually expressed in means and deviations of continuous distributions of measurements, are the object of study (14). The other, represented as mendelian, is analytic and reductionist; individuals and their families are the objects of study and the aim is to characterize the variations that set them apart. In medicine this latter line of thought is traceable to Archibald Garrod.

The Operational Gene

Fisher's resolution of the ancestral-mendelist contention in 1918 was based on an operational definition of the gene elaborated by T. H. Morgan and his colleagues. This definition accommodated the mendelian principles of segregation and independent assortment of units that bore a one-to-one relationship to segregating phenotypes. It was observed that the segregants could be mapped to chromosomal loci and that alternatives due to mutations, called alleles, could exist for each such locus. So the gene was defined operationally as (a) a unit of mutation; (b) a unit of recombination and segregation, characterized by orderly exchanges between chromosomes of indivisible genes arranged one by one along the chromosome, like beads on a string; and (c) a unit of function in which alleles controlled alternative phenotypes. It was an adynamic image. Genes could change position when chromosomes were altered, as in translocations or inversions, but these were aberrations; for the most part, genes had their place and stayed there.

This operational, mendelian, concept of the gene set the context for genetic thinking for upwards of sixty years, giving way only in the 1970s to discoveries of an unsuspected flexibility and dynamism in the genome. But there were inklings before that. Unequal crossing over, discovered in the 1920s, was known to duplicate genes to produce what were called pseudoalleles, or complex loci, within which the recombination seemed to be intragenic (15). A second adumbration of the future was that of McClintock, who observed phenotypes in corn that could be explained only by postulating genetic elements that moved around and altered the actions of the genes they came to adjoin. Although a few of McClintock's colleagues fell in with her line of thinking, most could not conceive the relevance of her observations. But when her experiments were repeated in a molecular context, their significance became clear (16).

The Functional Gene

However precisely defined operationally, the gene remained an abstraction. In 1935 Morgan said that although it was likely that genes were molecules of some sort, the geneticist had little need to be concerned with what they were because "at the level at which genetic experiments lie, it does not make the slightest difference whether the gene is a hypothetical unit or a material particle" (17). But other geneticists had wondered from time to time how the abstract gene could influence development or metabolism, a study they labeled "physiological" genetics (18,19). This movement culminated in the demonstration by Beadle and Tatum that what the still-abstract gene did was to specify proteins, specifically enzymes, later extended to any peptide, and that each gene, defined operationally, expressed a unitary relationship to one such protein (20).

Biologists received this "one gene–one protein" idea with indifference, even hostility (21). It did not fit with current ideas of metabolism and development, which proposed a mysterious interactive complexity in which each gene affected the work of all others, while each, in its turn, was influenced by all. This criticism was made by Delbrück, who maintained that the method of Beadle and Tatum could not rule out the possibility that several genes could influence one protein or that one gene could influence several proteins (22). So while devising experiments to meet the criticisms, Beadle rounded up precursors to support the one-to-one idea and found them in forty-year-old reports of Wright's work on the influence of genes on coat colors in guinea pigs and in Onslow's, Scott-Moncrieff's, and others' studies of variation in anthocyanin pigments in plants (18,23,24). So it wasn't that no one had perceived the biochemical role of the gene; rather, it was that the work could not give the one-to-one answer.

Although Wright speculated that the genetic effects he saw were mediated by enzymes, there was little biochemical evidence, and although the biochemistry of the anthocyanin differences was very advanced, no mention was made of enzymes in the reports. Perhaps the precursor most useful to Beadle was Garrod, whom he generously proposed as the originator of the one gene–one enzyme idea (20). Here again we have an attribution by a later observer to a predecessor of an idea that was compatible with the time of the former but alien to that of the latter. In fact, Beadle was too generous: Garrod never used the word gene, retaining throughout his life the detachment expressed by the early geneticists who did not distinguish traits from genes (25).

The influence of the one-to-one principle, as exemplified in the inborn error of metabolism, was nowhere greater than in medicine. The advent of chromatography and electrophoresis in the 1950s made it possible to detect genetic individuality in disease and health, and as a result of these and other technological advances, together with the rise of medical genetics as a career, the list of inborn errors and protein variants increased at an exponential rate (25–27). These events have led to the proposition that the inborn error, in the guise of variations in unit steps of homeostasis, occupies a central position in

What Is a Gene?

the concept of disease, and it is the thinking based on this principle that might be called Garrodian.

The Structural Gene

The one-to-one principle did nothing to make the gene less abstract; its structure remained uncharacterized. For a long time everyone assumed that genes were proteins that could specify other proteins. For example, as early as 1917 Troland proposed that proteins had both autocatalytic and heterocatalytic functions. The former involved duplication of proteins acting as genes; the latter included catalysis and other functions mediated by proteins in the living cell. And as late as 1945, H. J. Muller cited his preference for protein as the genetic material because of "its possibilities for different permutations and combinations of its amino acids," as opposed to nucleic acids whose "basic structure is everywhere much the same" (28). The idea had taken hold that nucleic acids consisted of long chains of the four bases, repeated always in the same order—obviously an unlikely repository for the required diversity of information. The idea was not easily given up, but that it should go was suggested by Chargaff's observation of the equivalence of guanine to adenine and cytosine to thymine. On these grounds Chargaff concluded that there was something special about the DNA, and the base ratios were critical to Watson and Crick in their formulation of the structure of DNA.

Muller's 1945 paper was a comprehensive summary of operational genetics together with such speculations about function and structure as could be accommodated within the operational context. But even as the paper was being written, four independent currents of inquiry were converging to lead to a structural definition of the gene, a description transcending, but still compatible with, its statistical, operational, and functional predecessors. This structural definition did emerge, but the methods that evolved to do the work led to observations unanticipated by the mendelian mentality.

What were these currents? There were four, and none of the participants in any of them began with any mendelian bias; none came into the work from classical genetics (23,29) (Figure 2). The first current consisted of observations by physicists. X-ray crystallographers observed the structural patterns of nucleic acids and proteins, studies initiated without genes in mind but directly antecedent to the ideas of Watson and Crick, whose model of DNA was based in part on the results of such methods (23,29). So there was a purely structural current that was necessary but that was not seen to make a conceptual contribution until DNA had been identified as the genetic material. A second current began, again without reference to defining genes, in Griffith's observation of the transformation of pneumococci from one polysaccharide capsular type to another. Avery, McLeod, and MacCarty undertook to identify Griffith's "transforming principle," and it turned out to be DNA (30).

Avery started with the assumption that the transforming principle might be the type-specific polysaccharide itself, and it was only after years of work that he and his colleagues accepted their discovery that the DNA was the genetic material. It was a hypothesis that they did their best to falsify, but in the end they accepted it with enthusiasm, understanding thoroughly its general implications. But when in 1944 they published their results, they were restrained in generalizing the role of the DNA. They were right to have muted their claims since the idea was not immediately accepted. The principal objection was that however purified the DNA, there might still lurk a few molecules of protein to serve as the transforming principle (31). Avogadro's number was evoked in evidence of this idea. But, as everyone knows, Avery's views were substantiated by Watson and Crick, who in 1953 published a model of the DNA that accommodated the principles of physics as well as the biological necessities of replication and the storage and transmission of information. The discovery of the various RNAs and the triplet code followed.

A third current of inquiry had begun as early as 1935, when Max Delbrück, a physicist, was drawn to think about what genes are because he saw that thereby he might solve "the riddle of life" (32). Biology, he said, was unlike physics in being historical. As opposed to atoms, which have no history, "the essence of life is the accumulation of experience through the generations." Accordingly, "the key problem is how living matter manages to record and perpetuate its experiences." And since this record is stored and transmitted in whatever is reproduced, it is reproduction that is "the elementary phenomenon of living matter." So Delbrück cast about for an organism ideal for the study of replication as the key to the riddle of life and found it in bacteriophage, which he and Luria exploited, meeting regularly in the summers at Cold Spring Harbor, together with their numerous associates and pupils, to work, teach, and think. Among the many attainments of Delbrück, Luria, and the "phage group" were the demonstration by Hershey and Chase that the genetic information was carried only in the DNA, and experiments by Benzer that gave structural refinement to operational definitions of genes as units of function, mutation, and recombination (33,34). For example, the unit of mutation could be as small as one base pair.

A fourth current was generated by Tatum's extension of the idea of the inborn error to *E. coli,* an observation used by Lederberg to demonstrate sex and recombination in bacteria, which, in turn, enabled Yanofsky, as the beneficiary of all four currents, to demonstrate in the same organism a colinear relationship of sequences of base pairs in DNA with sequences of amino acids in proteins (35,36).

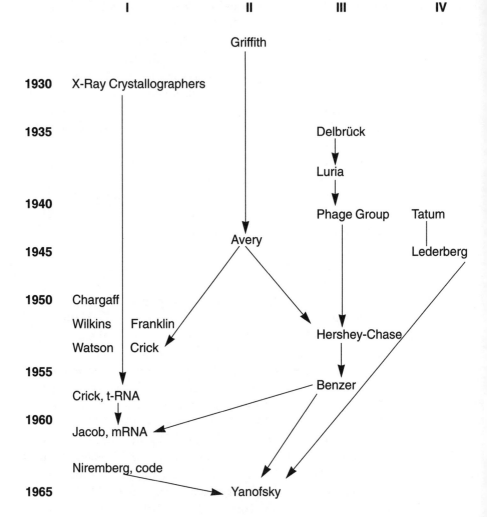

Figure 2 A time diagram of investigators in four disciplines whose work led to a structural definition of the gene.

Thus the structural definition of the gene was completed, and thus the critics of the one gene–one peptide rule were silenced. Now the statistical, operational, and functional versions could be integrated into the structural definition of a gene as a strand of base pairs in the DNA whose arrangement is reflected in that of the amino acids in the single peptide it specified. The order and quality of base pairs in the strand is susceptible to change by mutation and crossing over, and the strand itself represents the basic unit of recombination. This concept was gratefully received by the medical genetics community. It was

Descent with Modification

precisely complementary to the idea of the inborn error and explained it. And it represented fulfillment of an important medical principle: the establishment of a direct relationship between symptomatology and cause. Now one could visualize pathogenesis as a result of an abnormality of a unit step of homeostasis, with consequences directly traceable to that abnormality and to insufficient homeostatic efforts to compensate for it. In this form the inborn error could become central to medical thought.

THE MOLECULAR GENE

At this point there was a generally held belief that this structural definition would stand and that the progress from the statistical to the structural gene had been straightforward, even inevitable. Mendelism had been given molecular affirmation. Many of the participants pronounced the job done and set off to breach what they called "the last frontier": the organization and function of the central nervous system.

But almost immediately the structural definition of the gene began to seem incomplete. The first incompatibility was the description by Monod and Jacob of a part of the DNA of E. coli that appeared to regulate coordinately two structural genes engaged in the metabolism of lactose (37). While this operator locus could be shown to undergo mutation, it was not transcribed and it made no protein product. So there were exceptions to the structural definition; DNA, in this case the operator sequences, could function usefully without transmitting the information to make a protein. But were such sequences genes? Next it was observed that molecules of nuclear mRNA were much larger than those of the cytoplasm, which led to the discovery that the nuclear transcript contained exons that were later translated and introns that were removed before translation and so had no influence on protein specificity (38). Now the structural gene was redefined to include transcribing DNA and its local regulatory appendages, and this is the definition that appears in the authoritative textbooks of molecular genetics and biology (1–4). But some genes have additional regulatory sequences located at a distance, and the whole unit is contained within domain boundaries that insulate one or more genes from the influence of neighbors (39). So why is not everything within the domain boundaries defined as a gene?

Perhaps the gene could be defined as a smaller, rather than larger, unit. Introns isolate the exons, thereby reducing the likelihood of unequal recombination within them, which would constitute a destructive mutation. But when the recombination is within introns, there is opportunity for shuffling of intact exons, even to the extent of forming quite new genes (40). A famous case is the low-density lipoprotein receptor gene that has one exon derived from factor XII of the clotting cascade and another similar to one found in epidermal growth factor. The latter appears also in fibrillin and other proteins (41–43). So perhaps, since it is the unit that endows the transcript with the information to characterize its product as a protein, the exon, wherever it appears, should be called the gene. But then what we now call one gene would consist of several—perhaps dozens—of genes.

And there are more exceptions (13,44,45):

(a) DNA exists in cells in the form of a double helix, transcribed normally in only one direction. But occasionally a transcript is made from the other strand, which, of course, specifies an entirely different protein (46). Both could be called genes, but they come from one sequence of base pairs.

(b) One transcript may contain the information to specify two or more proteins or peptides (47). Do they derive from one gene or two? One transcript may also produce an enzyme with multiple active sites, so that it has several activities (48,49). One gene or more?

(c) One RNA transcript may be processed in such a way as to produce two or more different proteins, doing further violence to the one-to-one principle (50).

(d) The DNA sequence of the genome is not static. Repetitive sequences, varying in number, abound. One class is the rRNA genes; many others have an unknown or no function. Some repetitive elements have the property of increasing their number by transposition or by first being transcribed into RNA and then reverse transcribed into cDNA, which inserts randomly into the genome. The site of insertion may be the exons or regulatory sequences of another gene, with the result of alteration in the expression of the target gene. Other examples of this dynamic nature of genes include trinucleotide repeat sequences in the transcribed portion of genes. These repeats vary in number in normal people and increase dramatically in certain disease genes, such as those for myotonic dystrophy, fragile X, Huntington's disease, and others (51). No one calls these transposable or repetitive elements genes, but they are a part of the genome and they may influence transcription. It is ironic that the wrinkled-seed mutant reported by Mendel was a result of a transposable element (52). Much of the DNA, apart from the repetitive elements, is both noncoding and untranscribed. What is it? Evolutionary baggage? Remembrance of genes past? Certainly some consists of unusable duplicates called pseudogenes and some is the residue of viruses that invaded the DNA in the distant past. But whatever it is, it appears not to be accommodated in any traditional concept of the gene.

So, we seem to have been pursuing a fantasy, a human construct that we are trying to impose on nature. We have been facing a paradox: the more detailed the description of whatever we suppose ought to compose the gene, the more difficult it has become to know what to include in the definition. And when the whole of the genome is known, new insights are bound to surface. Fogle suggests that a source of our uncertainty is that we have been conceptually constrained by basing the quest on the principles of mendelism, principles derived from distributions in families of visible or otherwise measurable traits that cannot predict events in the DNA (44). That is, there is a dissociation between the organizing principles of the DNA and the one-to-one vision of mendelism.

With hindsight this dissociation makes sense. Life at meiosis and life after fertilization are things apart. At meiosis, the diversity required by a species for adaptation to an uncertain environment is generated by both mutation and recombination. And because the meiotic process is uncoupled from what goes on after gametogenesis, anything goes—nature is free to tinker without check. But from the moment of fertilization, the constraints of development are imposed and variation of whatever kind, if it is to be observed in surviving organisms, must be expressed at some phenotypic level as a mendelizing alternative to the prevailing mode.

So what is a gene? We have before us a definition of a molecular gene that includes a DNA transcript plus its regulatory accouterments. If this definition is not completely satisfying it is only because it defies our expectation by omitting some nontranscribable, and including some nontranslatable, DNA; that is, we were comfortable with the structural gene that bore a one-to-one relationship between sequences of DNA and amino acids in gene products. But despite its omissions and excesses, the molecular gene attains the same informational link between DNA and homeostasis as did that "structural" gene. It is a remarkable invention of nature that represents a compromise between the economy of the mendelizing "gene-to-phenotype" relationship so necessary to an efficient homeostasis and the profligacy of molecular events at meiosis so necessary to evolution. And it accommodates no less satisfactorily the integration of the statistical, operational, functional, and structural definitions.

These latter are integrated, but not lost. A practical demonstration is given in the study in drosophila of gene clusters called "bithorax" and "antennapedia." Genes in these clusters, or gene families, control the antero-posterior segmentation of the fly. The details of the arrangement of genes in these families were worked out beginning in the 1940s, principally by E. B. Lewis, using a classical genetic analysis appropriate to the operational definition of the gene. Bithorax genes were shown to control the lower segments, while antennapedia influenced the upper region. More recently, these gene families, now called "homeotic" genes, have been subjected to molecular analysis that showed them to be regulatory genes containing homeobox domains specifying transcription factors. These homeobox genes are much conserved and appear in many organisms, including human beings. Here the operational analysis was essential to the molecular scrutiny.

In medicine, the position is much the same. Practical necessity requires that we continue to use all of the definitions, and we shall probably do so even after the anticipated revelations of the Human Genome Project are in hand. We shall need them because they accommodate the physiological complexities of interlocking homeostatic systems characterized by emergent properties not necessarily predictable by knowledge of the structure of each of numerous component genes and their proximate products. For example, we know that heredity plays some part in the cause of a disease when the recurrence rate in families is above that of the incidence in the general population. Twin and adoption studies may help to establish the extent of the hereditary contribution, but without offering insights into what is inherited or how. Scrutiny of pedigrees, perhaps followed by formal segregation analysis, suggests a gene to account for the trait when distributions of affected persons are found to agree with some mendelian mode of inheritance, while evidence of linkage of the disease trait with a locus of known position in a chromosome adds rigor to the idea of an operationally defined gene. These are statistical and operational definitions and they can be raised to a functional level by finding some biochemical attribute that segregates with the disease trait. Then, if the biochemical variation can be assigned to a mutant protein, the outlines of a structurally defined gene have taken form. But no one is satisfied with so indirect a definition any more, so the final phase, often carried out even in the absence of other evidence, is the characterization of the sequence of base pairs in the DNA. As it happens, in sorting out the diagnostic heterogeneity of complex syndromes we proceed in just this way. Beginning with the abstract, we move through the operational to functional and structural levels of genetic definition, ending with positional cloning of specific genes. Thus does the ontogeny of diagnosis recapitulate the phylogeny of definition.

And in this recapitulation we see how the two independent lines of thought have coalesced in conformity to Fisher's theoretical construct, now being resolved by the methods of molecular genetics. Galton's continuously distributed phenotypes are a consequence of Garrod's chemical individuality, and both are outcomes of how selection has dealt with an exuberant variation generated at meiosis. Both are associated with genes whose qualitative primary effects are discontinuous, each charged with specifying a protein that is integral to a unit step of homeostasis. In medicine, we perceive the variant genes that contribute to continuously distributed variants as risk factors. Those that produce discontinuous effects are observed to promote the phenotype directly. But quantitative measures of all genes are continuously distributed. Even the most penetrant gene effects are likely to be modulated by those of other genes as well as by individuality of experiences, while some of the genes contributing to multigenic disorders, also influenced by other genes and experiences, approach the penetrance of those that cause the classical inborn errors, occasionally reaching our notice in the form of some version of disease. So in a sense, the drosophiline notion that one gene affects many and many affect one, the basis of Delbrück's criticism of Beadle's one-to-one principle, is turning out to have substance, and what began in dispute ends in agreement and enhanced understanding for all.

What, then, is the answer to the apparently simple question "What is a gene?" For the practical pursuer of genes and grants the answer is likely to be the molecular version. Such a gene is concrete, can be manipulated and moved about, and will turn out to be an agent of treatment (53). And it represents a satisfying fulfillment of the quest for proximate causes. But educators must conjure with other meanings of the concept—for example, with the implications and consequences of the information latent in the molecular structure of the gene. It is the genes that identify each of us as whoever we are and at the same time connect us to relatives and, more distantly, to the species of human beings and even to the whole of life. And as inheritors of the genetic experiments at meiosis, we are each an individual participant in the grand scheme of selection and evolution. So an educator's answer to the question "What is a gene?" might be the following: the genes represent the options and constraints within which each individual forms the developmental trajectories that prepare him to face adaptively his experiences of the environment. In describing the identity of the gene, this definition includes function, the focus of the next chapter.

15

The Paths of Gene Action

But the term code-script is, of course, too narrow. The chromosome structures are at the same time instrumental in bringing about the development
they foreshadow. They are law-code and executive power—or to use
another simile, they are architect's plan and builder's craft—in one.
—Erwin Schrödinger, *What Is Life?*

The path from gene to phenotype is as open to interpretation as are the
definitions of the gene. Gene action is implicit in these definitions, in
which the genes are distinguished by their phenotypic outcomes, whether functional or structural. Action is also implicit in the three time frames. One action
is that of self-replication and reproduction of individuals, a second is embodied in the flowering and decline of individual organisms with time, and a third
resides in the specification of the proteins that constitute the unit steps of homeostasis that assure the moment-to-moment integrity of open systems. This latter catches the attention of medical people, but all are actions for which genes
are responsible. How do they help to describe the path from gene to phenotype?

In the history of this description two polar positions arose from antithetical views of development expressed by the early geneticists and by embryologists of the same time (1). In one of these positions, the gene is supreme. It fills,
as Schrödinger saw it, the office of both "law-code and executive power." Executive power is, in this case, the means by which the "law-code" is imposed
and enforced. That is, all the acts that fulfill those decisions are determined by
the front office—here, the genes. The genes propose; the cytoplasm disposes.
This orientation, which is compatible with the drosophila agenda, is the basis
for genetic determinism (1).

At the opposite pole are those who perceive the DNA as an inert molecule
that, although fulfilling the requirement of the "architect's plan," requires the
cytoplasm to supply the "builder's craft" (1). And indeed, the act of transcription does depend wholly upon a complex of proteins without which nothing
happens, a complex activated by other proteins, which transmit signals from

within and without the cell. In fact, all of the business of the cell is transacted by proteins without reference to the genes, whose only business is to specify the structure of those proteins. And it is the proteins that promote development and metabolism spontaneously and without participation of the genes, except that they respond to signals to promote or retard the rate of transcription. This view is compatible with the thought of embryologists who envisioned the cytoplasm as doing the business of the cell.

But for medicine, the genes have a special meaning. No one denies that without the cytoplasm, the genome is inert. Nor can it be denied that diseases are associated with experiences. But we reserve for the genes a central place in medical thinking because their presence in the chromosomes of an individual is invariant; they are always there, always projecting the same information. They are present from conception and gone only in the dissolution of death. So they are permanent markers of individuality—usually of health, sometimes of vulnerability, occasionally of disease. Their potential for promoting disease must vary from one individual to another, from one developmental stage to another and in modification by the products of other genes and experiences, but they themselves are always there. As for the experiences associated with disease, we cannot see them in the same way; they are shadowy, usually unknown. The only evidence for their existence may be heritability coefficients of less than 1.0, so they are not permanent markers, stamped from the start into individuality. No doubt they vary in kind, intensity, and duration in the lives of individuals, but they are so often lost to memory as to be unreliable markers.

So it is not for ideological reasons that we accord the gene capabilities that actually reside in their products. Had we an equally detailed record of the experiences and developmental history of the individual whose genes we know in some detail, there might be less emphasis on "genes for" and less genetic determinism.

THE PATH FROM GENE TO PHENOTYPE

It was to elucidate the path from phenotype to gene that the physiological, biochemical, and molecular geneticists worked to define the gene, which acquired new meanings with each new level of definition. The word *phenotype* originated in response to the necessity for an expression of an affinity between an observable trait and an abstract "factor." Mendelian segregation and independent assortment required it, and the word acquired a new meaning with each new definition of the gene, elaborating a hierarchy that begins with whatever embraces the whole of the being of an individual organism and ends with the DNA.

But today we engage in another kind of thinking. We prefer, where possible, to reverse the path so as to go from gene to phenotype. That is, now that we are able to isolate and characterize genes, we try first to determine the nature of their protein products and then to fathom the roles of those proteins as unit steps in some homeostatic system. Such a designation constitutes the point of union between a gene and its several phenotypes and at the same time gives some inkling of what treatment might be.

The path is illustrated in Table 3, which shows that a gene provides the information for a transcript, which is translated into the specificity of amino acid sequence in a protein that assumes a conformation appropriate to its function as an integral component of some homeostatic system. So far the relationship of gene to both product and function is one to one, and we may speak of a gene "for" both the specificity of the protein product and its function within its homeostatic system. But beyond this point there is a change in the relationship. Now, while in no way losing its identity as a product of a gene, the protein must identify itself with the purposes of the homeostatic system of which it is only one component. This means that its gene is now a gene "for" whatever it is that the system, or "integron," does. That still may leave a fairly straightforward relationship—the factor VIII gene is a gene for clotting as well as for factor VIII—but the path becomes tangled when one integron is articulated with others that fulfill a number of functions and they with still more. Of course, none

Table 3 **The Path from Gene to Phenotype**

Representative Disease	Gene	Abnormality
PKU	DNA ↓	Deletion, substitution
	mRNA ↓	Regulatory mutant
	Protein ↓	Mutant protein, protein deficiency
Gout	Metabolite ↓	Accumulated metabolite, metabolite deficiency
	Tissue injury ↓	Pathogenesis a consequence
	Homeostatic system ↓	Accumulation or deficiency
Hypertension	Multiple homeostatic systems ↓	Further consequences of the preceding gene modification
Schizophrenia	Final phenotype	The disease

Descent with Modification

of these articulations is of genes; all are of gene products exerting their primary, modifying, or epistatic effects on the summary functions of the systems to which they are relevant. Indeed, we are catapulted into physiology, into what one student of complexity has called "homeodynamics" (2). In the end the gene becomes "for" so many characteristics that it gets lost in the shuffle and eventually, when facing such phenotypes as height, intelligence, or capacity for esthetic experience, we are no better off than the drosophilists who proclaimed that each gene affects all phenotypes and each phenotype is affected by all genes.

So the longer the path from gene to phenotype, the more likely is its impulse to be subject to modification and to be affected by the evolving developmental matrix, and the greater is the influence of the environment on the traits to which it contributes. That is, the measurable influence of a gene is inversely proportional to the complexity of the phenotype to which it makes a contribution; homeostatic integration brings phenotypes that cannot be predicted by their individual parts. One is reminded of a jigsaw puzzle, in which the picture formed by assembling the components is a mystery until at some point in the articulation of the parts it begins to emerge, but it is only when the last piece is fitted that the whole of the artist's intention is divulged.

Homeostasis represents the adaptation of open systems to their environment, so the conditions of the environment must be reflected in that adaptation. These conditions vary all the way from the force of gravity, which is much the same the world over, to the most idiosyncratic tastes and habits, a product of variations in culture and individual propensity. So again, the more complex the phenotype, the more elements needed to attain it and the more it must be described as an adaptation to experiences. Intelligence quotient is an example. It is a much abused phenotype, capable of many descriptions and definitions. To some it is more or less inherited, to others it is largely cultivated. But since what we measure as IQ comes into being only in relation to experiences, it is a word we use to describe how those experiences are met; it is clearly a product of adaptation to the environment. At the same time, there are kinds and degrees of that adaptation that must be influenced by endowment. So the only important question generated by the contention is not whether nature exceeds nurture in the genesis of intelligence, but that of society's obligation to see that potential—of whatever degree—is cultivated.

THE PATH FROM PHENOTYPE TO GENE

Even with the resources promised by the Genome Project, we may not always be able to penetrate this complexity to discern the roles of genes or experiences in the origins of the most complex phenotypes. At best, we will work out some sort of story for the species, but the exact path that each individual human being has taken to whatever he or she has become is likely to remain forever unknown. Still, for medical purposes that is not necessarily a handicap. In medicine we usually describe a different path: not that from gene to phenotype, but the more traditional route from a disease phenotype to the mutants and experiences that engendered it. Here the complexity of phenotype is less of a deterrent because the stricken homeostatic system is likely to call attention to itself by the quality of the signs and symptoms it evokes. The path is further narrowed when some physiological or biochemical abnormality draws attention to specific aspects of that system, properties that lead in turn to protein elements that serve as "candidates" for a gene search. This search ends in the description of one or more molecular aberrations in genes that specify one or more unit steps of homeostasis that give grounds for a plausible account of the origin of the clinical expression. So disease cuts through the complexity of the normal integration of systems to define a new one-to-one relationship of phenotype with gene.

Under these circumstances it is possible to think of a gene (or genes) "for" a disease because the step or steps in homeostasis that have broken down to make the individual vulnerable have become identifiable. It is a little like a battlefield promotion of a private soldier to a position of command. Like that of a private soldier, a gene's contribution to a unit step in homeostasis is made anonymous by the complexity of levels of integration. Its service to such grand goals as physiological, developmental, and genetic homeostasis, however essential to all, goes unnoticed because it is integrated. That is the role of the private soldier—to serve unnoticed. But in a fiercely contested action there is a sudden decimation of ranking officers and the private assumes command, becoming a salient figure charged with the disposition of others, no longer insignificant but easily identified "for" good or ill—for ill in the case of the mutant gene—and a magnet for medical attention.

Conclusion

To return to the path from gene to phenotype: it is not the gene or its product that causes the phenotype, or the disease, but the concatenation of events that conspire in some contingent way to bring about the outcome. Sometimes the gene effect overrides all other components and produces the disease willy-nilly, although with individual variation in just how it does so. More commonly the intervening events impose variability, even to evade in one person what is inevitable in another.

For treatment, the physician's job is to find a point of entry that offers the best chance of amelioration or cure. That point may differ according to heterogeneity of both genes and provocative experiences, but in the end it will turn out to be some component part of a homeostatic system that is abnormal. Similarly for prevention, the goal is discovery of points of vulnerability. But for prevention, contingent variation clouds the prospect for prediction of outcomes in different people who express the same vulnerability. Uncertainties posed by these variables are a subject of concern later in the book.

In the meantime, having defined the gene both in concept and in action, and having, in the course of doing so, employed, with abandon, the word *mutant,* it is time to define this word in the context of the gene. This the next two chapters will do.

16

Whatever Is, Is Variable

E Pluribus Unum
—Motto displayed on the great seal of the United States

The motto, which means "Out of Many, One," is intended to express the unity of a federation of states, but it is no less applicable to other organisms composed of many parts. Indeed, it is a description of nature. An example is the developing organism, whose cells, after repeated divisions, differentiate variously and form distinctive parts that coalesce into a unified whole, an individual in whom everything is in touch with everything else; none of the parts is sufficient. Nor can the whole be independent, "entire of itself"; necessarily, individuals seek community with families, friends, and acquaintances.

As it happens, nature also reverses the motto to read, Ex Unum Plures— Out of One, Many. Having settled on a single mechanism for the replication of the cells of which all living bodies are composed, in a stunning paradox nature makes a virtue of imperfections in its scheme to create through reproduction the wherewithal for the variation expressed in trillions of unique organisms and millions of species. Mistakes were never so well rewarded. But although the scheme has been an incontestable success, there is a minor proviso. Evolutionary success is measured in hundreds of millions of years, but in the shorter perspectives of generations and lifetimes that bring individuals into focus, we see that nature has been inefficient; its instrument is a little blunt. For every adaptive advance there are disadaptive mistakes, most of which are disposed of by what evolutionary biologists call "purifying" selection. The necessity for such selection is a consequence of mutations in the DNA that account for the variation observed in all organisms, some of which are marked for oblivion. The irony of the qualifier "purifying," suggesting the necessity to purge the gene pool of whatever is undesirable, is not lost on physicians to whom all people, including the handicapped, are "created equal" in regard to the opportunity to participate in life, liberty, and the pursuit of happiness.

It is at just this point that biology and medicine are most polarized. The biologist seeks to understand the optima for species but neglects the fates of individuals, while the physician concentrates on the ills of individuals without regard for species. It is a matter of emphasis on different time scales. To the student of evolution, biological history is paramount, while to the doctor, it is the moment that matters, a moment in a lifetime of the experiences of a single individual. But of course these time scales are inalienably connected; it is the mistakes of replication, together with unique combinations thereof, that furnish at once the wherewithal for adaptive evolution and the origins of diseases that afflict individuals. It is one more instance of the tension between the welfare of the species and that of individuals, and one more evidence of the ulterior hand of remote causes at work.

Some Questions

It is plain enough how these antithetical positions can be a consequence of the same means, but many questions arise as to relationships of one to the other. First, is it true that whatever is, is variable? This question is not worth the effort to answer it if framed in the context of every single nucleotide in the genome, but if posed as "Is the specification of every unit step in homeostasis subject to mutational or recombinatorial variation?" it is more reasonable. We assume the answer is yes: in the interests of species, all such homeostatic devices must have been the object of mutation—else how did they come into being? We owe to prokaryotes many of the metabolic properties of our cells, but it was by mutation, especially by the creation of new gene families by unequal crossing over and duplication followed by further mutation, that eukaryote evolution proceeded.

Indeed, it proceeded at so stately a rate as to suggest an evolutionary clock (1). But amino acid substitution is too slow a mechanism for creating the complexity exhibited in higher organisms. For this, gene duplication serves the purpose, not only by increasing the number of genes capable of further mutation and divergent function, but by reshuffling exons to create genes that specify proteins with new functions. These gene families, clusters, or complexes, sometimes called supergenes, represent a fundamental characteristic of the genome, and one that Bodmer has suggested may allow us better to grasp the genome's diversity (2,3). That is, rather than attempting conceptually to construct the whole organism from its sixty to eighty thousand genes, each with its separate role in homeostasis, the job may be facilitated by starting with the families and grasping their integration into complexes of families, and so on. The immune system is an example. Its various arms are served by related genes presumed to have arisen in duplication in the phylogenetic past. Protein kinases, the globins, collagens, and several kinds of adhesion molecules are other well-studied families. But possibly, as Bodmer suggests, analysis by gene families will be most helpful in understanding behavioral phenotypes that could never yield to an analysis that begins with single genes.

So, by inference, we conclude that everything is open to mutation. In any case, it is a hypothesis we continue to do our best to falsify. Perhaps it is one more question that can be answered only after the exposure of the whole genome.

Individual Variation in Mutability?

If whatever is, is variable means that all steps in homeostasis are subject to the effects of mutation, a second question is, are there individual variations in mutability? Are there nonrandom individual differences in kinds and numbers of mutations? Are there conditions of the DNA, or of its protein accouterments, that make one individual more prone than another to mutation in general or to particular kinds and frequencies thereof?

Chromosomal aberrations have been known or suspected since the heyday of drosophila genetics. Now we understand them in molecular detail. That is, the chromosomes themselves consist of molecules of DNA protected by molecules of protein that contain and condense them, form nucleosomes, and then at replication, expand them, separate their helical strands, and induce and control replication, scanning, proofreading, and editing the new strands to correct the vast majority of the mistakes made. Other proteins are involved in timing the cell cycle and, after inducing replication, moving the chromosomes to the two poles, redistributing the cytoplasm, and dividing the cell into two new self-contained units. These processes require dozens of proteins, each with specific sites for attachment to the DNA, to receptors, and to each other. Many of the proteins of replication assemble into a single instrument, the better to proceed rapidly along the DNA.

Now, having recounted the number of different processes undertaken in DNA replication and cell division, and recognizing that each such process includes numerous steps and that each step is mediated by one or more proteins, the question of individual variation seems to answer itself. That is, if all unit steps of homeostasis are mutable, so must be those of the processes of replication and cell division. We have empirical evidence of the individuality of mutation in repair enzymes in the several kinds of Xeroderma pigmentosum, where at least nine complementation groups, implying products of genes at nine different loci, have been detected (4). Why should we imagine that other enzymes would be spared?

So how do we answer this second question? We have the empirical evidence of the rare Xeroderma pigmentosum families in whom some aspects of DNA repair are imperfect and we reason that if there are mutants that make for serious disease early in life, those same loci are capable of harboring alleles promoting less severe abnormality—including, and perhaps hastening, some aspects of aging. And unless the genes and enzymes involved in the Xeroderma disorders are in some way different from all the others involved in replication and repair, the answer to the question could be yes, mutability may indeed be individual, and if this is so, more mutants might slip through into the gametes of some people than others. Still, given that mutation must always be a rare event and that its products are usually disadaptive, individual genotypes with very many new mutants must be infrequent.

A Gradient of Selective Effect

A third question is, is there a gradient of selective effect, a distribution of mutational influence on homeostasis? Once it was axiomatic that all new mutants must be harmful and were quickly dispensed with. But we now know that mutations in introns and in the third base pair of transcribable codons do not lead to amino acid substitutions and that many mutants that lead to such substitutions are selectively neutral. So the axiom is in need of modification. We assume that most new mutants do disappear, whether by selection or by chance, but plenty are left to constitute the common variation in human populations. The extent of this variation and how it was attained has already been reviewed, and although most of such polymorphism is apparently neutral, common alleles presumed to be neutral are known to be associated with multifactorial diseases.

So there seems to be the start of a gradient among genes widely spread in the population. Most of the genes that account for human homeostasis must have been fixed in the gene pool by selection, but some—including many or most polymorphic alleles—will have arrived by chance, but did so only as harmless additions to the gene pool. Others may be harmless except under exceptional stress; not the best homeostatic material, but acceptable for all but very unfavorable conditions. Beyond these are genes that narrow homeostatic resiliency even under ordinary conditions, past them are others that disrupt it in varying degree and contribute to the numerous monogenic diseases, and finally come mutants so disruptive as to interfere with the earliest life, or even the formation of viable gametes.

Given that the processes of gamete formation and of their union to form zygotes are governed by proteins, the idea of such lethal mutations is inescapable. Further, since embryogenesis is characterized by the interactions of proteins, lethals are to be expected here as well. So, at one end of the gradient are mutants so damaging as to make them unlikely ever to be seen, and about whose individuality we can only guess. In the middle, and with a very wide range of influence when measured by reduction in lifespan, curtailment of reproduction, and residual handicap, are most of the rest, while the symmetry of the gradient is preserved by proposing that at the other end of this progression are the mutants that are selectively advantageous. But how to detect the latter, given that their advantage lies in some slight improvement in some individuals in a mechanism that already works? Such mutants are like an orchestral musician of outstanding sensitivity and distinction, who, when playing superlatively well, raises the quality of performance of the whole orchestra to a level—for which the conductor is given rave notices. In solos the musician's extraordinary skill is apparent to all listeners, but for the genes there are no solos, except when they wreak havoc or at the very least contribute to such a degree of disharmony as to make themselves apparent. There is in addition a gradient of mutational effect within loci, with alleles that vary widely and distinguish individuals and families, and each of these is further graded depending upon the concatenations of the other genes among which they find themselves. So the gradient is represented in a continuous distribution of selective effect, and the position of any gene in it must vary, even if only slightly, from one individual to another.

The known mutants and the diseases they cause are listed in *Mendelian Inheritance in Man* and in the several editions of *The Metabolic and Molecular Basis of Inherited Disease*. So an affirmative answer to the question of the existence of a gradient of mutant effect is amply supported by unassailable data, and the variations, which are usually familial, easily distinguish individuals.

Is Mutation Random?

A fourth question is, can we expect that all of an individual's DNA is equally open to mistakes of replication, and are all mistakes equally likely to be discovered and repaired when they occur? The answer is again partial and uncertain. Cooper, Krawczak, and Antonarakis have examined point mutations associated with disease, taking biases of reporting into account (5). Transitions outnumber transversions two to one, and there are "hot spots" at which mutations turn up more frequently than expected. The most salient among the transitions is that of CpG dinucleotides, which is presumed to be a consequence of the ease of deamination of 5-methylcytosine. This dinucleotide is, in fact, underrepresented in the genome but accounts for more than a third of all mononucleotide substitutions. Hot spots for other dinucleotides exist, too, offering further evidence of nonrandomness. There are hot spots for deletion as well, and unanticipated differences in the incidence of deletions from gene to gene. So, for genes involved in disease at least, mutation seems to be nonrandom.

Are Phenotypes Predictable?

A fifth question is, can we predict phenotypes when we know the following about the mutants: either (a) their description (i.e., aneuploidy, deletions large and small, point mutation, insertion, triplet repeat, trisomy, and so on), or (b) the gene product and its function as an enzyme, a structural protein, a transcription factor, etc. This question comes up in other parts of the book, so it suffices here to say that there is a very rough correlation between the kind of mutation and its phenotype—but only very rough. For example, some deletions are well tolerated and some point mutations are lethal.

CONCLUSION

There is some reason to suppose that much, or all, of the DNA is mutable, that there may be individual differences in mutability, and that there is a gradient of intensity of mutational effect that distinguishes individuals. Some parts of the DNA may be more mutable than others (but whether this is a property of individuals is not known) and finally, there is a very rough correlation between kinds of mutation and phenotypes.

What this means is that in creating variation and then exposing it to selection, nature gives with one hand and takes away with the other, and does both with a fine indifference to individuals. As representatives of Homo sapiens, nature requires each of us first to be receptacles for variation and then to be objects of the tests of natural selection. We accept this endowment, recognizing that life is a game of chance. But because we know that for some individuals the dice are loaded, we have organized ourselves in medicine and through other cultural means to ensure such equality as we can. For most of us, though, the virtues of this capacity to vary are easily observed in the diversity, health, and vigor of our species, and among individuals, in the wherewithal for each to seek a destiny marked with an individual stamp, to have a life of choice and even sometimes to have powers commensurate with aspiration.

The partial answers to the questions posed in this chapter show something of nature's scheme for giving and taking. If everything is variable, even including the individual capacity for generating new variation, and if there is a gradient of mutational effect both within and between loci, then it is certain that individuality will prevail no less in sickness than in health. Nature's proliferative powers, exerted in the interest of adaptive variation and constrained by natural selection, in producing the mutants that lead to evolution, act as remote causes of disease. So, for the physician, the moral of the story is that even while gathering cases of disease into macroscopic, typological categories, the populational microscope must be applied to discover how individuality in disease leads to groups within groups, and finally how treatment is after all to be a matter of what suits each patient's needs.

It is also possible that some of the unrest among medical educators is due to a tension analogous to that between the needs of species and those of individuals. In biology the species requires new variation for adaptive purposes and attains it by a means that is beneficial in general but indifferent to imperfections that fall randomly upon individuals. Similarly, medicine embraces eagerly new knowledge and technology that are of inestimable benefit to the whole enterprise but is less innovative in working out how best to use these novelties in advancing those qualities employed in the doctor-patient relationship that once differentiated individual practitioners of the art of medicine. But, as in the case of mutations, to discover the imperfections in the doctor-patient understanding is to find ways to prevent or to treat them.

17

The Semantics of Genetics

Scientists usually assume that only their data and theories matter for scientific progress, that how they talk about these data and theories does not matter, that it is irrelevant to their actual work. But in introducing this particular way of talking, the first generation of American geneticists provided a conceptual framework that was critically important for the future course of biological research.

—Evelyn Fox-Keller, *Refiguring Life*

Fox-Keller refers to the language the drosophilists used. It became the standard language of genetics, regardless of organism, and it is still employed in human and medical genetics. But now molecular genetics is changing the meaning of old words and coining new ones, so the question for this chapter is, what is, or will be or should be, the lexicon of genetic medicine.

The Classical Lexicon Meets Molecular Genetics

All the definitions of the gene reviewed in chapter 14 represent steps in the fulfillment of a genetic agenda, so it is no surprise that the language employed and the imagery of the gene and its behavior reflect genetic rather than medical missions. This genetic agenda originated in Mendel's rules, which formed the basis for the elaboration by Morgan and his colleagues of the mechanics of heredity in drosophila. Kohler has described how the drosophilists came to organize their program of research (1). He tells how, in the beginning, Morgan tried to use the fly to study development. Mutants were named according to the organ system to which the phenotype seemed to belong, but as more and increasingly diverse mutants turned up it became less evident which developmental system was involved, and in the end, the developmental approach was abandoned. It could not thrive because the rules of genetics had not been worked out and the rules could not be elaborated in the study of development.

In the meantime, Morgan's students were attracted to the relationships of phenotypes to one another in their chromosomal position, and a program of study of chromosomal mechanics and gene mapping began, in which genes were named according to visible departures from the usual. Kohler shows how, to facilitate the work, the investigators used many ingenious tricks to standardize the fly—even to reconstruct it—to serve the mapping analysis. And, of course, the mapping work led to what we know as the physical basis of heredity, including the rules of segregation, recombination, linkage, and chromosomal behavior in mitosis and meiosis. Although new words were added by the drosophilists, much of the language they used—gene, genotype, phenotype, dominance, allele, mutant, and so on—was adapted from what already existed.

These words, which at their inception were necessarily vague, now took on a new precision imparted by a deeper understanding of what they could mean. For example, Bateson understood the word *allele,* which he invented, to mean the presence or absence of what he called a "unit factor" and, along with DeVries, he reserved the word *mutant* for the major departures they both believed to be the stuff of evolution. But as the mapping work prospered, alleles were defined as hereditary units capable of occupying specific chromosomal loci. It also became plain that there were sets of "multiple alleles," each presumed to have arisen as a mutant version of the "wild type." Multiple alleles could not be accommodated by presence-absence, and so the idea was dropped by all but Bateson, who clung to it to the end. The mutants among the sets of multiple alleles were abnormal but often had only a minor impact on life or activity. So to the drosophilists, the word *mutant* took on a meaning opposite to that of DeVries and Bateson, to whom the word meant a major departure, a saltation, and a selective advantage.

These words, along with the rest of the vocabulary of the drosophilists, are still with us, although they have acquired nuances to fit our more penetrating understanding of the meaning of the word *gene.* They are entirely appropriate for the phenotype-to-gene analysis that dominated drosophila and physiological genetics—and that has been compatible with the development of medical genetics. But now, the direction of the analytical path is shifting and new words are being added by those who work with the genes themselves. These investigators are evolving a new language to fit new observations—for example, transcription, translation, cDNA, tandem repeats, intron-exon, transposon, recombinant fragment—and the literature of today identifies genes with letters and numerals, designations even more inaccessible than the abbreviated names of the phenotypes of drosophila.

These words and designations accommodate to new definitions of the gene. Where the drosophilists named their genes and loci for the mutant phenotype, the molecular biologists name them for the molecule they specify. Some, however, are named first for an abnormal phenotype and later, when it becomes known, for specificity. Examples are the oncogenes and their loci, which were initially designated according to the cancer they cause and then were found to represent loci engaged in producing molecules that control growth. Some molecules, and so loci, are named for the disease (i.e., huntingtin), but when it is clear what huntingtin does, it may be renamed for its function—or not, according to how deeply rooted the name is; the CFTR locus has not been renamed even though its specificity is known. Practical necessity requires naming genes and loci, and whether the drosophiline or the molecular convention is used depends upon what is known. Specificity is preferable, however, if only to demystify such locutions as "modifying" and "epistatic" genes as well as to curb abuses of the concept of "genes for" in relation to distant phenotypes of such complexity that the exact role of each of several, or many, genes is uncertain.

The Vocabulary of Genetics in Medicine

In medicine, wherein the whole range of gene definitions is used, words are employed to fit each of the several levels of distinction. For example, when, as a preliminary to further steps, the statistical approach is taken, the gene appropriate to that level of investigation remains an abstraction, no matter what visions of DNA sequences dance in the heads of observers. And when the level is operational or functional, the language used to describe the phenotype is limited to words and images no less suitable for drosophila than for human beings with "genetic" diseases. It is only at the structural level that the words begin to change, that the term codominance is introduced, that we distinguish structural from enzymic mutants, and that usages such as "presence or absence of cross-reacting material" (CRM^+ and CRM^-) tell us that the mutations are variable. In addition, at this level we begin to dispense with such words as penetrance and expressivity as genetic heterogeneity emerges with refinement of biochemical analysis. Finally, as we have seen, when the gene is defined as DNA, new words appear—dominance and recessiveness become gain of function, loss of function, dominant negative, and so on—giving the concepts an image both concrete and physiological (2).

But even though more suitable for use in molecular genetics, the words are still reminiscent of Bateson's presence-absence. And since so much of genetics in medicine revolves around the description and disposition of phenotypes at some distance removed from the genes, even when the DNA composition of the latter is well known, our discourse is still consonant with the drosophila agenda, and as long as our thinking and our locutions remain so compatible with that agenda, we will be constrained by it and inhibited from new ways of thinking and talking, especially about individuality. It is well, at this point, to recall that the drosophilists had no interest in individuality. Matings were arranged to test hypotheses about characteristics of the organism, not individual flies. The latter, who had no individual identity, were counted only as representatives of the contrasting classes among the offspring. And as long as the drosophilists worked within this operational context, their thinking and their language did not embrace individuality. It is also germane to recall that the idea of genetics entered medicine from without, and that those who accomplished this intellectual invasion were steeped in the lore, not of medicine, but of drosophila genetics. In fact, the first textbook of human genetics widely used in the United States was that of Curt Stern, a well-known drosophilist. The first edition appeared in 1949, the third and last in 1973 (3). So it is not surprising that genetics in the medicine of today continues to reflect the thinking of the drosophilists.

A characterization of how this heritage restricts our thinking is revealed in Table 1 (chapter 7), where the alternative forms of thought are contrasted. As long as our minds are dominated by the machine mentality, then in that degree we are typological, individuality is that of the class, and stress is given to reductionist analysis and its uses in illuminating the mechanisms of the diseases that make medical genetics one specialty among all the others that medical students must reconnoiter and even consider as possible for their life's work. Genetic medicine calls for something in addition: the populational approach to individuality and the idea that genetically determined variation of the unit steps of homeostasis must inform all disease—just as it does the variations of human structure, form, and behavior that we all take for granted. This requires an emphasis that draws as much attention to remote causes and to the individuality of the victims of hereditary disease as that accorded proximate causes and the disease itself.

MEDICINE AND POPULATION THINKING

Individuality is usually given a secondary emphasis in textbooks and courses, which, although alluding to the terminology of polymorphism and population genetics, do not weave these themes into the intellectual fabric of medical genetics. They are not always represented as germane to the diagnostic-prognostic-treatment missions. But, in fact, they are. They offer answers to the "why" questions: why this person, why this disease, why now in the lifetime, and so on. And, although the word gene is no less prominent, the point of view—and so the vocabulary—is different. Here the primary object of scrutiny is the individual, a human being endowed with a unique aliquot drawn from a gene pool composed of the genes of variable individuals and whose constancy and variation are a consequence of the patterns of the reproduction, migration, and mortality of those individuals. So how the genetic composition of populations is attained or, more generally, the identity of the forces that drive evolution, is a question of no small interest in medical education.

And the lexicon we have contains words suitable for working with these questions: natural selection, genetic drift, migration, mutational load, molecular evolutionary clocks, and the various theories of evolutionary change—classical, balance, neutral, and others more molecular. Pretty far from medicine? Paradoxically, the connection is in fact very close because the dynamics of population genetics tell us how it is that specific sets of genes come together in individuals to make them vulnerable to—or proof against—disease. So population genetics, far from being a separate aspect of human genetics, just one among many and to be accorded a lesser position in a textbook, supplies a framework within which to construct the details of diseases not perceived as "genetic."

MORE DROSOPHILINE LANGUAGE: MUTANT–WILD TYPE

Chapter 10 on genetic homeostasis reviewed the means whereby the composition of the gene pool is maintained, and there it was apparent that, among all the genes available to the species, there is a gradient of selective effect that varies from lethal to neutral to beneficial genes that confer a new advantage. That chapter was devoted to the collective genome of the species. Here the focus is on the composition of individual genotypes, each a reflection of the distribution of genes in the pool of which each is an aliquot. There the issues were phrased in the drosophiline language of wild-type versus mutant, at least until polymorphism and the neutral theory of evolution revealed the polarizing, typological meaning of these words, words we must understand if we are to break out of our drosophiline constraints (4).

A polymorphic locus is defined as the seat of more than one allele with a frequency of more than 1 percent, and empirical observation reveals that few of these are outliers in distributions of measurements of function. In such a case, which is the mutant and which the wild type? In the lexicon of drosophila genetics, *wild type* is defined as the standard, the normal, the naturally occurring allele. And such a definition must represent a large proportion, perhaps most, of human genes; we are all presumed to be homozygous for many standard genes that have demonstrated their worth over the millennia and are little tolerant of alternatives. So the mutant is the nonstandard, the abnormal, a changed gene. But how and when and where did the standard become the standard, given that it must have originated in some distant past where it was . . . what? A mutant no doubt, and one that contributed some extra bit to survival and reproduction. Standard genes are like aristocrats: people of substance, good breeding, superior, and well turned out, but necessarily the descendants of aggressive, no doubt vulgar, eccentrics who attained their station as a result of the unscrupulous vigor with which they pursued it.

But these definitions are ambiguous, especially when applied to polymorphic loci that harbor two or more alleles each qualifying as normal, and so we call them all "wild type" in consonance with the designation by the drosophilists as "isoalleles," those whose effects fall within the normal range. Isoalleles were so called because they could be distinguished only in relation to one another, which raises the question of which is "iso" to the other. In fact, all are isoalleles until one is shown to depart, however slightly, from wild-type effect, at which point it becomes a mutant.

But where, exactly, do wild type, isoallele, and mutant meet? Where does one become the other? Where there are several wild-type alleles, which is the original, the standard, and which of the others were derived therefrom by mutation, especially if there are demonstrable functional differences even when all are defined arbitrarily to be within some normal range? If one allele has a frequency of 90 percent, a second 9 percent, and a third 1 percent, which is the standard? In fact, the gene with the frequency of 1 percent could be the original, now all but replaced for reasons of drift or a new selective pressure, and that 90 percent gene could be the mutant that is replacing it. No doubt every gene was once a mutant and each attained its frequency by virtue of its role in some evolutionary scheme or other. The source of the ambiguity is in the typological uses of the words. Wild type and mutant are easily distinguished when the former is represented as that which in becoming the latter is so grossly changed in form and function as to be readily associated with disease.

And that may be all we have to know as long as we contemplate only segregating monogenic diseases. But we are going to have to think more about diseases in which two—or several or many—genes introduce homeostatic limitations that predispose individuals at certain times in development to the effects of experiences that test or exceed those limitations. We can live comfortably enough within such homeostatic constraints except in the face of testing experiences. So now how do we define wild type and mutant? It may be that the defining experience is rare and the limiting genes are common, so can such genes be wild type in the context of ordinary life and mutant in the extraordinary condition? The position becomes less and less tenable as the testing experience is more and more frequently encountered. If frequent enough, then wild type becomes mutant because it is not normal under the frequent condition; if less frequent, then mutant is wild type because it contributes under usual conditions to normal homeostasis.

The limitation of these terms is demonstrated by defining preventive medicine as that which makes wild type out of mutants by changing the conditions of living. So in confronting disease of complex origin we might dispense with these typological terms and, calling them "alleles" or "variants," think more of how gene products are disposed throughout a lifetime of development and experience. Furthermore, we must do so in the context of particular lifetimes in the expectation that the uniqueness of genes, experiences, and lifetimes will be reflected in the particularity of signs, symptoms, and outcomes. The virtue of blurring the typological distinction was perhaps first proposed by Schrödinger, who saw that the words differentiated heretics (mutants) from orthodox (wild type), a position that could be avoided by calling both "versions" (5).

Neither genes nor experiences are of themselves harmful. Disease ensues when these two influences coincide to constrain the powers of one or more homeostatic systems, a state expressed in an array of genes that, in concert with a singular set of experiences, has promoted a particular pathway of development to make an individual unique. That is a definition of individuality free of the shackles of typology, and one that is supported by the evidence of genetics. When sequences of base pairs in genes associated with monogenic disease are examined, extensive genetic heterogeneity is usually observed. In the case of relatively frequent monogenic diseases, the usual condition is that of one or two common variants and then very many unique ones, so that on occasion the cases with novel variants outnumber those with the usual. And were it possible—or useful—to detect the sequence of all the base pairs of the usual variants, who can doubt that an occasional additional variation would be turned up even in the translatable exons, while variability in the introns or flanking sequences is a certainty. One purpose of so detailed a definition of individuality, one that sometimes goes beyond the useful or even practical, is to give the strongest emphasis to a constructive way of thinking, a way that is a part of everyday experience when it comes to the appearance or behavior of individual human beings, each of whom is recognized as unique by everyone else, but that has been constrained in medicine by typological thinking, which in medical genetics has been informed by the concepts and vocabulary of the drosophilists.

18

Classification of Disease

Classifications have been the way physicians and other healers have abstracted common qualities from otherwise unique sick individuals, no doubt doing violence to the special features of each person's experience.
—Stephen J. Kunitz, "Classification in Medicine" (1)

The human mind is attuned to classification. Books in libraries, food in supermarkets, archival data, all are assorted and arranged in the interest of coherence and accessibility. Living organisms are sorted out by nature into millions of forms that are identified by biologists who arrange them into phylogenetic classes and species. In this enterprise, the work of paleontologists and systematists, based on morphology and function, has been vindicated and their classes have been generally validated by molecular testimony to the coherence of the phylogenetic structure they erected. This classification could be said to have existed a priori and so has been discovered, while the assortments of librarians or archivists have been created to serve some cultural end. Today's classification of disease includes both; it is a mixture of the fruits of discovery as well as those of invention, but because diseases are expressions of living organisms, we have reason to suppose that a classification compatible with physiology must exist and will be discovered.

MEDICAL CLASSIFICATION

In medicine, diseases must be classified for the sake of both practice and research; information about diseases must be ordered, the better to retrieve it for diagnosis and treatment. To these ends there has evolved a system of great practical utility, capable of assimilating new entities into existing classes in consonance with the medical thinking of the time (2,3). It is not especially logical, but it is inclusive. At present the system is based on the following: (a) etiology—as infections and diseases due to genes and toxic substances; (b) anatomical organ systems—lung, nervous system, cardiovascular, renal, endocrinological, and so on; (c) age at onset—as diseases of the neonatal period, infancy, or aging; (d) therapeutic—as medical or surgical; (e) developmental—including anomalies and disorders of growth and development; (f) reproductive—that is, obstetrical and gynecological; (g) behavioral—psychological and psychiatric; (h) a growing class called "metabolic" that is based on function and includes the classical inborn errors; (i) other—some textbooks list a few conditions that seem to defy classification.

This is the order observed by the International Classification of Diseases and that appears in textbooks of medicine, surgery, and the various specialties (4), and these classes have not changed much since the first edition of Osler's *The Principles and Practice of Medicine*. They are represented in the organization of medicine, including the departments and divisions of medical schools and hospitals and the segregation of practice into the various specialties. And it is natural that they do so. The classes are based on biology in that organs represent outcomes of the differentiation of cell types, and they appear to offer no resistance to new interpretations of disease based on physiology, biochemistry, and molecular biology. The rubrics are flexible and seem capable of accommodating all sorts of novelties. But the classes are both typological and entirely consonant with the essentialist view of disease so compatible with the machine mentality. Indeed, the position is that pictured by Holton, of a taxonomic scheme consisting of classes that "in the absence of some 'first principle' to which to rise and from which to derive an ordering matrix, they may simply fall back on the production of pigeon holes with plausible labels which invite one to disaggregate the incoherent vastness of possible observables" (5).

THE SYSTEM IS IN FLUX

However lacking a "first principle," we have been satisfied with our system for a long time, and I know of no agitation for a new one. The many calls for revisions in medical education do not include anything so revolutionary. In any case, this way of assorting diseases has stood for so long and is woven so intimately into our thinking and behavior that modifications are likely to be resisted. But the changes that are coming are not the product of anyone's idea of reform. Even as we see it as a given in medicine, the present classification is being undermined by the advent of detailed insights into pathogenesis that expose the molecular qualities of homeostatic steps that have been overridden.

Classification began with an assortment of patients by signs and symptoms to make diagnostic categories, names of diseases that came to be identified with certain treatments. Changes came with new knowledge based on morbid anatomy, and the pace picked up markedly when infections were sorted out according to microorganisms and the principle of making new diseases out of old was consciously established. Then, all sorts of novelties were brought to light, first by biochemical analysis and then by a combined biochemical-genetic approach. Now we are in the age of a biochemical-molecular-genetic process that comes down to variations in molecules that represent steps in homeostatic systems. At every step in this analytical descent from phenotype to genotype, new diagnostic categories and diseases have been discovered.

Today, the story of pathogenesis is perceived as incomplete until there is a precise description of the steps of homeostasis that are disordered, as well as of the proteins that officiate at those steps and the genes that specify them, and more and more are diseases classified accordingly. And since derangement in several points in a homeostatic system may produce a similar pathogenesis, but each in a different patient, each is given a new name and appears separately in the textbooks under an already existing heading. The several diseases of the urea cycle are examples. Together on the one hand they are called the hyperammonemias, and on the other each is named according to the enzyme deficiency that characterizes it (6).

The conventional wisdom is further assaulted by discovery of metabolic disorders that are expressed in the cells of one organ with consequences that characterize the disease appearing in another, a quality often observed in inborn errors of metabolism. An example is PKU, wherein the homeostatic defect occurs in the liver and kidney but the disease is most obvious in the nervous system. This anomalous position is accommodated in the present system by naming the disease for its most salient quality and classifying it accordingly, and the organ in which the disease originates is neglected. For example, PKU was once classed among other types of mental retardation, and so it was a disorder of the central nervous system. Later it was perceived to be an inborn error of metabolism and so a "genetic" disease, but it is seldom classed with disorders of the liver. Today it is classed among the hyperphenylalaninemias (7).

Other diseases with biochemical attributes are accommodated in the current system as inborn errors that fit into a class called "metabolic disease," a category with which the classifiers have been uneasy for a long time. But now that category has become too comprehensive, so that all sorts of subgroups have made an appearance—disorders of amino acids, for example, or of lysosomal enzymes or peroxisomes and so on, all categories not readily reconciled with convention. The well-known book *The Molecular and Metabolic Bases of Inherited Disease* exemplifies this trend (8). Seventy percent of the seventh edition is devoted to disorders assorted by homeostatic function, transcending academic departments and specialties and without reference to any of the standard taxonomic classes. The remainder, which includes, among others, cancer, congenital anomalies, and diseases of the blood and immune systems, all easily accommodated by the current system, are also perceived in the book as inborn errors—that is, disorders of homeostasis. So the implication of *MMBID* is that when the truth is known, all disease will turn out to be represented as defects of one or more homeostatic elements, and if so, the rubric of metabolic disease, in including all, is rendered useless. So one outcome of *MMBID,* so subversive of the old way of classifying diseases, might be a new system based on the "first principle" of the specificity of homeostatic disorder.

A Basis for a New Classification

Such a basis has a strong appeal not entirely because the old is awkward and lacking in elegance, but because in today's analysis of disease, emphasis is placed on the molecular and diagnostic individuality of the patient. These qualities are wanting in the present system, which is typological. That is the meaning of the epigraph heading this chapter. Kunitz is saying that the classes of disease, in representing all victims, have ignored the individuality of each. In the opening paragraph of his paper, Kunitz cites Alfred North Whitehead thus: "'Classification is a halfway house between the immediate concreteness of the individual thing and the complete abstraction of mathematical notions'" (1). That is, in our scheme of classification we are likely to serve ideally neither the individual nor the species. The classification is neither wholly typological nor wholly populational; it is not based altogether on either molecular evidence or on signs and symptoms, and it fits neither the essentialist nor the nominalist definition of disease.

But are we to be trapped forever in the halfway house, or can we escape by the application of a new "first principle," a new system based on the unit step of homeostasis? Is this possible—or practical? The wherewithal to fulfill homeostatic function is the proteins, and since all proteins are specified by genes, perhaps we are moving unmindfully toward a genetic classification of diseases. That is an attractive proposition, but an unlikely one. All a gene does is specify a protein or determine when in development it appears and in what amount; it plays no part whatever in what the protein does and so may be absolved of immediate responsibility should its product fail in its homeostatic mission. But though the product itself is variant in amino acid sequence, conformation, or amount, there is not necessarily any disease. The latter is a consequence of how incongruent the variant protein is in its homeostatic setting.

The gene is not altogether irrelevant since it specified the culprit, but although for a long time we have been able to classify diseases according to homeostatic aberration without knowing the genes, it will never be possible to classify according to genes without knowing their protein products and their homeostatic missions. So it is the homeostatic derangement upon which a new classification might be based.

A Catalogue of Vulnerabilities

Such a classification must begin with a list, not of the phenotypes we call inborn errors, but of the names of the variant proteins responsible for the unit steps in homeostasis that are altered in those inborn errors. A list of this kind constitutes a catalogue of vulnerabilities that is always provisional because limited to proteins known to be involved in some people and at some time and phase of their lives in disease. Homeostatic steps omitted from the list will enter when shown to be associated with disease, so the roster is likely to grow until it embraces all homeostatic steps that can be the seat of disease. Presumably redundancy in metabolic systems is such that even ablation of some steps may leave the whole unperturbed. But even these will be associated, under appropriate conditions, with symptoms. Such appropriate conditions may be particular concatenations of other genes or special experiences of the environment—or both. Either way, whether the inborn error is monogenic or multifactorial, the proteins will enter the list of vulnerabilities.

Classes of Vulnerabilities

But such a list is not a classification. Were there only a few such vulnerabilities, no classification would be needed or they could be a class of their own, but since there are already hundreds and there will be thousands, some means of access will be required. At this stage we cannot predict precisely what form the classification will take. No doubt it will retain some ties to the old; many homeostatic systems are organ specific, so there are likely still to be vulnerabilities for diseases of the eye or the brain or other organs. But its ultimate logic is not easy to discern given our present knowledge of what must be only a few percent of the whole. For example, new families of genes with hitherto undisclosed functions turn up all the time. So how can we compose a coherent structure until much more of the unknown has been fathomed? For the moment, we could do worse than to follow the sorting out that is emerging spontaneously in the evolving editions of *MMBID,* where functions are emphasized over organ systems.

Monogenic Inborn Errors

Obviously, cell differentiation leads to organ specificity in the action of the products of the variants associated with the inborn error, but each class comprises disorders of homeostatic systems without regard to the organ wherein the inborn error occurs. For example, while classes labeled "carbohydrates," "peroxisomes," "purines," "pyrimidines," and so on may conjure up visions of the organs in which these processes transpire, the classes are of the functions—the processes transcend the organs. Toward the end of *MMBID* and occupying only a few of its pages there is a minority of disorders that, however hereditary and metabolic, are listed under the old organ-system headings. But even though embraced within such rubrics, the conditions included follow the pattern that characterizes the rest of the book: the inborn error as a consequence of the incongruence of the protein product of a variant gene and its homeostatic system.

Multifactorial Inborn Errors

Almost all the conditions included in the seventh edition of *MMBID* are monogenic inborn errors. But these conditions, no matter how many they are today or how many they will be tomorrow, must always affect a minority of the human species. How can the majority be accommodated in this incipient classification based on unit steps in homeostasis? Their diseases do not fit the mold of the classical inborn error and yet some—for example, types I and II diabetes and gout—have been included in *MMBID*'s list of inborn errors since the first edition. There is an intuitive wisdom in doing so. Both forms of diabetes as well as gout are by common consent heterogeneous and multifactorial in origin, and all three represent the continuity of the inborn error with Garrod's concept of chemical individuality.

We know that both monogenic and multigenic phenotypes can be heterogeneous, but is the multifactorial model of disease compatible with a classification based on the inborn error of a unit step of homeostasis? In fact, there is no difficulty whatever. If genes contribute to multifactorial phenotypes (or diseases), they can do so only by way of the specification of proteins, themselves unitary components of homeostatic systems. So the only difference between a monogenic inborn error and a multigenic phenotype is that the latter is a consequence of two or more genes specifying two or more unit steps in one, two, or more homeostatic systems. The difference is one of degree rather than of quality. This point will be developed more fully later, when it is shown how all phenotypes are in some degree multigenic in that variation in monogenic phenotypes is sometimes demonstrated to be due to the effects of the protein products of what are, under the circumstances, called "modifying" genes. So we are again troubled by semantics. What is the difference at the level of gene action between a "multigenic" phenotype and "modification" of a monogenic phenotype? Obviously, in observing that, at the level of the unitary relationship between genes and their products, all genes are created equal, we must argue that there is none: the difference is in the phenotype. Since one segregates and the other does not there is utility in such a distinction, but both can be defined in the same way as two or more genes specifying two or more proteins, each fulfilling unit steps in homeostasis.

So, the two or more unit steps in homeostasis that comprise the multigenic set may join the catalogue of vulnerabilities as qualitative equals of those associated with monogenic disease. And all of these may be classified as inborn errors of the unitary steps in the homeostatic systems to which they belong. But unlike the monogenic phenotypes in which the relationship between a unit homeostatic step and a disease phenotype is unequivocal, the association of the several unit steps with the multifactorial disease may be obscure. So how we classify the multifactorial units of vulnerability will depend upon how those units are deployed to produce the multifactorial disease. Table 3 (chapter 15) revealed the several levels of integration leading to a final phenotype and gave examples of diseases described at the various levels of complexity. At the level of homeostasis, each unit of vulnerability is complete of itself and may contribute to more than one aspect of other levels and so to more than one disease. It can be at once a modifier of a monogenic phenotype or contribute with others to a phenotype that emerges at a particular developmental stage.

Classifying by vulnerability rather than by disease allows us to use both new and conventional classifications at once. It allows us to reconcile the need for separation of diseases into discrete entities even while recognizing the continuity of their origins in the same mechanism. Each such unitary contributor to a multigenic vulnerability is likely to be classified in more than one way—on the one hand as an inborn error of homeostasis and on the other as contributory to a disease that is itself classified in one of the rubrics employed in *MMBID* or even in the old classification by organ system. So until the list of vulnerabilities is several times its present number, we will continue to classify in provisional ways or revert to the conventional wisdom. The point is, we have not yet finished the historical evolution of the classification that began with phenotypes and is now moving toward definitions of diseases as aberrations of unit steps of homeostasis. So again and again we fall back on whatever is the best we can do.

It might be supposed that infections will create a problem. But all that is needed is an extension of what is already in *MMBID*. There we find a section devoted to deficits of "Defense and Immune Mechanisms," and these are authentic inborn errors. But how do we classify, say, pneumococcal infections? If it can be shown that human beings are differentiated in susceptibility to the pneumococcus, we are faced with no anomaly in classification. But suppose, however unlikely, that everyone is equally susceptible. Then vulnerability is no less molecular for being defined by the pneumococcus; the organism has devised a way to infect by means of aspects of the human cell for which it has evolved an affinity, and that is the vulnerability that might enter the list. This question of infections is given more attention later in the book.

THE UTILITY OF A NEW CLASSIFICATION

How can this list and classification help us? First, in contrast to what we now employ, it has an attractive logic. All disease is based on inborn variations of homeostasis. Occasionally, as in scurvy or deficiency of other essential metabolites, the hereditary differences distinguish species rather than individuals, but in either case it is the genetically determined incongruence that makes for susceptibility. So the list and classification are based on the elements of structure and function that all human beings share. Second, it is flexible enough to accommodate new knowledge about genes, gene products, homeostatic steps and systems, and all degrees of integration thereof. The list and classification represent an elastic grid with unlimited space for admitting new entries without endangering the logic.

Third, the list and classification of vulnerabilities is more compatible with the nominal than the essentialist version of disease, is populational rather than typological, and focuses medical attention on the individual rather than the disease. Each individual's list of vulnerabilities is sure to vary in detail from all others, even while some components are shared. Typological thinking about a disease emphasizes the qualities shared by many while neglecting the variety of the combinations of qualities that characterize individuals. The ultimate in typology is attained in the diagnosis-related groups (DRGs) that classify exclusively for economic reasons, and that in their indifference to individuality would squeeze the last drop of humanity from our profession. This revision of justification for classifying is echoed in the latest edition of the International Classification of Diseases (4). Originally intended to "provide access to medical records for medical research, education, and administration," it now proclaims its use "to facilitate payment of health services, to evaluate utilization patterns, and to study appropriateness of health care costs." Whatever the worthiness of these goals, in their adherence to typology they do nothing to free us from Whitehead's halfway house.

Finally, the principal utility of a new list and classification is in prevention. As they appear in the list, the vulnerabilities represent substrates for disease, not the diseases themselves. So, in principle, the primary role of medicine ought to be to act first upon the information inherent in the vulnerability rather than to await the symptoms of the disease it warns against. I have been careful to say "in principle" here because experience has shown us time and again that the same variant and inborn error may have a very different impact in different persons, so that we are learning to be circumspect in the indiscriminate application of preventive measures. Here it is enough to suggest the utility of a list of vulnerabilities in prevention and to imply that any such use would be likely to bring about significant changes in medical thinking. Chief among these is the recognition that in prevention it is always a person, classified by individual vulnerability, that is the object of attention, while in treatment it is usually the disease, classified by pigeonhole, that is the object of the therapy.

WILL A NEW CLASSIFICATION CHANGE ANYTHING?

What change might occur as a result of a new system of assorting diseases? Perhaps not very much very soon, but given that we are comfortable with what we have at present, whatever happens will be evolutionary and adaptive rather than revolutionary and destructive. But some things might occur visibly and soon. For example, reductionist explanations of pathogenesis will ensure that the classes of disease will continue to change in the direction marked by *MMBID*. That is, the various cancers may be assorted into defects of growth factors or abnormalities of transcription factors, while others may be named according to whatever homeostatic steps are involved. Heterogeneity will continue to divide complex diseases into simpler entities, the trend being downward in the level of identity on the path from phenotype to homeostatic unit and its gene. So, old names might gradually go and we may see a time when hypertension seems as archaic as dropsy. In its place might be disorders of renin, angiotensin, and so on. But hypertension will not disappear until we have a firm grip on its heterogeneity and the validity of its treatment according to type.

Would the gradual adoption of new classes change the organization of medicine? Not likely very soon. Oncology centers will continue to cater to patients with tumors, whatever their disorders are called; obstetricians will still deliver babies; and the prostate gland will continue to command as imperiously as ever the conjunction of old men and urologists. And pediatrics is likely to persist if only because grownups don't like to consort with squalling babies in waiting rooms. The point is that a new classification will be a reflection of new ways of thinking in medicine and of recognition by students and doctors of the implications of what is happening around them. But the most important impact of a classification based on unit steps of homeostasis will be in moving us out of Whitehead's halfway house to compel us to think first of the individuality of vulnerabilities and then of how they may be assembled to compose a category.

Will attention to individuality cause the doctor to look beyond the uniqueness of vulnerability to its implications for each person on life, family, and society? It will do that when the uniqueness of both individual and vulnerability are uppermost in the doctor's mind, when we think first of sick people and then of disease.

VI
Reproduction, Frequency, and Continuity

The definition of the gene (part V) in structure, function, and variability makes possible in part VI a review of the remaining aspects of the definition of evolution offered in chapter 7. The reader will perceive immediately, however, that the definition of the gene depends upon the processes to be reviewed in this section, just as they depend upon the definition of the gene. We are always describing the same thing from different perspectives. That is, the gene would not have become what it is were it not for diploidy and mutation. And were it not for mutation there would be no variety to submit to selection, and without selection the phenotypic nuances that constitute the gradient of selective effect would not exist to be observed as unity and continuity in expression of both health and disease, themselves traceable to variations in gene frequency and heterogeneity. Perhaps heritability, at once the most abstract of the qualities described in part VI and the most succinctly expressive of medical aims, summarizes it best. Heritability is a variable that, in subsuming all the other processes, exposes as nothing else can the origins of human variation—including disease—in the meeting of nature and nurture at the node of the unit step of homeostasis.

Chapter 24, the last of this part, is a summary pitched in the context of infections. Nearly anything else would have done, but nowhere else could the logic of genetic medicine be more usefully displayed than in relation to the archetype of environmental disease.

19

The Diploid State

If it be true that the essence of life is the accumulation of experience through the generations, then one may perhaps suspect that the key problem of biology . . . is how living matter manages to record and perpetuate its experiences.

—Max Delbrück, "A Physicist Looks at Biology" (1)

As a young man, Max Delbrück perceived the "riddle of life" as a goal to pursue. He sought the answer in reproduction, which he concluded was at its starkest in bacteriophage, an organism that he studied to the great benefit of genetics and biology. But the riddle has ramifications. No one would deny that reproduction is central to life and its continuity or that it is at its least complex in bacteriophage, but higher organisms need complexity in reproduction to attain the intricacies of their function, so it is no surprise that along with the advantages of the scheme that nature settled on there are some disadvantages. In this chapter, these virtues and violations are examined in the context of genetic medicine.

THE DIPLOID STATE

After establishing that a disease is familial, our first question is whether its distribution in families satisfies some mendelian hypothesis. Is it a dominant? A recessive? Sex linked? Or none of these? A decision is of interest because each category evokes a different set of characteristics, different diagnoses, and different outcomes.

But although we are aware of the relationship of these familial distributions and our diploid state, we seldom reflect that they are a consequence of the evolution of biological complexity. Prokaryotes carrying only one set of genes are the oldest organisms, having appeared billions of years ago. Since we know that in nature anything that can happen, sooner or later will happen, we cannot be surprised to learn that even prokaryotes have a diploid stage. Evidence of this sexual phase in bacteria was demonstrated in 1946 by Lederberg, who discovered a strain of *E. coli* wherein intact bacteria conjugated and the DNA of one was transferred to the other, after which the two DNAs paired and recombination took place (2). A reduction division followed, and the haploid state was resumed. This kind of conjugation is infrequent, so most representatives of the strain never attain diploidy; it is the haploid condition that characterizes the species, with occasional ventures into diploidy to reinvigorate the strain. Further evolution led, perhaps by way of heterokaryons of prokaryote haploids, to diploid cells that aggregated to form increasingly large and complex organisms composed of differentiated cells, among them gametes in which a reduction division had occurred to restore the haploid state. Thus, although no organism appears altogether to have given up its haploid heritage, complex organisms spend little time in that condition.

How was the diploid state established? Maintenance of diploidy requires reversion to the haploid state followed by re-establishment of the diploid. This requires some sort of differentiation into sexes, a feat attained through the evolution of sex chromosomes, a transition that resulted in human beings in the familiar X and Y chromosomes, in which feminizing properties reside in the X, masculinizing in the Y. As the process went on, the Y lost substance as well as the ability to recombine at all but a small part of the X. Efficiency might have led to chromosomes containing genes devoted only to the business of sex determination, and the Y generally fulfills this criterion, but the X chromosome of mammals, however, failed to evolve in that direction so that numerous genes unrelated to sex reside there.

What sets sex determination in motion? The mechanisms are similar to other developmental processes. There is a homeostatic system constituted of proteins each specified by a gene and consisting of a cascade of regulatory elements, a hierarchy of transcription factors that activate genes for the development of primary sex differences. And, as in all other homeostatic systems, there are mutants, inborn errors that in this case result in sex reversals that have helped immeasurably in elucidating mechanism.

After fertilization male cells are haploid with regard to X-linked genes and are exposed to the rigors of whatever mutants there may be. Female cells with their extra dose of X-linked genes are saved from imbalance by the expedient of permanent inactivation of one X. But still the two sexes differ since X inactivation is random in each cell and in all daughter cells the same X is in the active or inactive state, so the organs of the female are mosaics of the two Xs. This mosaicism imparts phenotypic variability not available to the male with his single X.

ADVANTAGES AND DISADVANTAGES OF DIPLOIDY

These features of sex determination have been presented as preliminary to a contrast of the virtues and handicaps of diploidy. What are the advantages and disadvantages of paired chromosomes and genes? More particularly, what are the implications for individuals in their experience of disease? There is a central tendency about species that limits individuality. Since it is in the nature of individuality to be expressed in diverse ways, almost anything suitable for most will be undesirable for some. And the diploid state is no exception. It is one more example of the tension between the welfare of species and that of individuals.

Advantages

Advantages and disadvantages of the diploid state are listed in Table 4. No doubt the most important advantage is the variability conferred by the opportunity for the species to call upon sets of multiple alleles and for the individual to be heterozygous at many loci. Recombination to form new combinations adds to the fund of variability and promises that each gamete—and, a fortiori, each zygote—is unique. So to the species is given the wherewithal to adapt in changing environments, and to the individual is imparted a particularity denied haploid organisms that reproduce in clones. The special case of heterozygote advantage is a further source of variation, though of unknown extent.

A second advantage is dominance, in which variants in one chromosome are muted by the "normal" alleles of the other. Population geneticists see this protective device as having been a prominent selective force in promoting the spread of diploidy. Competing ideas about the origins, or "evolution," of dominance sparked one of the numerous controversies in the development of genetic thinking. The controversy began with agreement that new mutants would be nearly always destructive, just as they are in haploid organisms, so the advantage in dominance would lie in the presence of homologous genes that could negate the mutant effect and so make it tolerable. It was around how this state desirable state had been attained that ideas differed. R. A. Fisher held that the recessive condition was reached by selection of modifiers to suppress the threat of mutants, while J. B. S. Haldane concluded that selection would give preference to those wild-type alleles that opposed them (3,4).

Sewall Wright's explanation was more physiological. He reasoned (in the late 1920s) that the reduction in function due to the mutant should be about one half, and that for most gene systems the effect of the normal allele should suffice. But since so many loci were characterized by sets of alleles of varying competence, there would be some wild-type genes that would be insufficient to counter the mutant effect and so a heterozygote effect would be observed. In addition, there were other variables, genetic and nongenetic, so that the same allele might exert dominance in one individual and express a more or less recessive effect in another. To Wright, dominance was a product of interactions, and selection acted to preserve phenotypes that expressed such interactive relationships rather than upon genes one at a time. Dominance, he said, is "a phe-

Table 4 The Diploid State

Factor	Advantages		Disadvantages	
	Populations	Individuals	Populations	Individuals
Increased variability	Recombination, variability in function, heterozygote advantage	Individuality, adaptability, protection against mutant effect	Accumulation of mutants, wide range of mutants tolerated	Recessive diseases, heterogeneity, range of severity of disease, consequences of sex linkage, consequences of imprinting
Sexual reproduction	Biological differences, cultural differences	Cultural variation		
Evolution of complexity	Gene families, multicellularity, complexity of function, dominance			

nomenon of the physiology of development to be associated with the various types of epistatic relationships among factors" (4). So in emphasizing one gene at a time, Fisher and Haldane were thinking typologically, while Wright, whose initiation to genetics involved a physiological approach, thought of the whole of the variation embraced in populations of individuals, each of whom represented a special phenotype.

Diploidy also allows the formation of multicellular organisms with differentiated cells and the elaboration of new genes in gene families with consequent novelty in functional complexity. These developments are entirely conditional upon the protective margin provided by dominance. For example, the shield of gene dosage is clearly demonstrated in the necessity for multiple somatic hits required for homozygosity of the mutants that lead to cancer. Haploidy could never be depended upon for the long run.

However manifold its advantages, the maintenance of the diploid state has been no minor job for selection, which has evolved an elaborate apparatus of cell types, structures, organs, hormonal signaling systems, and behaviors of differentiated sexes to ensure the perpetuation of the species by sexual reproduction. And human beings, ever ready to make a virtue of necessity, have created a variety of cultures in which not only reproduction and the nurture of offspring but the processes of pairing and mating are truly central preoccupations.

The advantages recounted so far are those of the species or of populations. What of individuals? Here the chief advantage is the variation that provides opportunity to express diverse selves in an uncertain, often unfriendly environment. Such flexibility is denied the haploid organism, to whom eccentricity is death. And an aspect of this crowning attribute of diploid individuals is dominance, which allows individuals to harbor alleles that in homozygotes cause recessive disease. It is possible to demonstrate that, on average, everyone must have some of these genes. But that is not the point. The point is that individuality requires that although some people have the average number, others have many while some have few.

As to whether the behaviors and practices surrounding reproduction are of advantage to individuals, the vast majority of people would say that sex and gender had been cardinal features of their lives, and an observer of human society would agree, adding that the range of individuality in these is no less than in other behaviors.

Disadvantages

The disadvantages of diploidy, implicit in its advantages, are significant in the genesis of disease (Table 4). Dominance allows the accumulation in the population of genes that in homozygotes promote disease or that, in the heterozygous state, represent vulnerability. Such accumulations, which are fed by new mutations, must be balanced by losses, whether in homozygotes with recessive inborn errors or in heterozygotes susceptible to multifactorial disease. Fortunately, the pace of both accumulation and loss is, by human reckoning of time, remarkably deliberate. The double set of chromosomes also expands the range of mutations; translocation is impossible when there is only one chromosome, and trisomies and other aberrations commonly observed in diploids are unlikely to be observed in haploid organisms.

As for disadvantages in individuals, gene dosage expressed in heterozygotes, compounds, and homozygotes—to say nothing of modifiers in both chromosomes—broadens the range of variability of symptoms, signs, and outcomes among all disorders. And the complexity of interactions among gene products and between such products and experiences is raised exponentially in multifactorial disease. Opportunities for genetic heterogeneity both within and between loci are much enhanced, contributing to the individuality of disease.

We are given a glimpse of the hazards of haploidy and the protective powers of diploidy in the stark contrast of effects in the two sexes when affected with X-linked mutants. Ornithine transcarbamylase deficiency is an example (5). There are numerous mutants that produce a devastating disease in hemizygous males, with perinatal onset and early death. Treated survivors may be mentally retarded or die early in life, but a few male patients who have onset later, even in adult life, are helped by treatment. In comparison, most female heterozygotes experience nothing or only some discomfort after eating what is to them an excess of protein. But some have symptoms, occasionally rivaling those observed in the hemizygous males. Presumably the latter are victims of an unlucky lyonization; here dominance is a property of the number of active X chromosomes carrying the wild-type gene in the active state.

A further form of haploidy is observed as a result of imprinting in which genes derived from one parent are suppressed, leaving those from the other parent to stand alone (6). If the latter are mutants, disease may be a consequence. Several such disorders have been described. What distinguishes them is the uniparental origin of the affected patient.

Conclusion

Size and complexity require the diploid representation of genes; the haploid state is too exposed to adverse selection. And diploidy has been an overwhelming success. The emphasis here on the minor snags in so efficient a mechanism derives only from the purpose of the book. That there are flaws in this ingenious solution to the problems of complexity is only one more evidence of nature's willingness to settle for something less than perfect. It does so in the interest of species and at some cost to individuals. But since the health and survival of individuals is the object of all medical aims, it is our business to know and understand just where and how nature is settling for something less than the ideal and so to anticipate which individuals are going to be the cost. And to that end, we must ask how that cost is to be exacted, and how often. These questions form the substance of the next two chapters.

20

Gene Frequency

Think of the field of visible joint frequencies of all genes as spread out in a multidimensional space. Add another dimension measuring degree of fitness. The field would be very humpy in relation to the latter because of epistatic relations, groups of mutations which were deleterious individually producing a harmonious result in combination.
—Sewall Wright, from a letter to R. A. Fisher (1)

While Fisher saw evolution as a process in which all members of a species participated and which moved at a majestic, unvarying pace, Sewall Wright saw it as a sometime thing, varying in speed from place to place and population to population. He envisioned it occurring more here than there in a "shifting balance," according to the average selective fitness of small populations. On a map, high-average fitness would constitute a rise in the contour, low-average fitness a valley, and because of variable mating systems, migration into and out of local populations, and chance, the contours are always in flux. It is something like a series of town meetings held throughout a state. Decisions are positive here, negative there, but when averaged, constitute the will of the people of the state.

The distinction between these two visions must have originated in fundamental differences in outlook. Fisher began his career as a mathematician and saw genetics statistically. Wright learned genetics by studying the inheritance of coat colors of guinea pigs, whose individuality was plain to see in the variable patterns of colors of their fur. It was known that the colors arose from chemically characterized pigments, which caused Wright to imagine the variations to be associated with genetic differences in the enzymes by which such pigments were formed and degraded (2). He was a physiologist through and through! So it is no wonder that he saw evolution occurring in a local, piecemeal way. It had to be so because it was living individuals who were its instruments, living individuals who, in comprising the selectively fit who reproduced and the selectively unfit who did not, accounted for local variations in frequencies of genes and diseases. Furthermore, local evolution could be rapid here even when slow somewhere else, while when the evolving population was the whole species, the pace was necessarily slow.

The Fisherian view of selection and change has little appeal in medicine; it is too remote from the individual, who is the object of scrutiny in a medical encounter. But Wright's idea of local fluxes in small populations is comfortably accommodated in medical genetics, where founder effects, migration, and concentration of traits in population isolates are all standard fare. Indeed, they are standard fare because of Wright's ideas, and they are clarifying ideas for students coming into medicine. For example, if a disease is represented as a consequence of vulnerability in one or more unit steps of homeostasis, each of which is specified by a gene, then the likelihood of encountering that disease in a given population is correlated with the frequency of that gene in that population. So, when thinking about diseases, the genetic constitution of a population is critical for an understanding, not only of distributions of morbidity, but of potential disease, and we may wish to characterize populations according to the frequencies of their genes. Ashkenazi Jewish populations are an example. They are known for high frequencies of genes for Tay-Sachs, Gaucher disease, Bloom syndrome, dysautonomia, and the BRCA 1 gene for breast cancer. And there are others: a high frequency of adrenogenital syndrome among Aleuts in Alaska and tyrosinemia in Quebec, and the concentrations of thalassemia among Mediterranean populations are well known. There is a large literature on the subject, including several books (3–6).

The point is that, in these interpopulation variations in frequencies of disease-associated genes, there are echoes of Sewall Wright's fitness contour map. In reducing the fitness of their victims, these genes detract from the average fitness in the population and so draw that parameter down toward a valley. In reality it is unlikely that the genes associated with rare and noxious disease detract much from the average fitness even of the populations where they are most in evidence—the diploid state sees to that—but they are informative in revealing in molecular detail how selection and evolution work through physiological properties, through the influences of genes on the proteins of the unit steps of homeostasis. And if the average fitness of populations is little affected by rare genes, it is surely more responsive to others that are more frequent and that act in concert to lead to vulnerability to diseases more frequently experienced. So the frequencies of diseases and their genes are a practical application of population genetics, itself representing a confluence between Darwinism and Mendelism.

DISEASE FREQUENCY, GENE FREQUENCY

What does it mean when we ask the frequency of a disease? If we approach the question in a typological frame of mind, the answer seems straightforward:

it is expressed in incidence and prevalence, the figures that appear in annual tables and statistics and that raise all sorts of questions. How and under what conditions was the diagnosis made? Is there a point at which the disease is so mild as to be subclinical and so not included? What populations were studied, which ethnic groups, which cultures, and where in the world? And what is the mortality, expressed per annum, per case, and per unit of the population? Does it vary from year to year and place to place? All these, and others, are conventional epidemiological questions that bear on disease frequency.

Such questions are asked by geneticists, too. They have importance, for example, in counts of people with inborn errors; one must know the incidence of an inborn error before committing state resources to screening programs. Other questions are asked: Is the disease observed principally in one ethnic group? Is it concentrated in communities and population isolates? Is the frequency affected by assortative mating or consanguinity? All of these questions, both epidemiological and genetic, probe the origins of Wright's map of peaks and valleys, where fitnesses (and diseases) vary with distributions of genes and the experiences with which their products are in varying degree congruent.

Disease Frequency

When thinking typologically, we ask about the frequency of a disease, but the population thinker adds the question of why frequencies are what they are. Why is one disease rare and another common? For both questions, we must know something of the qualities and the quantities of genes and provocative experiences and of the qualities of the affected homeostasis, but the why questions are most comfortably answered if asked in an evolutionary context. Given a species that is well accommodated to environments commonly encountered, rare diseases must be a consequence of (a) breaches of adaptation due to rare genetic variants that invariably make their victims unfit—that is, many of the conventional inborn errors of metabolism; (b) chance encounters with environments infrequently met and that are inimical to us all—for example, cyanide poisoning; or (c) chance encounters in which a rare genetic variant meets an infrequent and alien environment—for example, paralysis and apnea in patients with atypical cholinesterase alleles, when succinylcholine is used as a muscle relaxant.

As for common diseases, at least for those where provocative experiences are known, they are due mainly to encounters with environments that have been systematically altered from those to which the species had, in evolution, become reconciled. These changes have occurred in response to social and cultural imperatives that are at odds with genetic adaptation and so lead to diseases either of deficiency of that which is needed for development and maintenance or of intolerance, a consequence of experiences that overtax aspects of the genetically constituted homeostasis. Some of these provocations are (a) socioeconomic status, both high and low; (b) increased population densities that have altered the population dynamics of microorganisms; (c) dietary and other social habits for which human beings are not genetically prepared; and (d) toxic byproducts and effluvia of industrial societies unknown and undreamed of when the human genome settled into more or less its present state. And each of these provocations varies in kind, intensity, and duration, and is mediated by a homeostasis made variably vulnerable or resistant to it by one or more variant unit steps, which means that some people are more likely than others to express consequences in the form of disease, and among these, some more severely than others.

So, what enters into the estimation of disease frequency? A mathematician might say that the frequency of a disease would be the product of the probability of the relevant genes appearing together in one individual times the likelihood that such an individual would encounter a provoking experience. But there would be qualifiers having to do with, for example, the relative importance of the genes in bringing the pathogenesis to overt expression. Which is the "main" gene and what is its frequency as opposed to modifiers? And there is the kind, intensity, and duration of provocation. A further qualifier not unrelated to these is penetrance.

Variable Penetrance

Penetrance is a conventional drosophila usage; a gene known to be present fails to be expressed. Typically the concept was invoked when a gene skipped a generation, identifying flies of the intervening generation as nonexpressing carriers. The word had the same meaning in the early years of medical genetics, but it more or less disappeared in the era of biochemical genetics because nearly always minor clinical differences could be found or some expression could be elicited in a tolerance test. Now, in the molecular age, the word is again in common usage in connection with the models designed to test for linkage.

But although it was always a descriptive word and conjured up no visions of mechanism, paradoxically, in these times when genes and their actions appear in molecular guise, it may have some conceptual virtues. A disease is usually counted only if it is in evidence: the factors of pathogenesis have come together to generate the symptoms or signs that bring a patient to a doctor or a hospital. But what of individuals who appear to have the same factors but have no disease—or have so little as to escape the notice of patient and physician? "Appear to have" are the governing words here. For example, the unaffected may not have precisely the same alleles, a difference readily detected by a sensitive homeostasis. Or it may be the same allele, even to the last nucleotide, but the powers of the homeostatic system to which the gene contributes its product may be such as to compensate—that is, the other elements may enhance the flux through a pathway. Or still other systems may act to degrade or excrete an accumulating metabolite, or otherwise to galvanize the system to preserve the steady state—that is, the impact of the same allele may vary with the qualities of the developmental matrix. Another possibility is that a dose of the provocative agent sufficient to precipitate symptoms in most genetic susceptibles fails to overwhelm a genetically resistant homeostasis, and to maintain the symmetry, we might say the provocation is "impenetrant."

These qualifying circumstances are of far less moment in the classical inborn errors in which the gene effect is usually easily observed with only modest modification and there is no need for provocative contributions from the outside. But the worth of a descriptive concept such as penetrance is more evident in the never-never land of multifactorial disease. There the full range of penetrance is likely to characterize each disease.

Individuality is a principal quality of disease. That is, the outcomes of a given agent of proximate cause vary from expression overt and severe to something trifling or even undetectable. What, then, is the frequency of the disease? To the machine thinker who adheres to the essentialist version of disease, the frequency is measured by counting the number of cases with the signs and symptoms that bring the patient to the notice of the doctor. But for the population-preventive thinker who subscribes to the nominalist concept, incipient disease, or just the assembly of the factors of cause, assume the importance of the overt version. So what is there to count? The genes most closely associated with pathogenesis? The modifiers? The kinds, intensities, and duration of provocative experiences?

It is perhaps not surprising that medical practice has been more or less limited to the management of overt disease observed by physicians only when patients present themselves with complaints. And yet if we would have a comprehensive understanding of disease, we have to include in addition to that which is readily enumerated: (a) that which is expected to be but is not; (b) that which is only barely detectable, and (c) that which, in time, may be detected. The genes associated with these conditions that do not enter counts of frequency will surely be exposed by molecular analysis, and they are equally sure to be among the most vexing problems facing physicians in the age of genetic medicine because how are we going to know what, in the absence of intervention, their outcomes will be?

Occult Disease

A different influence on frequency is revealed in intrauterine disease (7). When counted at birth, frequencies of trisomies, deletions, and other chromosomal anomalies are always manifold fewer than those for the same anomalies when counted among abortuses. Evidently there is strong selection against these deformities in utero. As for the variations in aberrations between chromosomes, they could be telling us that the unrepresented trisomies are lethal. Monosomy of any chromosome, for example, is the least common—indeed, is limited to the X. Are we to believe that monosomy never occurs? Or that when it does, it blights the embryo, perhaps even before implantation? If it is true that a large proportion of conceptuses never get to term, most must be lost before implantation.

Now, in the medicine that is confined to self-announced patients, fetal wastage is of interest mainly to couples who complain of infertility, but it is unlikely to be perceived as throwing light on any comprehensive concept of disease. But if our concept of medicine is to be based on logic, we have to go beyond patient complaints to describe the subclinical, acknowledge the lethal, and even, if we would grasp its limits, to understand what disease is not.

The lesson for medicine is that what is unobserved is as illuminating of the logic of disease as what is evident. That there is some amount of genetic material we cannot do without is intuitively self-evident, but that losses are going on in utero may be telling us things not so obvious. That is, these unseen losses of conceptuses that lack critical genetic substance are subject to the earliest and harshest onslaught of natural selection. And if there is chromosome loss, why not also mutants that lead to classical inborn errors of critical unit steps of the expanding homeostasis of the embryo, steps that involve conserved molecules critical for the most rudimentary processes—chromosome replication, cell division, energy metabolism, and the like? And both, representing the earliest onset of disease, demonstrate the beginning of a progressive narrowing of its repertory; its range is never again so great as at conception.

Multiple Diseases

Why don't people have several diseases at once? The answer is that some do, but where genetic differences are influential, the frequencies are multiples of those of the genes involved. So there should be a frequency distribution in the whole population of human beings in which unlucky outliers on one side have several or many genetic susceptibilities, some or several of which will be overtly expressed in the lifetime, while their more fortunate brethren at the other end have none at all. The former die in utero or otherwise prematurely; the latter are privileged to experience the decline of a healthy old age. Since it is the nature of such distributions to drop off from the mean, outliers are infrequent. The modal position is at the moment unknown. So, do we all have some genes that put us at risk for something? No doubt, but the risk must often be contingent, dependent upon the simultaneous presence of other genes of certain type and requisite number, upon developmental qualities, and upon experiences, perhaps at particular phases of the lifetime. It is a promise of the Human Genome Project to provide lists of genes that constitute risk. But what we do about those risks has yet to be decided.

CONCLUSION

If disease is to be perceived as a consequence of incongruence between homeostasis and experiences of the environment, the forces that account for the qualities, frequencies, and effects of both the specific genes and the experiences that have conspired to produce disease are the remote causes that engendered the proximate causes that set the stage for pathogenesis. It is remarkable, even humbling, to observe how thoroughly medicine is shaped by those forces. We are a reactive profession. We dance to a tune played by biological and cultural evolution. Molecular genetics has shown how the music was generated in phylogeny, and how it constrains the dancer. Unlike artists who give life to what never existed before, our creativity is devoted to learning how we must adapt to and blunt those remote causes. And to that end we have erected medical schools, departments, specialties. And medical education.

21

Heterogeneity

It is this that draws us back and back to the Greeks; the stable, the permanent, the original human being is to be found there . . . we understand
them more easily and more directly than we understand the characters in
the Canterbury Tales. These are the originals, Chaucer's the varieties, of
the human species.
        —Virginia Woolf, "On Not Knowing Greek" (1)

Mrs. Woolf has acutely drawn the difference between the essence and
the variant. The Greeks are stable, permanent, and original, and
they are a standard, a type, and a model for human aspiration. In contrast,
Chaucer's motley band of pilgrims exemplify human variation. They exhibit
the range of human heterogeneity.

Webster's dictionary defines *heterogeneity* as "differing in kind, or made
up of dissimilar ingredients." In medicine the word is most often used in relation to dissimilar causes of similar phenotypes. Heterogeneity of cause can be
genetic—the same phenotype can have genetically diverse origins—or it may
arise in different experiences of the environment; or versions of the same phenotype may be a result of variation in both.

Why should it be necessary here to define a word so frequently used in medical genetics? It is necessary precisely because of its infrequent use wherever typological thinking holds sway. Recall that the typologist relies on abstract qualities such as means and dispersions, where emphasis is given to the parameter
rather than the individual. Who has not observed the intellectual contortions
of clinicians who wish to label discordant cases with well-established diagnoses? The cases are acknowledged to be variants, but they are believed to be
variants of that which is already well known. But why could they not equally
represent something new—that is, different causes of phenotypic similarities,
perhaps causes not previously described? That requires population thinking,
wherein the concrete reality of individuality is uppermost. When each individual is perceived as unique, then diversity of both cause and phenotype comes
to mind first, not last.

Genetic Heterogeneity

The first evidence of genetic heterogeneity was Mendel's observation of alternative forms of the traits of peas; heterogeneity was observed even when the definition of the gene was only statistical. This was followed by the drosophilists' definition of systems of multiple alleles, a definition based on an operational gene. Later, when biologists began to take an interest in the genetics of disease, reference was made to different genetic causes of the same disease; for example, J. B. S. Haldane alluded to dominant and recessive forms of retinitis pigmentosa in 1941 (2). But the idea of heterogeneity did not enjoy wide use in medical genetics until there was a functional definition of the gene. An early example is that of the recessive and dominant forms of methemoglobinemia described in the 1940s. The recessive form was attributed to reduced activity of the enzyme NADH dehydrogenase, while the dominant type was associated with an abnormality of globin (3). Further heterogeneity of this inborn error has been uncovered since; many allelic variants of NADH dehydrogenase have been found, and there are mutants in both alpha and beta chains of globin to account for the variety of the dominant disease. A second early example is cystinuria, described by Harris et al. in 1950, an inborn error which the reader may recall was one of Garrod's original four (4). Two forms of the disorder emerged, both inherited as recessives, but families differed in whether heterozygotes excreted lysine and arginine. In the heterozygotes of one set of families these amino acids were easily detected, while in those of the other set there were none. The conclusion was that the families were characterized by mutants at different loci, and the principle of within-family likeness and between-family difference was demonstrated clearly.

Later, when genes had been given a structural definition, variants in the structure of protein products were observed in all sorts of inborn errors, revealing more allelic variation than had been suspected. And today, when he molecularly defined gene can be characterized in sequences of base pairs, the variation is beyond anything imaginable at any other level of definition of the gene. Thus it became the rule to look for genetic heterogeneity on the assumption that it might be found, and today the rule is that it exists unless shown not to; molecular analysis of inborn errors invariably exposes genetic variants.

This idea of heterogeneity has been cultivated mainly in the medical sphere where precision in describing relationships between expressions and their causes may make a difference in management. It is not that biologists are unaware of, or uninterested in, say, allelism. Rather, the problems they study do not necessarily call for a molecular analysis of all possible variants of the genes whose properties they study. In contrast, journals reporting work in medical genetics are filled with just such descriptions. In medicine, wherever there is evidence of gene action, the search for heterogeneity is mandatory.

MONOGENIC DISEASES

What forms does genetic heterogeneity take, how is it detected, and how does it make a difference? The concept is best illustrated in monogenic disease, wherein allelic heterogeneity is easily contrasted with that of mutants at different loci. An initial clue is provided by clinical variations, sometimes rather subtle. For example, intrafamily likeness is high and interfamily difference is great in such clinical expressions as age at onset, sex differences, severity, or response to treatment.

So today genetic heterogeneity is the rule, a consequence partly of the incursion of genetics into medical thinking and partly of our detailed knowledge of cell structure and function. If gene-specified proteins are the basis for structure and function, and if it is acknowledged that all genes are not only mutable but subject to change in all of their parts, then genetic heterogeneity is inevitable. It is allelic because mutation is random and multilocal wherever several proteins serve one or allied functions.

Allelic heterogeneity is everywhere to be found. Abnormalities of the enzyme glucose-6-phosphate dehydrogenase are exemplary. Three hundred seventy-six variants are associated with expressions that run all the way from congenital and unvarying hemolytic anemia to no discernible effect. And in between is variable susceptibility to the adverse effects of drugs and other agents that provoke a reversible hemolysis differing in degree according to the variant - (5). Evidence for multilocal heterogeneity is given in tabular form in *Metabolic and Molecular Bases of Inherited Disease*, which lists, for example, ten genetic and physiologically distinct forms of glycogen storage disease, twelve hemolytic anemias based on mutants of the enzymes of the glycolytic pathway, and a half dozen distinct disorders of enzymes in the urea cycle, among much else.

Molecular analysis of allelic variation in any inborn error reveals a far wider range of variants in both kind and number than could be predicted on clinical grounds. When the disease under scrutiny is relatively frequent—cystic fibrosis and phenylketonuria are examples—most of the families share two or three common mutants, while those of the remainder are unique. So, since the diseases are recessive, many of the cases are true homozygotes while others are compounds; some include one of the common mutants and others two rare ones. But when the disease is rare, all, or nearly all, of the mutants are unique and all of the cases are compounds. These conditions were predicted by J. B. S. Haldane on the basis of the principles of genetics elaborated by the drosophilists. And they make sense. The common variants aggregate because of aggregation in ethnic or cultural group, heterozygote advantage, or chance, while the rare ones are either new mutants, necessarily rare, or old mutants which, despite selective disadvantage, have been carried along for generations, awaiting their extinction in the lotteries of gametogenesis and fertilization. Or they may go down in the flames of recessive disease in consequence of a consanguineous mating or after migration into a population that carries one of the common variants, or simply in an offspring of a union occurring with a chance of one in a million or less. Nowhere is the normally unobtrusive hand of remote causes more plainly revealed.

These outcomes, as so much else in genetic medicine, are based on principles elaborated in the context of monogenic disease and therefore strongly influenced by the drosophila agenda. But most disease is not monogenic; in most disease the genetic contribution is multiple. So the question arises, what forms does genetic heterogeneity take in multifactorial disease?

MULTIFACTORIAL DISEASES

The single gene disorders that have so preoccupied the medical geneticists are Virginia Woolf's Greeks. They are, for the most part, straightforward. They segregate in families and, in principle, when we understand one, we have a good basis for understanding others. But the diseases of complex origin are something else; they are as variegated, as multifarious, as Chaucer's pilgrims. That is, while necessarily variations on the theme of the monogenic inborn error— the genes of multifactorial phenotypes segregate and specify unit steps of homeostasis, too—the range of phenotypic variability and of genetic heterogeneity are multiples of those of their monogenic homologs. So how do we think about them (6)? To begin, we must recognize a continuity that dissipates the typological separation inherent in the prefixes *mono-* and *multi-*. The complex disorders are variants of the monogenic which, in their way, are also multigenic. So, to bring unity to the concept of both, we must again shed our drosophiline thinking and concentrate on the unit step of homeostasis.

The monogenic disorders are perceived as bona fide diseases because of the apparent one-to-one relationship between gene and phenotype; they are segregating effects of variants of a unit step in some homeostatic system. But other genes explain some of the variability, and the only way they can influence the expression of the disease is through their impact on the unit steps they specify, which in turn influences those of still others. When one step in a system is deficient or otherwise perturbed, others will try to compensate, and whether and how they do so is a property of the qualities of the molecules specified by the genes involved. Some compensators will be robust but some may be less competent or even deficient themselves, and, failing in their compensatory duties, they only enhance the failure of the first. In this the genes will be said to interact, or to be epistatic. But there has been no interaction of genes; rather, the integration of homeostatic steps has been compromised by the qualities of the proteins specified by both "main" gene and modifiers.

How Do Monogenic-Multigenic Phenotypes Differ?

The differences between monogenic and complex disorders arise principally from the position of the relevant genes in the gradient of selective effect. The genes of the former are apt to be high in the gradient and to impose great burdens in the form of early mortality, reduced reproduction, and permanent disability, while those of the latter are scattered widely throughout the midportion so that main genes, defined as those specifying the most critical homeostatic damage, and modifiers are more nearly equal in their influence, and each imposes less burden than the single gene in the monogenic inborn error. These genes are likely to be more frequent than those of the monogenic disorders, and are often polymorphic and tolerable in homeostasis except when hard pressed by experiences. Theoretically we might even conjure up a disease involving very numerous unit steps presided over by very numerous genes, each with so little more or so little less impact than the others as to characterize the disease as a consequence of a chorus of modifiers. The point is that the disease, in its pathogenesis and its signs and symptoms, is caused not by the genes themselves but by their influences on specific protein unit steps of homeostasis. The modification is mediated in every instance by a protein performing either to compensate for the inadequacy of another or to weaken it still more.

Models

We have good models for the monogenic disorders, but is there something to guide our thinking about the complex? A brief digression into the past is illuminating here. Until recently, theories of multifactorial disease were largely typological—perhaps perforce, since they were based on the operational gene which meant that data for genetic analysis of individuals in families were lacking. A popular approach was that of Falconer, who envisioned a continuous distribution of measures of susceptibility to disease. These were composed of influences of both genes and experiences of the environment, and included a point representing a threshold beyond which appeared affected individuals (7). The data could be used in the calculation of coefficients of heritability that assigned relative contributions to the variance of genes and experiences.

There are many variants of Falconer's model, with and without thresholds and often including recondite mathematics, but in none can any individual human being be distinguished, so we are left with a strongly typological description; all those above the threshold have the disease, while those below do not. The model offers no inkling of what influences accumulate and conspire to push an individual up to or beyond the threshold, nor any understanding of what differentiates such an individual from another who remains below it. The genes invoked in this model were "main genes" and "polygenes," entirely operational concepts. The former were presumed to give the disease its character, and the latter constituted a background upon which the main genes imposed their stamp. Polygenes were endowed with the mysterious power of "additiveness," which hints at some quantitative influence, and initially it was the number of polygenes that boosted the phenotype up to and over the threshold. In time the polygenes became modifiers, in deference to the structural definition of genes as specifiers of protein components of homeostatic systems.

Something like the above appeared in most textbooks of medical genetics published as recently as the late 1980s and early 1990s, in which attention to multifactorial disease was directed mainly to recurrence risks. But in all of these books, reference is also made to new developments that emphasize "risk factors" in the form of genes found in some or many individuals with "diseases of complex origin," a new name signaling a passage from mathematical models relevant to populations to biochemical and molecular analysis suitable for individuals and families. It is another example of the transition from the operational gene to the molecular version, in which the drosophila-appropriate, typological mentality gives way to molecular, population thinking.

So today, the gene hunters, those dauntless Nimrods of the DNA, are strongly disposed to include the complex diseases among their prey, and the outlines of molecular ideas and models are emerging. Detailed description of the methods used in the search for genes is outside the purview of this book, but it must be said that they are based squarely on—what else?—the ideas of linkage of the drosophilists and the operational definition of the gene. But only the searching methods are influenced by the drosophila agenda; the variants the methods discover serve to illuminate pathogenesis and, as risk factors, they take their places for each disease among an array of "genes for." Such arrays are already impressive. For type I diabetes there are a dozen or more, most of unknown homeostatic provenance. There are even more such genes in the list of risk factors for atherosclerosis, and such rosters are being assembled for type II diabetes, high blood pressure, Alzheimer's disease, and others (5,8–11).

A Model of Complex Disease

What sort of model is emerging, however dimly? First of all, it cannot depart entirely from Falconer's statistical distributions of susceptibility. Those distributions were based on intrafamily correlations, so any model of multifactorial disease must account for susceptibility based on both genes and experiences. One way of accommodating both the old and the new is to think of the complex disorders as arranged in a distribution of increasing variability, continuous with that of monogenic diseases. That is, there is a progression based on increasing numbers and kinds of contributors to the phenotype. At first and in closest proximity to disorders called monogenic, are two major genes that give a disease its character, plus some modifiers and experiences to add variability, but the heterogeneity that counts most here is that of the major genes. This trend is continued with increasing attenuation of the contribution of each individual gene and a progressive augmentation in the role of experiences. Here the heterogeneity of both genes and experiences is increased and may confound the investigator by appearing within families as well as between. Finally, the distribution ends in conditions in which experiences, as the major contributors, play over a diverse array of genetic heterogeneity to account for a high degree of individuality. In this progression, the definition of disease becomes more and more nominalist, approaching in the end the definition of every case as his or her own disease.

This description accounts for sources of genetic variation but omits the elements of ontogeny and aging. Mutants high in the selective gradient promote the eruption of disease forcefully and quickly, while those lower in the gradient are likely to be a party to a pathogenesis of deliberate progression, beginning sometimes in infancy or even in utero and moving through ups and downs of intensity to emerge after decades as signs and symptoms, perhaps in old age and promoted by aging. Cancer is the prototype for this mode of origin. Cancer of the large bowel is well known to pass through a series of stages, covering many years from the formation of benign polyps to metastasis (12). And each step is characterized by different genetic variants. Some version of this protracted pathogenesis might explain other conditions as well.

In this abstract treatment, changes in unit steps of homeostasis have played no part, but here I wish to emphasize how the discovery of such variants is changing the way we define and classify disease, including new entities that emerge from old. The old, which were based on signs and symptoms and then on pathophysiology, are giving way to new conditions defined by their genes and their cognate unit steps in homeostasis. For example, several forms of hypertension have been differentiated as single-gene disorders, while other cases, called "essential," have been found to be associated with numerous alleles of polymorphic loci (9,13).

Whether lesser variants at the loci that distinguish the monogenic types of hypertension participate in the essential variety is unknown. It seems plausible; weaknesses, individually of no great moment, may conspire to augment one another's failings to lead to vulnerability. Atherosclerosis and heart attack may be products of such interactions. Variants of the cholesterol transport system, the clotting cascade, the endothelins, and other molecules constitute vulnerabilities that, separately and together, increase the probability of disease. And curiously, some of the loci involved are shared with other diseases: variants of fibrinogen, for example, contribute to clotting disorders as well as, in the form of at least one particular polymorphic allele, to coronary thrombosis (14). And even alleles may be shared. Polymorphic alleles of angiotensin-converting enzyme (ACE) are associated with both hypertension and coronary artery disease (9,15). Perhaps it should be no surprise that given the integration of homeostatic devices, variants in unit steps turn up in more than one disease. We find the same sharing of alleles in different cancers: variants of the p53 repressor gene turn up in many forms of cancer, both inherited and somatic (12). Here the variant fails to regulate the manufacture and use of growth factors that, unrepressed, transcend the otherwise tight integration of cell growth in other physiological systems.

At this point, enter the epidemiologist to correlate clinical expressions with specific genes and homeostatic variants. The question is, are particular alleles associated with particular signs and symptoms and, if so, do they create such divergent clinical expressions as to constitute subtypes or new diseases? In either case, the individuality of the pathophysiology might be such as to require some specificity of both prevention and treatment. Further, the dissection of complex phenotypes and their resolution into the genotypes of origin is likely to hasten the reclassification of disease into something more compatible with its genetic characteristics. Once dropsy and consumption were diseases; now we are traveling rapidly a reductionist path in which variation in the unit step of homeostasis is the central feature of disease. Variants of the unit steps are recruited independently in the lottery of meiosis and fertilization into genotypes, where they put at hazard the homeostatic systems of which they are a part. In some diseases, one such step—or misstep—is enough. In others, it is the concatenation of missteps that lead to disease. Given the opportunities for variety in the replication and assembly of chromosomes, it is no wonder that the same variant steps turn up in diseases that in the present system of classification are perceived as different disorders. Just as domains of genes can be shuffled to produce new genes, so unit steps of homeostasis can be shuffled into combinations that characterize subtypes or even distinct diseases. At the same time, the same unit steps may exist as harmless variants in assemblies of other genes.

So, not only does the discovery of each additional contingent variant constitute yet another nail in the coffin of the essentialist definition of disease, but the name of a disease as it is applied to outcomes of specific constellations of variant unit steps will continue to need reevaluation as more and more of the individuality and heterogeneity of pathogenesis is exposed. That is, we must be open-minded in our use of a name when it is used to embrace all cases sharing similar phenotypes. Perhaps new names or subtypes are required when the resolution at the level of unit steps of homeostasis reveals a heterogeneity in which unrelated cases are unique. And when all relevant unit steps are counted in, heterogeneity may even be intrafamilial. No doubt necessity requires pragmatism in retaining inclusive names, but in understanding proximate cause and pathogenesis we are obliged to pursue a nominalist course.

At present, in naming diseases, we are faced with a hierarchy based on how precisely correlations among causes, pathogenesis, and expressions can be defined. At the top of the list appear conditions of unknown cause, each a product of pathogenesis vaguely understood or not at all, and poorly linked to signs and symptoms. Most behavioral disorders, including psychoses, are in this category. Fifty years ago heart attack and stroke were as enigmatic as psychosis is today, but biochemical and molecular insights into causes and pathogenesis promise to clarify the abundant genetic heterogeneity that is emerging. Such an analysis, while unlikely to reduce these diseases to a level in the hierarchy equivalent to PKU or pneumococcal pneumonia, might result in several overlapping versions of, say, hypertension, each of which, because of clinical differences, might bear a different name, even though some of the genes might be shared. Such inroads into the classification of diseases is likely to be a principal benefit of the Genome Project.

NONGENETIC HETEROGENEITY

The nongenetic causes of disease are no less heterogeneous than the genetic, but they differ significantly from the genetic in two ways. First, genes are discrete, unitary, and present from conception, and every individual of a species is presumed to have the same set of loci, however heterogeneous each individual set of alleles may be. Elements of the environment also have discrete entity, but experiences of them may differ from one individual to another in kind, intensity, and duration of exposure. That is, as opposed to only two doses of a gene at any one locus, whether , alike or different, elements of the environment affecting the function of the product of a specific gene may be very many and can vary widely in amount as well as in whether exposure to it is brief or prolonged, limited to once in a lifetime or intermittent.

This leads us to the second difference. The homeostasis specified by the genes and conditioned by development determines which experiences individuals can tolerate, to what degree, and for how long; the genes, as the instruments of development and adaptation, limit the tolerable heterogeneity of kind, intensity, and duration of experiences of the environment. Not that these limits are for the human species especially narrow, but the concept is important in lodging responsibility for intolerance of the environment with the products of the genes. It could not be otherwise. The individuality of structure and function that characterizes homeostatic design specifies also what the design is for—what it can do and what it cannot accommodate. So while the heterogeneity of the environment that can be experienced by any species is set by the varieties of ecological interactions among the animate and inanimate elements of the earth, the opportunities and limitations of tolerance for each species are set by its genes and its development. The capacity for increasing tolerance, or otherwise escaping pressure, is what evolution is all about, and no doubt every species has within itself the potential to adapt. But such a change in a species is always at the expense of the individuals who do not have that potential. And since in medicine our primary concern is for those who cannot adapt, the principle of limitation of tolerance to an exuberant heterogeneity of the environment is uppermost on our agenda.

So in the end, the genetic evidence has it that there are no Greeks. Essential, permanent, and representative human beings exist only in the poetic imagination. And while we need and value them there, we are all Chaucer's pilgrims, variegated and individual in genes and experiences as well as in the development that is a consequence of how those genes and experiences direct our homeostatic devices. And we are no less variable in our incongruities and in how they dispose us to disease. Who can doubt that, when all is known, it will be seen that one's experience of disease is as characteristic of one's self as the nose on one's face? But however individual, we are still subject to the limitations of species; even Chaucer's band of individuals comprehended only human beings. So human variation, however exuberant, is limited, and in this limitation is an element of unity in disease. But within the limits, the range of disease is both expansive and continuous, qualities that further characterize human disease, and these form the substance of the next chapter.

22

Unity and Continuity of Disease

There are not many differences in mental habit more significant than that between the habit of thinking in discrete, well defined class-concepts and that of thinking in terms of continuity, of infinitely delicate shadings-off of everything into something else, of the overlapping of essences, so that the whole notion of species comes to seem an artifice of thought not truly applicable to the fluency, the, so to say, universal overlappingness of the real world.

—Arthur O. Lovejoy, *The Great Chain of Being*

The differences between typological and population thinking were never more elegantly expressed than in this excerpt from Lovejoy's book. We have observed that the former is characteristic of medical thought when dominated by the machine mentality; the latter is the path of genetic medicine. The chapter on classification is an attempt to reconcile these polar thought processes in a classification that accommodates at once to entities and to individuality. Here this line of thought is pursued in the search for evidence of unity and continuity in medicine.

We begin, as so often in other parts of the book, with a comparison between medicine and biology, in this instance purposes expressed in textbooks. Textbooks of medicine are pretty much alike. They are above all practical—they seldom deal in concepts, and they tend to dispense their information in tight compartments. Obviously they cannot include everything, so what they omit must be that which the editors perceive as less critical for a general understanding, and among these omissions are the concepts of unity and continuity as they apply to disease. Textbooks of biology, in contrast, begin right at the start to elaborate principles that unify the whole subject, and as evolution is their guiding principle, continuity is everywhere in evidence. Logic suggests that what is possible in biology can be done in medicine; if biological congruence exhibits unity and continuity, so must incongruence.

Unity

The unity of disease has been demonstrated in the chapters on the path from gene to phenotype and on classification (see Table 3 in chapter 15). There it was suggested that, ideally, all diseases be described in a hierarchy of expressions along a path from gene to phenotype, and that when the whole of the pathogenesis of all diseases is known, the patterns will, in principle, resemble one another, even when there is much complexity, as in disorders in which numerous elements feed into proximate cause. The central unifying feature of such a principle is, of course, the variant unit step of homeostasis , and today, this kind of unity is exemplified in those inborn errors in which information is available at every level in the hierarchy. How can it be otherwise? If congruence can be described in the hierarchical path from gene to phenotype, then incongruence must be represented as due to one, several, or many variants within in the same hierarchy.

The reason diseases are conventionally described in separate compartments are also revealed in Table 3. They are the same as those that have compelled us to organize information around a classification that precludes generalizations about disease. The factors that unify disease are not apparent when few descriptions can include all levels of the hierarchy, so the most practical path is to treat them all as if there were no common themes, to make do with what comes to hand, and, acknowledging the exigency of medicine, to do what we can. This exigency puts the textbooks of medicine in the position the committees concerned with medical reform do not like. While the description of each disease is coherent and complete—indeed, a casual reader must be impressed by the labor and care that go into the assembly of so much, and such diverse, information—the editors are generally at less pains to emphasize qualities that bind the whole together.

Still, in some recent editions the existence of, even the need for, unity is recognized in two ways. One is in the uniformity of the presentation and description of diseases. For each disorder, etiology and epidemiology are followed by pathogenesis, signs, symptoms, the course of the illness, and, finally, management and prognosis. In this way it is acknowledged that all diseases can be described in the same terms—for example, all must have an onset, whether it be at fertilization or after a life of one hundred years, and all must have causes, frequencies, and distributions in human societies. Obvious, one might say. Yes, but we are concerned with education here, and the obvious that is left unspoken may remain unobserved.

Second, the books present introductory sections on, for example, symptomatology or common signs or general principles of growth and development and aging, all evidence of common properties of disease. The implication is, that since we are all human, it can be no surprise that pain, fever, anorexia, and rashes are symptoms and signs that transcend the classes of disease or that nearly all of the diverse disorders of the heart can end up in shortness of breath, edema, and other evidence of organ failure.

So, unity is not absent from the plans and lucubrations of the editors of textbooks of medicine, but they could go further; other indications of unity could be brought to the consciousness of the student. First, the texts could include a reminder of the inborn vulnerability in all disease that has been emphasized again and again in this book. A second unity is revealed in the definition of disease as a consequence of incongruence between a gene-specified homeostasis and experiences of the environment expressed in a developmental matrix. All three time frames—phylogeny, ontogeny, and the moment—are represented in all diseases. A third reminder lies in the realization that all of the diseases that could exist are latent in the genetic structure and physiology of the species. There can be no surprises. A mad scientist might design a drug of mass destruction or engineer a unique virus unlike any in nature, either of which might cause diseases previously unknown. But such diseases are diseases only because drug or virus has attacked their victims at some point or points in an existing physiological homeostasis that, however well adapted to the ordinary demands of the life of an open system, represents in the context of drug or microorganism a point of vulnerability.

Fourth, those same constraints limit the repertory of possible diseases. For example, although the human genome carries homeogenes similar to those of drosophila, human mutants of these genes do not produce a fetus with a leg growing out of the head, analogous to the anomaly caused by the aristapedia mutant in flies. No doubt the human genetic program rules such a mutant out of bounds. It is either lethal or the processes of development divert its effects into some other phenotype compatible with the existing plan. And a fifth unity is expressed in the manifest continuity both within and between diseases, a continuity that represents the plenitude of disease; both within and between diseases, all grades of disorder that can occur, will occur.

CONTINUITY

Having been at pains, in the chapter on classification, to find a scheme for assorting entities into discrete groups, it may seem a contradiction to advance here the idea that those same entities represent elements in a continuum of any kind. But continuity is, in fact, a further unifying characteristic. It is not that the diseases blend one into another to fulfill a continuous whole. That is clearly nonsense. Rather there are continuities, both within diseases and between them, in relation to causes, signs, symptoms, pathogenesis, and outcomes. And there are continuities in time and in relation to natural selection.

Continuity is a prominent feature of human ideas and experiences. There is a continuity of time, of phylogeny, of generations, and of ontogeny. Our biology, even that of the brain, partakes of the same principles of molecular biology, biochemistry, and physiology as other forms of life. It is true that there is a discontinuity of species; isolation allows populations to take different evolutionary paths and so to speciate. But we know that the continuity of physiological properties remains; bacteria can be persuaded to produce human proteins when human genes are inserted, and there is an extraordinary conservation of gene sequence that is reflected in amino acid sequences in proteins and in function. So there is a continuity of phylogeny that transcends the discontinuity of species as well as that which separates the individuals of which they are composed. And we have already remarked the continuity of genomes in which no completely new gene, unrelated in structure to any other, has been demonstrated to turn up all of a sudden. Rather, genes duplicate and form families that may diverge in function.

As for human individuals, we pursue our destinies through time from conception to a venerable end without the interruption of discontinuity. A woman's pregnancy, the onset of menses, the birth of her baby, and the menopause, however suddenly they come to notice, have all been in preparation for some time, and the genesis of these events has been latent in the inherited genetic program from the beginning. Perhaps the only discontinuities in a biological life are its beginning and its end. This is not to say that disease does not create discontinuities in the lives of individuals; anyone who has been sick knows that today's symptoms are worlds apart from yesterday's health. Rather, it is to say that the experiences of disease represent quantitative departures from existing norms and, as such, they are in no way released from the constraints of continuity.

Does disease (and do diseases) show this continuity in all of their qualities? Given that diseases are consequences of incongruence of some kind, their qualities must consist not of anything novel, but of distortion of the congruent state. Their signs and symptoms, which reflect a disordered homeostasis, are constrained by the qualities of the normal homeostasis, so if continuity is a property of life in general and of health in particular, it must be a property of disease.

The Characteristics of Disease

In this section we examine salient features shared by all diseases for evidence of continuity. The characteristics are set out in the left column of Table 5. Do these features show relationships with one another? Are there ways to analyze them together? Do they show the continuities just described? That is, can we say that they show gradations both across and within diseases?

Let's look at the list beginning with mode of inheritance and affected rel-

Table 5 Qualities of Disease Together with Correlated Normal Properties

Disease Character	Normal Property
Mode of inheritance and affected relatives	Distribution of habits, living styles
Age at onset	Developmental milestones
Latency	Genes and development
Frequency of disease	Frequency of individual qualities
Diagnostic specificity	Prominence of normal qualities
Number of diseases	Extent of individuality
Burden	Robustness, fecundity, handicap
Sex differences	Cultural
Influence of migration	Changes in mores, languages
Secular change	Aging, changes in ideas, habits, aims in life
Effect of socioeconomic status	Variation in disease and development

atives. Diseases may be dominant or recessive, show loss of function, gain of function, or other of the many dominant expressions—all seeming discontinuities. And yet these designations are possible only in relation to families. They represent, in addition to their physiological meanings, modes of inheritance, and their continuity within families is demonstrated in affected relatives. It might be said that the affected state represents a discontinuity, and so it is. But whether and how a gene is expressed in one person is, in part, a property of what else is inherited from the parental store of genes; disease allows no escape from the familial stamp.

Age at onset and latency are expressions of gene action in the developmental matrix which we know to be in continual flux. They tell us how pathogenesis has compromised the normal homeostatic dynamic to produce, early or late, the expressions of disease. If late, the process has been cumulative, perhaps even from the beginning of life, and the constant effort to adjust and repair has become a part of the pathogenesis itself.

The frequency of disease is a reflection of several familial properties: the mating pattern of the parents, their ethnic origins, and the social and cultural milieus wherein the affected have been exposed—or not—to provocative experiences. And obviously, the frequency of some diseases must vary with changes in the socioeconomic position of the family.

Why are there so many diseases, and why are some so easily diagnosed while others are nebulous in outline and elusive in description? These properties also flow directly from the mechanisms of congruence. The number of disorders that originate in defects in single steps of homeostasis is limited to the number of genes that specify and control the proteins that mediate those steps. Ordinarily these are relatively easily described because of their circumscribed pathogenesis. Diseases of more complex origins involving at the start more than one step in homeostasis are limited only by the number of steps and the kinds and degrees of their integration—not much of a limit. And diagnostic specificity varies inversely with the complexity of the web of causes and pathogenesis; disease phenotypes can be no less emergent than such normal qualities as stature, blood pressure, and behavior. And as complexity increases, so does the opportunity for individuality in the expression of disease. The logic of this continuity predicts that at some level of complexity, the expression of every individual within the range of pathogenesis and clinical picture that comprises a particular disease, will have been attained by a different path, and each person will be said to have his or her own disease. Even so, however distinctive, it is necessarily only a specific version of the disease because it is constrained by limits imposed by family, species, and phylogeny.

The burden of disease, as measured by threat to life, severity of symptoms, or residual handicap, varies from one disease to another as well as within each, the variation being a property of what has been inherited and experienced. Indeed, the variation may be such as to soften, or even to nullify, the consequences of proximate cause, and we say that the disorder is mild or subclinical, or, although the requisite genes and, therefore, homeostatic vulnerability may be present, without provocation there is no disease at all.

Sex in human beings is nearly bimodal, but not quite, as witness the many forms of intersex. But there is no such dichotomy in the effects of sex on the measurable expression of many diseases which, even while differing in means, show a good deal of overlap. And the scope for continuous variation in disease is at a maximum in relation to the influence of SES, migration, and secular change, where variable environments interact with the variable products of the numerous alleles of many loci.

There are other continuities expressed in the qualities of disease listed in Table 5. All are measurable—including mode of inheritance, which varies from monogenic to multifactorial as well as in phenotype—and all vary continuously both among diseases and within them. For example, since each disorder has an age at onset and a burden, they can be arranged in order from the earliest onset to the latest and from the most burdensome to the least. And there are correlations—for example, diseases of earliest onset are likely to be rare, inherited, numerous, burdensome, and uninfluenced by SES, while those of later onset are more frequent, multifactorial, less burdensome, and influenced by SES. These features vary within diseases, too, sometimes widely and often together. And so it is with the other qualities.

CONTINUITY WITH HEALTH

Variations within and among diseases that include mild disease, subclinical states, and lack of expression of latent cause suggest a variation that continues without rift into the healthy state to encompass normal counterparts of the qualities of disease. These are listed on the right in Table 5.

For each characteristic listed in the left-hand column there is a normal quality. If disease is actually a consequence of incongruence, then there must be a corresponding congruent state; if disease originates in an aberration of homeostasis, then it may be represented as the normal gone wrong. So we are likely to find its counterpart in the nondiseased. This is not to say that health is the absence of disease; health has its own qualities, its own definition. Rather, it is to say that since both engage the same homeostasis, there must be resemblances in how they do so.

To begin, mode of inheritance means familial aggregation, and although we expect, and do observe, mendelian segregation of monogenic polymorphisms that are unassociated with disease, we expect aggregation for such qualities as coloration, body size, cognitive qualities, and the like to be irregular and not to mendelize. But the variation in some of these—for example, body size—comes perilously close to disease or, as in extreme obesity, may be perceived as such or at the very least as contributing to other disorders. On the other hand, small stature tails off into dwarfism, while the other extreme, which may lead to fame and fortune as a basketball player, may also represent something of a handicap in a culture designed expressly for people who cluster around the mean.

Age at onset of disease has its counterpart in the ages of attainment of developmental milestones—talking, walking, puberty, menopause, and signs of aging. And, again, these may be familial traits and shade off into states that are hardly distinguishable from disease. For example, the fifteen-year-old boy who has not yet entered puberty but will soon do so may give the child, his family, and the pediatrician some uneasy moments. And the girl who has early onset of menses followed by early fusion of her epiphyses ending up at 4′11″ is not really abnormal but is on the brink; her height may be in some ways a handicap, depending upon conditions both of her choice and imposed upon her.

As to frequency, we have seen that the more extreme the burden, the rarer the disease. This quality is duplicated in nondisease, where all sorts of extremes are infrequent—for example, outstanding talents, aesthetic, athletic, mechanical, or intellectual. One has to doubt that everyone could gain employment as, for example, a tea taster, capable of distinguishing dozens, perhaps hundreds, of different teas. Nor can we all hope to excel in memory, mathematics, or manual dexterity, no matter what our opportunities. The hand of nature is here no less apparent than in disease. Measurable properties are distributed continuously; there are few bimodalities. This is a consequence of balancing selection: nature chips away at both extremes.

In health, latency is represented in the developmental trajectories that account for life's history in obedience to the influences of genes and experiences in the daily creation of a new developmental matrix. Since life is a dynamic process, whatever happens in its various phases must be outcomes of distant events or longstanding processes that shape the conditions for still later development. We have already seen how long is the latency for overt evidence of aging.

Diagnostic specificity has its equivalent in the prominence or mediocrity of normal characters—flaming red hair, for example, or a roman nose, great beauty of face or figure, and those talents cited earlier. All of these are qualities easily distinguished and that cause individuals to stand out from the rest of us, whose less memorable characteristics cause us, perhaps, to be easily mistaken for others or to be treasured by our friends for our "inner" selves.

As to number, since we are here comparing the expression of the ordered homeostasis with that of the disordered, the counterpart of the number of diseases exemplary of the latter might be the diversity of ways the ordered homeostasis can, as an open system, attain a steady state, a number we might suppose to equal that of individuals in the population.

Burden in disease is measured in threat to life, curtailment of reproduction, and residual handicap. Obviously, the antithetical qualities are robustness of health, fecundity, intelligence, and social competence. And there are degrees of health, energy, and resistance. Fertility can be uncertain, while reading and learning disabilities, neurotic behavior, and lack of opportunity can be handicaps that, while not perceived as diseases, may seriously constrain hope and expectations of a full life.

Sex differences in disease are due to the genetic and hormonal differentiation of the sexes, as well as to cultural properties of gender. Their normal counterpart resides in gender distinctions having to do with mating, reproduction, and child rearing. Some differences such as gestation, birth, and breastfeeding are biologically regulated, but many of the traits called masculine or feminine are now shared in varying degree. For example, the duties of child rearing and the maintenance of the household are now often shared, while women regularly aim for positions in industry, business, and professions that, in the past, have been more often attained by men.

Migration often leads to new modes of living, new languages, and new habits, with, as we have seen, new diseases as a result. But the fact that migration works both ways—that the health of the migrant is often improved—is little noted in genetic circles, even if emphasized by epidemiologists who stress the strong correlation between all aspects of life and socioeconomic conditions. The strength of the family, education, and opportunity all require some degree of social and economic security.

To summarize, we cannot overlook the fact that all of these properties of both health and disease are inherent in genetic, developmental, social, and cultural qualities expressed in families. Now, since families are the vehicles for the reproduction of the species and the development of individuals, the diseases expressed within them, in representing adaptive failure, are no less continuous with species and phylogeny than are the congruent qualities that represent adaptive success. If so, logic suggests that each episode of disease should be regarded as a familial problem and dealt with accordingly. Those who champion family medicine have already perceived this logic, which is antithetical to the mentality that sees each case as an isolated instance of mechanical dysfunction.

A Gradient of Selective Effect

I have referred in other chapters to a gradient of selective effect. Here it reappears as a cardinal example of the continuity of disease. There are several reasons that such a gradient should exist. First, the imperfection of mutational and recombinational events at meiosis is species business, and it is transacted in perfect indifference to the life or happiness of individual inheritors. And much of such novelty makes its heirs the object of "purifying" selection. So we human beings lead two lives: in one we are inheritors, generators, and transmitters of the variation that maintains the species; in the other, each of us uses a unique endowment to make a life of individual expression. It is a remarkable device and one that works well in the interest of the species and of most individuals, too, but sometimes these purposes conflict and incongruence arises. Second, since the mutations range in degree of damage to the DNA from losses of whole chromosomes to harmless base substitutions, their potential for impact on the developing organism must vary from lethal to none. Indeed, the impact should go beyond none to that which confers resistance to disease, to a homeostasis that defies provocation or compensates for it. Third, the evolutionary significance of variant genes may make a difference. For example, variations in genes specifying housekeeping enzymes, histones, chaperoning proteins, or the cyclins engaged in control of the cell cycle may exert more physiological impact than those, say, that differentiate the alleles of the blood-group substances. Fourth, since some genes are active only in some cell types, and then only at some times in ontogeny, the effects of disruptive mutants, although concentrated early in life, must be distributed throughout development and aging. And fifth, since it is the business of homeostasis to modulate less than optimal influences, incongruence may be buffered and overt consequences deferred until some change in development, experience, or both proves too taxing.

The logic is as follows. The most destructive phenotypes, measured by burden, reproductive impairment, and permanent handicap, must be the first to be selected against, then the next most destructive, and so on. In primitive populations such selection would be expressed in mortality, but in the developed world, onset of disease is a surrogate. Since at the beginning most variation is genetic, its contribution to mortality and disease declines continuously throughout the life of a cohort of individuals, even while exposure to experiences capable of promoting disease in the genetically vulnerable increases and their effects accumulate. The latter are accumulative because with time there are both new experiences and more of the old, and because of the historical effect of today's experiences building on a substrate of yesterday's, preparing thereby new conditions for what will occur tomorrow. This means that the cohort is at its most variable genetically at conception and at its least at its end, while variation due to experiences is least at conception and increases and accumulates throughout. Remember that the gradient is not a measure of genetic variation, but of selection against phenotypes. So, postreproductive disease is no less associated with genetic variation than prereproductive, but selection is less intense. To lose one's life at fifty or sixty years of age is no less disastrous to the individual than losing it at fifteen or twenty, but the biological burden of the latter is far greater than that of the former.

These reciprocal trends are shown schematically in Figure 3, which appears above a distribution of mortality rates by age (Figure 4). The latter is a continuous and U-shaped distribution that resembles that made by the intersecting lines of Figure 3. Everyone knows that the diseases contributing to mortality in the two arms of the distribution of mortality rates are quite different. Figure 3 suggests a reason why they differ, and Table 6 lists the characteristics that differentiate them. As it happens, the antimode of the distribution of mortality coincides pretty well with puberty, so the list distinguishes pre- and postpubertal disease.

Table 6 **Differences between Prepubertal and Postpubertal Diseases**

	Prepubertal	Postpubertal
Mode of inheritance	Monogenic	Multifactorial
Age at onset	Early	Late
Frequency	Rare	Frequent
Latency	Short	Long
Affected relatives	Numerous	Few
Diagnostic specificity	High	Low
Number of diseases	Very many	Fewer
Burden	Great	Less
Sex differences	Occasional	Frequent
Influence of migration	No	Yes
Secular change	No	Yes
Effects of SES	Some	More
Success in treatment	Some	More

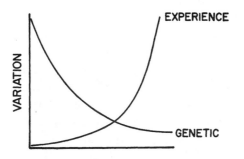

Figure 3   Reciprocal contributions to disease of experience and genes according to age at onset.
From Childs, B. Acceptance of the Howland Award. *Pediatric Research* 26(4): 392, 1989.

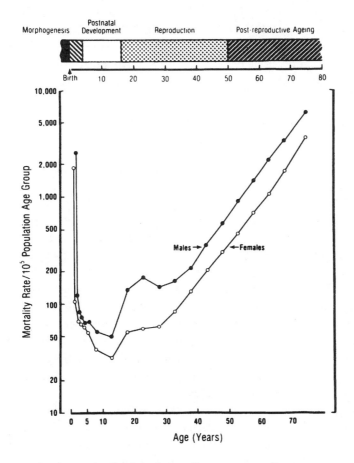

Figure 4   Distribution of mortality rates according to age.
From Costa, T., C. R. Scriver, and B. Childs. The effect of Mendelian disease on health: A measurement. *American Journal of Medical Genetics* 21: 231, 1985.

This description of the gradient of selective effect teeters on the brink of the typological, even though provisos as to the variable effects of both genes and experiences acting on homeostasis have been repeatedly affirmed. There is a danger that the gradient as described might be supposed to partake of the qualities of the great chain of being, which, as we saw, was complete, immutable, uninterrupted, and ordained from above. But we know that individuality always intervenes to confound such regularities. The same genes are associated with one effect in one person and another in another, depending on the qualities of the genes themselves, the variations of the experiences, and the influence of the developmental matrix. So the gradient is not of either genes or experiences, but of individual phenotypes, themselves a consequence of vulnerability deriving their specificities from the genes. If it were of either of the former, the same gene or experience would reappear at more than one point in the distribution, depending upon the factors enumerated in this book, and there would be only the loosest kind of gradient, unpredictable and not very useful. So let us keep in mind that it is a gradient of selective effect, and we know that nature selects not genes, but phenotypes that exhibit those "infinitely delicate shadings-off of everything into something else."

CONTINUITY IN MODES OF INHERITANCE: MONOGENIC DISEASE

The list of disease characteristics (Table 6) represents confirmation of expectations raised by the selective gradient. One obvious implication of the gradient is the strong association of monogenic disease with early onset and multifactorial with later onset. But, in fact, there is no discontinuity. There are multifactorial disorders of childhood and monogenic diseases with onset in late adult life, Asthma and type 1 diabetes are examples of the former, and some forms of Alzheimer's and Huntington's disease exemplify the latter. Further, monogenic conditions are subject to modification and some monogenic inborn errors are made overt only in specific circumstances, both qualities more commonly associated with complex diseases. So, in a very real sense, all phenotypes are multifactorial, and the multiple genes that contribute to multifactorial phenotypes are constrained by nature to behave qualitatively in the same way as those that contribute to mendelizing phenotypes; at some level of gene action they too produce segregating effects.

What do we find at the interface? One example is phenylketonuria. Is it caused by the variant gene that specifies an ineffective enzyme or by the phenylalanine that is toxic in doses unlikely to be attained by the unaffected? Obviously, both are required and in a quantitative balance; the treatment consists of reducing, not eliminating, the offending agent. A second example is G6PD deficiency in African Americans. Here the cause of the hemolysis in deficient individuals is a consequence of the inability of the deficient enzyme to produce enough NADPH to prevent it in the face of the oxidizing effects of several drugs. Favism also depends upon G6PD deficiency, but for hemolysis some other genetic factor is needed, too. So, if PKU and G6PD deficiency are prototypical multifactorial disorders, favism is a prototype of multigenic, multifactorial disorders.

But it is not only the genes that distinguish these prototypical examples; so do the provocative experiences. Phenylketonuria is precipitated by intolerance to phenylalanine and only phenylalanine—nothing else will do. So the environmental component in this disorder is unitary and everywhere prevalent. In this it is at one with most other inborn errors, in which the "environmental" component consists of the intracellular homeostasis with which the mutant effect is incongruent. For example, in Tay-Sachs disease the life of a neuron is imperiled by an "environment" of accumulating glycolipids and by nothing else. In contrast, the agents of hemolysis in African Americans with G6PD deficiency are neither unitary nor prevalent; in addition to some infections, they are mainly drugs with no counterparts in nature—and they are numerous. So these two interface disorders are embraced in a continuum in which incompatible environments, or provocative experiences, vary from intrinsic and unitary to unnatural and numerous. Phenylketonuria looks back in the continuum to, say, Tay-Sachs disease with its unitary cause and relatively invariant expression, while G6PD deficiency in African Americans looks ahead to conditions with causes that are likely to be more variable, multiple, and cumulative.

Typological thinkers may reject the idea that monogenic phenotypes could be multifactorial, perhaps on the grounds that the former mendelize while the latter do not. But even the typologist must accept that PKU and G6PD deficiency represent a prelude to complex interactions observed in other diseases and that they are unambiguous evidence of a seamless continuity between the mendelian and multifactorial modes of inheritance. And, if so, then phenotypes of the latter mode may be seen as special cases of the former: although the modes of inheritance differ, both are associated with mendelizing genes. So our approach to analysis is guided accordingly. We know that the genes will behave the same in both cases; they will specify or regulate protein products, act epistatically, vary in influence with gene dosage, and provoke dominant or recessive effects, and our aim is, no less in one case than the other, to discover the genes and to characterize them as to both their primary effects and their contributions to the complex physiological aberrations represented in pathogenesis. In all this one can sense the nodding of the (graying) heads of drosophilists as they witness the confirmation of their own recognition of the continuity of monogenic-multigenic phenotypes, a concept used by Delbrück to force a definitive proof of the one gene–one enzyme concept offered by Beadle and Tatum. Even more striking is the molecular substantiation of Fisher's 1918 entirely statistical evidence for the origin of nonmendelizing characters in the action of several or many segregating genes.

Other Characteristics

What of the other characteristics listed in Table 6? How are they accommodated in the selective gradient? That monogenic disorders should tend to be numerous, infrequent, have an early onset, carry heavy burdens, and be relatively impervious to the effects of SES, migration, and secular change is to be expected. They should also show sex differences when the mutant is sex linked and diagnostic specificity should be high, given how discretely the homeostasis is distorted by the mutants. And we are all aware that definitive success in treatment is not likely to come easily. But all of these qualities are variable. For example, Garrod's inborn errors, while rare, were low on the scale of burden; no one has yet found a disease manifestation in people with pentosuria. And single-gene diseases of late onset are well known.

An empirical test of these expectations was made by Costa et al., who in the early 1980s studied a sample consisting of every third entry in the fifth edition of *Mendelian Inheritance in Man (MIM)* (1). Only those marked with an asterisk to indicate sound evidence for mode of inheritance were included, and protein polymorphisms were excluded. So in the end the analysis included 351 entries. The literature reporting these disorders was then searched for such information as age at onset, affected organ systems, burden as measured by threat to life, curtailment of reproduction or residual handicap, and effectiveness of treatment. Burden as it is defined here had more to do with threat to life than severity of symptoms. Death early in life or life-long disability due to a congenital anomaly are more burdensome than, for example, the deterioration and death of Alzheimer's disease. No matter how much suffering the latter causes it comes after a substantial lifetime that excluded neither reproduction nor fulfillment of talents and ambitions.

A comparison of the first and fifth editions of *MIM* revealed no systematic divergence in the later sample, suggesting that there was nothing systematic by way of ascertainment bias. Results were as follows:

(a) While 85 percent of monogenic disorders are expressed by age ten and 90 percent before the end of adolescence, only 1 percent is expressed after forty years of age. Nearly all of the recessives and X-linked phenotypes are expressed early, while the distribution for dominants is trimodal with one peak before birth, one in infancy, and one in adult life.

(b) More than one-half of the phenotypes involve more than one organ system—recessives most, dominants fewest.

(c) Integument, nervous, and muscular systems were most often involved, while respiratory, endocrine, and immune systems were least represented.

(d) Lifespan was decreased for more than half of all entries—for recessives, three-quarters.

(e) A distribution of mortality according to age at onset was bimodal, with the first peak at birth and the second at early to middle adult life (Figure 5).

(f) The impact on reproduction and social adaptation was considerable: for 70 percent, fertility was impaired, and 60 percent had major handicaps.

(g) In regard to all three criteria of burden, recessives were the most profoundly affected, dominants least, and X-linked in between.

In an allied study, Hayes et al. examined outcomes of treatment for all 351 entries (2). Criteria for success were increased lifespan, reduction in reproductive curtailment, and improvement in social adaptation. In addition, success in treatment of sixty-five inborn errors of metabolism included in the sample was evaluated according to the same criteria. These inborn errors were better understood than most of the other entities, and because the deficient enzyme or other gene product was known in all sixty-five disorders and the pathogenesis was better understood, greater success of treatment might be anticipated.

For the whole sample, the response to treatment was disappointing; lifespan was increased for 15 percent, reproductive potential for 11 percent, and healthy social adaptation for 6 percent. When all but the sixty-five inborn errors were excluded, the treatment restored 12 percent to normal function. There was some amelioration in 40 percent—in most cases only slight—and for 48 percent no treatment was known, or what was tried was unavailing. The conclusion was that, in the 1980s, the idea that to know pathogenesis is to know how to treat was overly optimistic.

When the position with regard to the same sixty-five inborn errors was reviewed ten years later by Treacy et al., there was no increase in the number of disorders in which, after treatment, the patients could be said to be functioning at the same level as their coevals, but there was an increase in the number of disorders that were partially ameliorated: here, 40 percent rose to 57 percent (3). In addition, the percentage of those remaining impervious to all efforts was reduced from 48 to 31. Clearly this represents an improvement, but definitely not a feat akin to the miracle of antibiotics, and much of this improvement was attained by the most rigorous and expensive techniques, including organ and tissue transplantation.

A moment's reflection reveals why these inborn errors are so intractable. Evolution leads to increasing integration, complexity, and stability, but only at the expense of increasing constraint. So we cannot expect an easy conquest of imperfections of what required millions of years to construct. No doubt gene therapy will help, but the virtues of prevention are nowhere more evident than in contemplation of the treatment of monogenic disease.

What is the significance of these studies? Taken in the context of the body as a machine their meaning is very much of a piece with a study of, say, 351 cases of pneumonia due to microorganisms ranging from mycobacteria to viruses. The variable effects of the organisms would be shown in clinical expression, age at onset, threat to life, and residual damage to the lung. The intent of such a study would be to illuminate the problem of how the human lung reacts to many different organisms, and the results would be useful in diagnosis and, perhaps, treatment. But, however illuminating of the various pulmonary syndromes that comprise the infectious diseases of the lung, the study would have little to say about disease in general.

If, on the other hand, the work was intended to answer questions about how the whole range of microorganisms reacts with human beings according to such criteria as age, sex, social conditions, genetic qualities, and the like, then the study would have been designed to cast some light on the general question of relationships between two kinds of living beings, each pursuing the same reproductive and adaptive ends in the competition of life. Such a design, however, is not compatible with conventional medical investigations that aim to improve the diagnosis and treatment of particular diseases. That is, had the studies of Costa and Hayes been done in the context of the body as a machine, they would have only marginal significance. They would be seen as examining the qualities of one kind of disease—genetic diseases—all due to one kind of proximate cause, and although the results would have been helpful in a general way, if examined only in the vein of conventional thought they would not do much to excite the imagination.

But from the perspective of disease in an evolutionary setting, these papers reveal some useful insights. First, the data fulfill the expectation of the gradient of selective effect. Monogenic disorders are represented most strongly in the declining arm of the mortality curve; 70 percent have declared themselves by age three, 90 percent by the end of puberty, and only 1 percent have their onset after age forty.

Second, the gradient in not monotonic. Figure 5 shows the effect of mendelian disease on longevity according to age at onset. Here there are two peaks: (a) the mortality of diseases with onset at birth is greater than that of those that begin in utero or in childhood; and (b) there is a second peak in the curve in early to middle adult life. But these peaks are not reflected in distributions of mortality due to all causes because they occur early in each developmental stage and drop toward the end. Evidently, with the onset of each new developmental phase there is a fresh spate of selection against variants, a new pulse of the selective gradient that places emphasis on genetic causes of disease and mortality early in each such stage of life, leaving phenotypes of less obvious origins to prevail at the end. For example, while inborn errors predominate among deaths in infancy, accidents and mayhem account for the later mor-

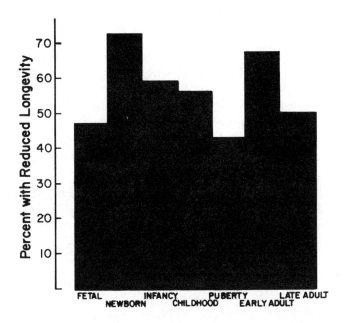

Figure 5 The effect of Mendelian disease on longevity in relation to age at onset.

From Childs, B. A logic of disease. In C. R. Scriver, A. L. Beaudet, W. S. Sly, and D. Valle (eds.). *The Metabolic and Molecular Bases of Inherited Disease.* 7th ed. New York: McGraw-Hill, 1995. Reproduced with permission of The McGraw-Hill Companies.

tality of childhood and adolescence. And the contribution of genes to the causes of premature death in adult life is far more intense than in later years, wherein mortality is more prominently associated with somatic mutations and the accumulated ravages of aging. All this is plausible enough; development brings new genes and new homeostatic adjustments that provide new contexts for the expression of genes present since conception.

Third, why does the number of life-endangering disorders with onset in the newborn period exceed that of those with onset before birth? In fact, as we have already seen, it does not. Disorders with onset in utero that come to term are only the backwash of a very much larger intrauterine mortality. So there is, in fact, a third peak in the distribution of curtailed longevity according to age at onset. Intrauterine mortality leaves only 20 to 40 percent of a cohort of conceptuses to take their chance with life after birth. Indeed, it is not too extravagant to say that the bulk of all the disease experienced by humankind has both origin and denouement, unseen and mostly unknown, and because out of sight, out of the medical mind. Admittedly there is little practical utility in knowing about the murderous climate of intrauterine life, or about the rise and fall of trends in distributions of mortality—that is, there is little that attracts the machine thinker. But for the kind of grasp of the nature of disease that is essential for balanced judgments about modern life, knowledge of this kind is the very basis of our warrant. Surely to include this most rapidly changing, most formative period of human life is to round out our view of human incongruence and to enhance our understanding of disease as it occurs later in life. Otherwise we are like those blind men who tried to describe the elephant by feeling its parts, failing thereby to describe the animal as a whole.

Fourth, what are the causes of this intrauterine mayhem? Apart from the losses of these embryos and fetuses due to chromosomal abnormality, the causes are unknown. But the molecular conditions required for early cell division, gastrulation, and blastula formation, and the precision of integrated gene action needed for embryogenesis, are such that there is certain to be an initial flushing out of mutants that threaten these intricate processes. It is the tip of the selective gradient and it begins, not at birth, but at conception—or even at failure to conceive. The products of mutational and recombinational extravagance are haled into court, as it were, where harsh judgments are rendered; indeed, they are the harshest of all since even the least such judgment may have to be paid in the form of a lifelong disability. So, in fact, health's tribulations begin not at birth but at conception, and the heaviest burdens are those borne at the beginning.

But perhaps the principal significance of these investigations of Costa, Hayes, and Treacy is their role as prototypes of what must come as a flood as the data of the Genome Project is released (4). In the 1980s the data were limited. Of the 351 disorders that constituted the wherewithal for the studies, molecular detail was known for only sixty-five (18%), and that only at the level of the deficient protein. So there were then very many questions that could not be asked with any expectation of a rational answer, questions of synthesis, of generalizations deriving from data composing lists of properties. The questions ask how the molecular details of mutants and their consequences relate to clinical expressions, and how both can be grouped in ways to draw inferences about homeostasis, human biology, and the entirety of disease. Since answers to such questions must await outcomes of the Genome Project, they will arise again later in a chapter devoted to that enterprise.

CONTINUITY IN MODES OF INHERITANCE: MULTIFACTORIAL DISEASE

Evidence tends to support the gradient idea in the case of monogenic disorders, but what should we expect of multifactorial disease? The genes engaged in the latter produce phenotypes farther down the selective gradient, so the diseases would be expected to have a later onset, fewer affected relatives, and lesser burden as measured by threat to life and fertility, to be fewer in number, to respond to variations in socioeconomic status, migration, and secular change, to show more variation according to sex, and to be more responsive to management.

The gradient of selective effect may be represented as a declining line, and we have seen that it is multimodal. But, in fact, each point represents a mean value, plotted against age; at any time of life there are more- and less-threatening disorders, and more- and less-threatened cases within each disease. So there should be a standard deviation for each point, and since experience tells us that the complex disorders are more variable than the monogenic, it should increase with age. Thus, multifactorial phenotypes would be expected to bear a reciprocal relationship to the monogenic and so to be infrequent early in life, to predominate late, and to have a broader range of ages at onset.

We have seen that monogenic phenotypes are in some degree multifactorial and that there is no discontinuity between phenotypes carrying these designations. What is the limit of the multifactorial case? How do we define a nongenetic disease? Presumably the latter is a consequence of some kind or degree of experience that causes disease regardless of any amount of genetic variation. But at the interface between the nongenetic and multifactorial diseases, there should be conditions under which some genotypes make it slightly more, or slightly less, likely for one person to get the disease than others, even when all are exposed to exactly the same kind, intensity, and duration of provocation. Also at the interface are the consequences of experiences of a lifetime, developmental trajectories that, keeping genetic variation constant, make it slightly more, or slightly less, likely for one person to express disease. There may be some experiences that cancel out or compensate for others, or there may be certain trajectories that lead toward and others away from injury caused by provocations. That is, why should there not be what we might call multifactorial resistance to disease? If genetic modifiers lead to nonpenetrance, so may experiences, treatments, and preventions reinforce the capacity for resistance of even normal alleles. So there is a continuity of the consequences of interactions between gene effects and those of experiences of the environment, and thereby do we account for the uninterrupted spectrum of disease from the genetic death of a conceptus that never implants to the demise of a centenarian as a consequence of the homeostatic chaos of aging.

All this is expressive of an increasing individuality in disease expressed along a continuum of diagnostic specificity. For example, although there is a modest variability in clinical expression of Tay-Sachs disease and no dearth of allelic variability, each patient is, within pretty narrow limits, representative of all. In contrast, when a patient is said to have atherosclerosis, no very particular clinical expression is conjured up by the name, and such is the degree of both multilocal and allelic genetic heterogeneity and such is the variation imposed by development, and such the variation in kind, intensity, and duration of experiences, that we can say that a patient given such a diagnosis is representative only of self.

A Test of the Gradient: Multifactorial Disorders

A test of the gradient hypothesis in relation to several multifactorial conditions has been reported (5). Several expectations were tested. In this trial no effort was made to arrange the diseases themselves in any order; the question was of the existence of a selective gradient within diseases. The assumption was that since such disorders are likely to be heterogeneous as to kinds and number of both genetic variants and experiences, the selective declivity should express itself in several ways:

(a) Age-specific age at onset should reach a peak and then decline. By some age or other, most of those possessing the requisite genes are likely to have the disease.

(b) Cases of early onset are more likely to have affected first-degree relatives, to be associated with "major" genes, and to express the disease with greater severity. That is, the most disadaptive mutants and aggregations thereof should stand out in cases with early onset, while those with late onset should be characterized by accumulation of experiences. As a result, the frequency of affected relatives should fall continuously. One expression of this trend is a decline in concordance of monozygotic twin pairs with increasing age at onset of the first twin.

(c) Family history and age at onset should vary with migration, secular change, and socioeconomic status. Where the homeostasis of a population is taxed by experiences of some new cultural environment, the prominence of the genetic contribution to the disorder in the population is likely to be reduced, but when the pressure on homeostasis is relieved, the apparent contribution of the genes in the remaining cases must rise.

(d) In diseases that show a sex difference in incidence that is not associated with sex linkage, the cases of the less frequently affected sex should have an early onset and more affected relatives. The idea is that a more powerful provocation—whether genetic, of experience, or both—is required to affect a member of the less frequently affected sex.

(e) Late onset cases should be milder, more readily prevented, and more responsive to treatment. An overtaxed homeostasis is bound to be easier to manage than one that was deficient from the start.

To provide a test of the hypothesis, nine diseases were chosen only because each had been a frequent object of epidemiological and genetic study. They were duodenal ulcer, non–insulin-dependent diabetes mellitus (NIDDM), Crohn's disease, gout, Parkinson's disease, celiac disease, systemic lupus erythematosus, rheumatoid arthritis (RA), and Alzheimer's disease. All but Parkinson's disease, Alzheimer's disease, and RA reached a peak for age-specific age at onset and then declined, but for each of these three, at least one study did show such a peak. Early onset of all diseases was more often accompanied by positive family history, and in all but duodenal ulcer, the cases of earlier onset were more severely affected.

The presence of some associated polymorphic genes was noted in duodenal ulcer (ABO blood groups), celiac disease, lupus erythematosus, and RA (HLA alleles). Major genes are demonstrated most prominently in the hyperuricemia and gout of early life. Three classical (monogenic) inborn errors have been distinguished: Lesch-Nyhan syndrome (H-G-PRT deficiency) and type I glycogen storage disease (glucose-6-phosphatase deficiency) have their onset in childhood, while PP-ribose P synthetase overactivity has its onset in early adult life. Gout also reveals the effects of gender. Women with onset at ages thirty to fifty, although greatly outnumbered by men, had more attacks of gout per year, higher serum uric acid levels, and more affected relatives.

The impact of experience in cases of late onset was illustrated in gout, where, hyperuricemia and arthritis were associated, in older males and females alike, with the use of diuretics in the treatment of hypertension, and in the effects of obesity and parity in type II diabetes. Lean patients with the latter are more likely to have affected relatives than obese, and parity follows the same pattern: nulliparous diabetic women are more likely to have affected relatives, a quality that declines with parity.

Data testing the idea of greater concordance of monozygotic twin pairs affected with these diseases were sparse, but the prediction was fulfilled for duodenal ulcer, lupus erythematoses, and Parkinson's disease—though not for NIDDM, where concordance was 95 percent. Although not included in the study under review, the prediction has been amply fulfilled for insulin-dependent diabetes (6).

As for the effects of migration, secular change, and socioeconomic status, although it is clear that cultural changes have greatly increased the incidence of type II diabetes and gout in certain populations, we have no data as to family history or age at onset before such changes and so can draw no conclusion. But the position apropos socioeconomic status was well illustrated in a study by Marmot and Rose, who contrasted mortality rates due to heart attack across four grades of civil servant in London (7). Although risk factors and mortality were inversely related to socioeconomic status, family history varied directly. Also, the very few of the highest socioeconomic status who did die were the youngest.

Success in treatment follows the expected pattern: there is an inverse relationship between intensity of selection against gene effects and successes. For example, dietary change alone often suffices in treating late-onset patients with type II diabetes, patients with iatrogenic gout, usually late onset, are relieved by a change in medication, and the generally mild rheumatoid arthritis of late onset is more susceptible to therapy.

This study suffered the handicap of looking for answers to questions that were never asked. The relevant investigations, in following the standard epidemiologic pattern, were not designed to ask them, and so the data are often nowhere to be found. In addition, the diseases included may not be representative—and, in any case, are a small sample of the universe. But there is no dearth of additional evidence. For example, there is an uninterrupted decline in affected relatives with increasing age at onset of major depression and schizophrenia (8,9). Recently, genes contributing to early-onset NIDDM have been discovered, as well as several genes associated with early-onset hypertension (10,11). Early-onset and genetically influenced forms of cancer of breast, prostate, and large bowel have also been described (12–14). The incidence among relatives of men operated on for benign prostatic hypertrophy before age sixty-four was four times that of those with later onset. Indeed, in the families of the early-onset cases, the disease segregates as a dominant (15).

Perhaps the idea of a gradient is nowhere better demonstrated than in the relationship between the number of triplet repeats and age at onset in Huntington's disease, myotonic dystrophy, and other disorders: the greater the number of repeats, the earlier the onset, the greater the severity, and the sooner the death (16). Although these phenotypes mendelize, there is no reason to suppose that such an origin must be associated only with monogenic disease.

Most of these properties are also demonstrated in the various syndromes of atherosclerosis and heart attack. Premature heart attacks in both men and women are associated with specific mutants, mostly involving genes specifying lipoproteins, and although women are far less likely than men to have heart attacks during their reproductive years, when they do, they are more severely affected (17). For example, the mortality from heart attacks in women less than forty-five years of age is nearly three times that for men. Individual women with premature heart attack were shown, on the average, to have more of the known risk factors than men, confirming the greater resistance among women to the effects of the same genes and experiences that in lesser individual concentrations bring down the men (17).

Cancer also qualifies as a multifactorial disease; indeed, in its requirement for variants of several genes to move the earliest changes to malignancy and metastasis, it is a model for understanding other diseases. But it is different, perhaps unique, in that proximate cause is sometimes hereditary, sometimes derived from somatic mutation, and sometimes both. This not at all apparent conclusion was reached by Knudson, who adduced mathematical evidence that supported the idea that some childhood cancers could be a consequence of one inherited allele together with a somatic mutant at the same locus, while some cancers with later onset could be associated with two somatic mutants (18). This imaginative thinking represented a new concept that informed the work of others in advancing and simplifying our understanding of cancer. The idea illuminates its age dependency and demonstrates its conformity to the focus in disease on unit steps in homeostasis as proximate cause—in this case, proteins that regulate the rates of growth.

All these studies confirm the decline in the gradient of the effects of genetic variation, the rise during life of the influence of accumulated experiences, and the interaction of the products of genes with those experiences in an ever-changing developmental matrix to produce an evolving individuality. That is, while our genes constrain us throughout life to be the same person we were at the start, our experiences explore and exploit the capacities for individuality those genes confer. It is no wonder, then, that the range of expression of disease broadens with aging or that the singularity of that expression increases.

This variety of individual expression of disease emphasizes the virtues of populational thinking. It is possible, perhaps forgivable, to be typological about monogenic disorders because the path from gene to disease phenotype, however complex it really is, seems so straightforward, and the apparent road to treatment seems simply one of filling in, or otherwise neutralizing, the homeostatic deficiency. But in multifactorial conditions any such typological interpretation is clearly out of place. Here the complexity of the path from gene(s) to disease phenotype is often unclear; indeed, we cannot always be sure of the role in each affected individual of the variants known in populations of affected patients to be associated with the disease. That is, some possessors of such genes live out a long life without ever experiencing any malign effect. We may suspect that each such person does so for an individual reason. For example, one lacks one or more of the other variants required for expression of the disease, while another has variants at all the requisite loci but one or two are milder versions that, however necessary, are insufficient to promote palpable disease. Still another has all the right variants but also the genes for a tightly knit and resilient homeostasis capable of adjusting to the variant effects; and some, while possessing all the genetic components needed, never encounter or never accumulate in just the right mix—or in the right order or chronology—all the experiences needed to attain the homeostatic failure that leads to disease.

As physicians, what we are all looking for are the most direct, the most unambiguous connections between proximate causes and the signs and symptoms of disease, and when we find such explicit relationships, we tend to emphasize them. And indeed, they are "the" cause—for some of those individuals in whom they are so singularly prominent. But given the gradient of selective effect, the variation in kind, intensity, and duration of provocative experiences, and the evolving developmental matrix, we must expect among populations of patients a continuity of pathogenesis that comprehends both those most unambiguous cases that resemble each other in both causes and expression and others in whom the clinical picture is, as it were, sui generis, deriving from a unique mosaic of vulnerabilities drawn from the menu that comprises them all.

Such a continuum exposes, as nothing else can, the dilemmas of education and training. The physician faced with the urgency of ameliorative need is likely to lay hold of whatever properties are shared by most of the patients, individualizing treatment empirically, while for the deliberative educator, each patient is of equal interest as a unique experiment of nature. Practical necessity requires grouping of patients for treatment regimens directed to the most-threatening expressions, but such empiricism need not exclude a populational basis; the inclusive treatment—and diagnosis, too—will be more quickly and appropriately individualized when approached in a populational vein. For example, treatment for high blood pressure is no doubt strongly influenced by the most recent reports in the literature of successes and failures of drugs new and old. But hidden in the generalizations of all such reports are the minorities that belie them, the cases that did not respond to that proclaimed to be most successful as well as the few for whom the drug said to be least successful was just what was required. Population thinking includes both.

IN THIS CHAPTER we have considered the idea of an unbroken continuity in the expression of disease. The intention was to explore the unity of medicine, to discover threads of thought about disease that can be woven into a comprehensive fabric. Each was an exercise in Garrodian thinking that began with the assumption that a student of medicine should examine that which holds medicine together before disappearing into one of its byways.

23

Heritability

Insofar as a balance sheet of nature and nurture has any intelligible significance, it does not entitle us to set limits to changes which might be brought about by regulating the environment.

—Lancelot Hogben, *Nature and Nurture*

There is a further dimension useful in defining the unity and continuity of disease: that of heritability. Heritability is an expression of the extent of the contribution of the genes to the variation of a trait observed in a population. It can be given mathematical expression as a coefficient of heritability based on correlations of measurements of a property between pairs of individuals—MZ and DZ twins, sib pairs, parent-child pairs, and so on. It is representative of no single individual, but of a particular population at a particular time. It has been sometimes misunderstood to be an expression of the extent to which a trait in a person could be attributed to genes or to experiences, a variation of the nonsensical question of the relative importance in an individual's makeup of heredity and environment. In fact, it is an abstraction that characterizes a population no less than an average value, and which, like an average value, can change from time to time even when the population consists of exactly the same individuals.

The heritability of any measurable quality can be calculated. If all the variation in expression of the quality were wholly genetic, the heritability would be 1.0; but if all the members of the population shared the same genes and yet the trait was variable, the heritability would be said to be zero. So, as Hogben says in the epigraph to this chapter, the heritability coefficient represents an expression of the variable contributions of nature and nurture to a phenotype in a population. But as he goes on to say, it is a quality that can be changed by altering the environment. This wisdom dates back to 1939, and yet the belief that heritability is a fixed property continues to be held in some quarters to this day.

The principle of heritability was invented by geneticists and has been most used to determine how genetic variation influences measures of crops and herds, with an eye to directions to be taken for breeding of desirable characteristics. It is useful in these fields because it is possible to control the conditions of the environment, the better to sort out and to manipulate the genetic contribution. But in human populations where neither contributor can be controlled and both are usually unknown, the concept has proved less helpful. Indeed, in medical thinking the concept has had no place at all. How could it, when medical thinking is so taken up with events that have befallen single individuals?

That is not to say that heritability has been ignored in human studies. It has been used most notoriously, and dubiously, in the ideological wars about racial differences in the results of IQ tests (1). To more profit, it has figured in work on such characteristics as height, birth weight, and obesity, as well as such diseases as diabetes, hypertension, and other disorders in which twin studies have been prominent. It has been useful particularly in convincing doubters that there is indeed a genetic contribution to unlikely traits—for example, in convincing psychiatrists that the psychoses have a heritable component at a time when psychodynamics dominated their thinking.

The method has been criticized as unable to make any genuine partition of causes; the interactions of gene effects, experiences, and development are too complex for any number to represent the actual role of any contributor (2). For example, the historical quality of development ensures that even if we could list all of the interactions that have led to a phenotype, we could never know their temporal sequences, a property we know to be critical in establishing trajectories in development that could have profound effects on measures of heritability. So is the principle of any use in medicine?

If we do not ask much in the way of numerical precision, there are two ways in which the idea of a more or less genetic basis for differences in susceptibility to disease in a population has a significant educational value. "Educational" is used here as elsewhere in the book to mean disposition of ideas, as opposed to "training," which in medicine always has to do with diagnosis and management of individual patients. I emphasize the word education also because in medicine heritability never had and never will have any meaning in regard to diagnosis or treatment of disease in any individual. A physician whose approach to a particular patient is informed only by epidemiological information is in serious trouble—or the patient is. Even when a choice of treatment has been shown in an epidemiological study to be effective in 90 percent of patients, the doctor has always to be prepared for the certainty that some patients must fall into the residual fraction. So heritability is of no more use in this regard than is epidemiology; both are too likely to represent typological thinking and to overlook the individual.

Within the bounds set by this warning, what educational use does the concept of heritability have? The first use was outlined in the previous section, where the decline in the gradient of genetic selective effect and the rise of that of the effects of experiences was noted. These combine to account for a decline of genetic vulnerability to disease throughout the life of a cohort of individuals born at the same time—a progressive drop in heritability.

What is the virtue of emphasizing these changes in vulnerability throughout life? It is simply that if you are to defeat the enemy, you had better know more than his tactics; you had better know his strategy. If nature can be said to have a strategy, it is that whatever reduces reproductive fitness is subject to adverse selection until reproduction is at an end, after which the species is, as it were, on its own. Such a strategy is reflected in the gradient of selective effect. To understand nature's plan we must cleave to the rules of the historian, for whom the remote past (phylogeny) and the developmental past are always in mind, no matter how detailed the description of the immediate events; in history, the past always informs the present.

As long as our sole aim in medicine is to score the tactical triumph of fixing the machine, strategies implicit in the reciprocal gradients that represent changes in heritability throughout life cannot become apparent. And yet, on what else are we to base a sensible preventive program? How else are the obstetrician, the pediatrician, the family physician to assist in the establishment in each individual of a homeostasis that takes advantage of favorable potential to skirt the traps that lurk within us all, traps that are a consequence of our participation in nature's larger plan? Forever to fix the broken machine rather than to anticipate its weaknesses is to respond reflexly to nature's tactics and to ignore her strategy, whereas to find the weaknesses and to remove that which defines them as such is to understand that strategy and so to nullify nature's tactics. The aim of preventive medicine is to raise the heritability of disease to a maximum.

The second use for the principle of heritability emphasizes individuality and population thinking. Epidemiologists have observed again and again that the incidence of many diseases varies with time. For example, in some countries the frequency of infections began to decline even before the advent of antibiotics, presumably in response to better public health, while nutritional diseases nearly disappeared as a result of better food and the availability of vitamins. Changes in particular populations have also been observed. For example, a sharp rise in type II diabetes and gout accompanied a rise in affluence among the Pima Indians in the United States and the Polynesians of Nauru, a result of their having assumed Western habits of diet, idleness, and locomotion by motor rather than foot (3). And it has been observed many times that when people move from one culture to another they take on the patterns of disease of the populations they join. Obviously the genes do not change; what changes in the individuals are their experiences, and what changes in the populations is the heritability. So heritability goes up and down. It is responsive to variations in exposure to cultural attributes of populations.

Heritability of Birth Weight

One example of the effect on heritability of easing of provocative experiences is the reduction, in the developed nations, of infant mortality as a result of affluence. These provocations are deficiencies of education, diet, housing, and medical care. Both birth weight and perinatal mortality are influenced by these deficiencies. Terrenato, Ulizzi, and colleagues have compared perinatal mortality according to birth weight of babies born in Italy in 1960 and in 1980 (4,5). Mortality was much reduced during these twenty years, and the distribution of birth weights among the dead babies showed two revealing differences: (1) the variance was significantly reduced, and (2) what had been a well-defined antimode of least mortality (or optimum birth weight) had flattened out. The reduced variance means that some among the outliers on both sides have been saved, and the flattening out of the antimode suggests a broader range of optimal weights due to reduced selection throughout the distribution. Since these effects are attributable to improvements in living conditions and health care, what has happened is that the babies with the least genetic vulnerability have been saved; the heritability of mortality has risen. Today, in the developed nations, much—perhaps most—disease and mortality among babies born at term of average weight is strongly influenced by genetic variation. Many of such babies have inborn errors. Ulizzi's most recent paper, which extends the study a further five years, shows that the rate of change in heritability has slowed as infant mortality approaches a minimum (6).

A further example is given by these same workers, who examined sex ratios among infants born in Italy and the United States between 1920 and 1980 (7). Male-to-female ratios of each year of this period were counted at birth, at one month, and at one year. This ratio at birth has been observed to vary between 1.05 and 1.07 in populations throughout the world. Since males are known to be more susceptible than females to infections, anomalies, and other life-threatening diseases, the ratio would be expected to fall from birth to one year in the direction of equality. And that is what Ulizzi and Zonta found for the year 1920. But thereafter the postnatal ratios tended to approximate, ending in the 1970s at something like the ratio at birth. That is, many babies that in the past died before reaching one year of age now survive. Better prenatal care, better medicine more broadly distributed, and better nutrition, housing, and the like have conspired to reduce the mortality generally and to equalize the edge females used to have over the more vulnerable males.

All this is compatible with a rise in heritability. As in the mortality and heritability of birth weight, the less vulnerable have been saved, leaving the minority of congenital anomalies, chromosomal aberrations, and monogenic inborn errors to be overrepresented among the babies who died in that first year of life.

The human body is capable of making active vitamin D, a hormone that promotes intestinal absorption of calcium. But there is a hitch: the conversion of dehydrocholesterol to vitamin D^3 in the deep layers of the skin is driven by ultraviolet rays, usually derived from sunlight. Prior and later steps in the biosynthesis of this hormone are carried out in other organs and are endogenously controlled, so that only insufficient exposure to sunlight leads to vitamin D deficiency and rickets. Nature has left this necessary chemical step to circumstance, rather than selecting for a fully self-contained homeostatic pathway; the sun has been incorporated into the homeostasis of calcium. But the sun is not everywhere equally available, so in the north, where it is a scarce commodity for part of the year, the active vitamin is supplied by the fish oil that abounds in the adjacent seas and so in the prevailing diet.

So the disease was no doubt rare until human ingenuity created clothes, dwellings, and cities, all of which shut out the sun, and rickets became a common disease of industrialized societies (8). But ingenuity heals what ingenuity hurts, so that after the virtues of fish oils were discovered, vitamin D was isolated, and a treatment was standardized, the incidence of rickets among infants began to decline. This drop was hastened in the 1940s by social agencies, including well-baby clinics that saw to the distribution of cod-liver oil and later synthetic vitamin D to the needy. So the cultural homeostasis kicked in to augment those of the physical environment (the sun) and the human body, and slowly at first, then rapidly, vitamin D deficiency rickets became a disease almost unknown to later generations of physicians. In the 1950s its decline was rapid. In one population in Baltimore, the number of cases dropped from 444 observed during the decade 1939 to 1949 to 60 seen during 1950 to 1960—a drop of more than sevenfold (9). The role of culture here is plain and instructive. The decline in incidence of rickets was hastened by the employment of women in the wartime industrial boom. They left their babies in care centers and were otherwise instructed in health care, and, for a change, they had money to pay for cod-liver oil!

Who were the sixty patients who remained in the Baltimore study? Some were certainly children who for one reason or another missed the opportunity. In the cliché of our time, they "slipped through the safety net." But in this population there was another change: as the number of cases dropped, the sex ratio of affected children rose from 1.65 to 2.16. It has been known for many years that boys are more susceptible to vitamin D deficiency rickets than girls; witness the ratio of 1.65 in the 1939–1949 segment of the study. But as vitamin D was ever more widely distributed, the first cases to drop out of the subsequent sample must have been the least vulnerable females, leaving the more vulnerable males to be overrepresented in what was left.

We do not know what this sex difference in vitamin D deficiency rickets is. It may have to do with variants in sex-linked genes that are known to be associated with some forms of resistant rickets, and if this is so, the decline in incidence of vitamin D deficiency rickets is accompanied by, or represents, a rising heritability. This thought is given plausibility by the proportional increase among the remaining cases of rickets of several forms of more severe disease, including so-called vitamin D dependent rickets and others, some resistant to any nontoxic dose of the vitamin (10). All are monogenic disorders that were always there to be counted as a small fraction, but were diluted to insignificance by the enormous majority of the vitamin-deficient cases. So the heritability of rickets rose substantially. As the provocation of deficiency was reduced, more and more of the residual variation was genetic; this certainly includes the monogenic forms and possibly the forms of lesser resistance.

The question these observations raise is, is there a continuous distribution of genetic vulnerability of all grades—in this instance to rickets, but more generally to other diseases, especially multifactorial? If there is such a distribution in regard to rickets and if all the individuals represented are given the same stimulus, including both irradiation and exogenous vitamin D, are those who get the disease anyway most likely to be drawn from that part of the distribution wherein lie the most genetically vulnerable? It is a plausible hypothesis. The emergence of the familial types and the change in sex ratio with the decline in incidence provide suggestive evidence; so does the greater susceptibility to rickets of premature infants and fast-growing babies in general who need more vitamin D for prevention. And although less thoroughly studied for reasons of ethics, a fairly wide range of requirement of vitamin D for prevention was recognized by pediatricians engaged in well-baby care. If four hundred units per day was the standard preventive, there were a few otherwise unremarkable infants who required as much as 1,000 to 2,000 units/day to prevent the disease. Such a dose is two to four times that normally needed, but is well under that required by the vitamin D–dependent children. Further, the patients who require moderately more vitamin D can be maintained by sunlight and dietary means while the dependent cases cannot. Similarly graded requirements have been demonstrated in the requirement for vitamin B^6 to prevent convulsions in infants (10).

If one assumes such a continuous distribution of vulnerability, an important concept of disease is illuminated. If there is genetic variation at the loci of whatever genes there are that bear on the homeostatic step or steps involved, then the threshold of overt disease depends upon the kind, intensity, and duration of provocations. When provocation is low, heritability is high, but when provocative experiences are applied generally and with intensity, heritability is low. When the experience is absence of ultraviolet irradiation of cells in the deep layers of the skin, then we are all equally susceptible to rickets, genetic variation notwithstanding. And if, in addition to that lack of irradiation, we are given no vitamin D, we will all come down with rickets. But when sunlight or vitamin D are irregularly experienced, then rickets will appear in individuals exposed to the same amount of provocation according to position in the distribution of genetic vulnerability.

In contrast to vitamin D deficiency and rickets are the experiences of the Pima Indians and those Polynesian populations to whom the life of abundance brought diabetes and gout. The same influences have also been responsible for unacceptable levels of heart attack and diabetes in the United States. Fortunately, recognition of such risk factors as diets high in calories and fat, smoking, and indolence has been accompanied by a gratifying decline in deaths due to heart attack during the past decade or two. Further, among the risk factors an increasing number of gene loci and alleles, often of polymorphic frequency, have been recognized, genes that predispose in various ways to atherosclerosis and these are often overrepresented among those who have heart attacks (11). So it may be that at the height of the epidemic a decade or two ago, heritability was at its least but is now on its way up; people dying today have more genetic reasons to do so. Again, as the incidence recedes there should be, among the residual cases, a greater genetic impact—more different genetic risk factors and more impressive family histories.

These two examples clarify a further principle. Heritability rises with reduced incidence of both rickets and heart attack, but there is a paradoxical effect: the heritability of rickets increases when something is supplied, while that of heart attack rises when something is withdrawn. It is the difference between deficiency and intolerance, and it is an illuminating example of nature's central tendency and of stabilizing selection. Adaptation is characterized as neither too much nor too little, and individuals whose attributes make them outliers in frequency distributions are subject to selection; they are picked off, the better to preserve the parameters of the distribution. So it would seem to be the business of medicine to steer the people on a course between the Scylla of deficiency and the Charybdis of excess. We know how difficult that is, but to the cultural, economic, and behavioral obstacles to the attainment of such an aim must be added some biological ones. In the examples already given we have seen that there are genetic causes of deficiency amid plenty (resistant rickets) and of excess in the presence of want; for example, in those parts of the world where diet is less dependent upon fat and where atherosclerosis is infrequent, the causes among the few who have heart attacks are likely to be diverse. The point is that the cases observed where the disease is infrequent represent outliers in distributions of vulnerability, and the outliers may be flanked on the side toward the mean by individuals whose propensity goes unexpressed in prevailing conditions but is easily raised to overt manifestation by changes in experience. So, the study of deficiency in excess and intolerance in want is one way of learning causes of disease.

Heritability

OTHER EXAMPLES

Reye's syndrome and infantile cortical hyperostosis are conditions of uncertain origin and are usually nonfamilial. For reasons that remain obscure, the incidence of both has declined, with the result that hereditary forms have emerged. For example, cases of inborn errors of the urea cycle have become prominent among residual cases called Reye's syndrome (12,13).

Iron-deficiency anemia, once so frequent among the undernourished, is now a relatively less common cause of microcytosis, which, in certain places is more likely to be found among heterozygotes for thalassemia or as a result of other, even less frequent genetic causes. And pellagra, now a rare disease in the United States, is occasionally to be seen in people who are homozygous for Hartnup's disorder and whose plasma amino acid levels, presumably under polygenic control, are on the low side of a Gaussian distribution of such levels (10). Such people are those for whom a modest deprivation is enough to precipitate the signs of vitamin deficiency. Also in this vein of nutritional deficiencies is cretinism, associated most frequently with a lack of dietary iodine. It is a deficiency now nearly universally supplied in the developed nations, and so the genetic causes of the disorder now predominate (10).

THE MEANING OF HERITABILITY

What is the meaning of heritability in the context of the logic of disease? Its traditional use has been as a measure of the genetic contribution to the variation in a population where it is often taken as evidence of both the presence and strength of heritable differences, a testimony to the lurking existence of allelic variation, however inapparent the genes might be. It is likely that this criterion for the genetic origin of a character will fall into neglect as the molecular biology of genetics becomes encompassing—or as the evolutionary view of disease comes to prevail. But as evidence for continuity in disease the principle of heritability cannot be surpassed. As heritability rises in response to the diminished prevalence of some experience(s) in a population, the first to leave the list of the diseased are the least vulnerable, and as heritability falls, they are the last to enter it. And further, as age at onset increases, heritability falls and with it, twin concordance and familial concentration. That is, heritability and incidence of disease are no measure of the state of the gene pool of a population; they are merely indicators of that part of it that is vulnerable to the current level of provocation.

Changes in heritability also tell us something about the contingent quality of vulnerability. Vulnerability is individual and contingent, a state of potential that depends upon a particular kind, intensity, and duration of a stimulus to raise it to overt expression or to suppress it. And if an individual and contingent quality, the rise and fall of heritability in populations is exemplary of continuity in disease. And above all, it must be evident that heritability of human disease cannot rationally be approached in a typological turn of mind. For diseases like atherosclerosis and heart attack there are many loci involved, many alleles and many varieties and degrees of experiences, so that each person arrives at the final point of a coronary thrombosis—or escapes it—for unique reasons. A statement that the heritability of a disease is this or that is typological until modified by recognition of the heterogeneity among the genes of the population, the ages of the individuals composing it, and the fluxes in provocation. It is one more evidence of the need for epidemiology to be pursued in a genetic vein.

Finally, a visceral grasp of the meaning of heritability in medicine brings the realization that words like *environment, experience,* and *provocation* actually mean the real, live social and cultural conditions within which individual human beings pass their lives, eating, drinking, sleeping, working, playing, traveling, loving, and producing children. It is the social mores that determine heritability, and, if so, it is the business of medicine to support the relevant social agencies in an effort to push the heritability in the direction of 1.0.

24

Infections

If microparasitism may be likened to a nether millstone, grinding away at
human populations through time, human-to-human macroparasitism has
been almost as universal—an upper millstone, pressing heavily upon the
majority of the human race.
—William H. McNeill, *The Human Condition:*
An Ecological and Historical View

This observation, made by a historian of note, brings infections into
history and history into the story of infections, a story in which biology and culture participate as equal partners, or perhaps in symbiosis. Among
microparasites, McNeill includes viruses and bacteria as well as larger organisms—trypanosomes, plasmodia, helminths, and the like. Macroparasites are
the organisms that head the food chain, of which Homo sapiens is the first. In
this graphic metaphor, McNeill has encapsulated the plight of the bulk of humankind in all but the most recent and enlightened human societies. Together,
the two millstones have kept the "majority of civilized populations close to
bare subsistence by withdrawing resources from their control." Emperors,
landowners, and marauding hordes traditionally took their "share," whether
by force or by tax, while microorganisms, capitalizing on the deprivation and
debility that was the inevitable result of such exploitation, took their toll in
disease and death. This is the position in some of today's third world, where
leaders use resources for personal ends at the expense of their disease-ridden
people.

The upper millstone is a property of human history, but the struggle between microorganisms and higher organisms must have begun early in phylogeny and so must be exemplary of co-evolution. And if of evolution, then
genes must be involved, and infections must participate in the logic of disease
as a consequence of the individuality of both contestants.

THE UNITY OF DISEASE

The idea of individuality is apparent in the thinking of those who investigate the homeostasis of microorganisms and who describe their individuality in the context of such qualities as virulence and antibiotic resistance. But in textbooks, infections are still perceived as the archetype of environmental diseases. And of course they are that, but when observed from another point of view, they resemble other diseases that derive from incongruence between the human genotype and the environment, the latter represented here by the microbial genotype and its works.

Archibald Garrod leaves us in no doubt about his recognition of infections as products of the individuality of both human and microbial species. In *Inborn Factors* he put it, "In our fight against the infective diseases we are not confronted with blind forces, acting at random but with the disciplined offensive of highly trained foes. Whilst on the one hand the weapons of attack have been improved by evolution, there has been a corresponding evolution of protective mechanisms of great ingenuity, and of no small efficiency, for the defense of the individual attacked" (1). So, human susceptibility and resistance are a consequence of the human genes that define individuals and account for variability in populations as well as those of the microorganisms that have "their own careers to work out." These careers are simply an aspect of nature in which one species preys on another, not out of spite or pride, but for food and the wherewithal to fulfill nature's requirement to reproduce. And as we know, when successful, these careers—the nether millstone—have a powerful impact on the numerical density and distribution of animals, including human beings. So, an infection must be seen as "a struggle of conflicting interests," and outcomes have to do with individual incongruities between these systems that evolve together, albeit at different rates.

Anthropocentrism causes us to see microorganisms as implacable enemies, and although we inherit an efficient means to oppose them, no small effort is devoted to enhancing our defensive weaponry by invention. But a deeper understanding of the position of man and microbe may be attained by entertaining, if only for a moment, an alternative view in which microorganisms are perceived as victims and the human immune system, antibiotics, and public health as offensive weapons, so that the human species is the bane and ruthless scourge of microorganisms who are only struggling to work out their own careers.

The genes of both agonists in the contest specify proteins, and as genes, they must vary. Accordingly, there must be variation in both the capacity of microorganisms to express virulence and the human partner to resist or to succumb. So virulence and pathogenicity are relative properties; if we say an organism is virulent, we must ask for whom, and if an individual is said to be susceptible, we should specify to what. As it happens, the organisms we recognize as pathogenic are likely to have adapted, not to infrequent individual human differences, but to the prevailing versions thereof—for example, to cell surface proteins that characterize the bulk of the population. What would be the virtue of adapting to a molecule unlikely to be encountered, as opposed to making a receptor of a molecule likely to be found in nearly all human beings (2)? Accordingly, what the organisms do is to define as a human weakness a molecule that is, in regard to its ordinary physiological function, a strength. For example, HIV uses the CD4+ receptor, some strains of *E. coli* attach specifically to molecules of the P blood group substance in the epithelium of the bladder, and streptococci have developed numerous adhesins that give them an advantage as they lodge themselves in the pharyngeal mucosa.

So, just as we define as a weakness in bacteria an aspect of their physiology that makes them susceptible to antibiotics, they define their points of entry into human cells as points of human vulnerability. And just as organisms vary in regard to sensitivity to antibiotics, so do the points of entry vary in sensitivity to microorganisms; inherent resistance to polio, malaria, and the tubercle bacillus, among others, has been described. So infections qualify as in no way different from other diseases. It is the unit steps in the physiological homeostasis, in this case of both adversaries, that constitute the battleground. The unity of disease is preserved. But what of continuity?

CONTINUITY

Continuity is expressed in infections, as in other diseases, in gradients of selective effect for both organisms. The gradient of virulence among organisms depends upon strategies employed for gaining access, for reproducing, and for ensuring transmission.

It is often supposed that co-evolution must end in an amicable coexistence in which human beings tolerate microorganisms without disease, even assisting in their spread. Some microorganisms might even pay rent in the form of vitamins useful in human metabolism, and many have attained this nirvana. But some have worked out no scheme to uncouple virulence from dissemination and so are doomed to infect so as to be transmitted (3). So co-evolution can attain any of many degrees of accommodation for species and, we may assume, an additional range of variation for individuals within the species. All of this means that our relationships with microbial life remain fluid; the latter can define new human weaknesses by mutating to forms for which our defenses are not prepared, even while we enjoy the advantage of an intelligence capable sometimes of inventing the means to thwart their designs (4,5). But invention is not always immediately successful—AIDS is an example—and the power to mutate, particularly of viruses, is great. So, as long as parasitic organisms continue to pursue their careers, the human species is under an unrelenting threat (6).

No doubt individual variation and selection have led through phylogeny to our high degree of resistance; for example, the adaptive immune response appears to have evolved after such primitive effector mechanisms as the alternative complement pathway and natural killer cells were already in place (7). Both depend upon gradations in resistance and susceptibility. Although Garrod acknowledged differences in these properties, he knew of no examples of either: disorders of immune defense should qualify as inborn errors but he knew of none. How could he? The very high prevalence of infection and their mortality would have made them inapparent; heritability was low. And the dominance, in his time, of the germ theory of disease would surely have excluded from most minds the idea of infections as a consequence of anything other than bacteria. The gap between alkaptonuria and pneumonia was simply unbridgeable by all but Garrod himself.

Now, of course, we know of many straightforward monogenic defects in human defense against microbial infection, including deficiencies of antibodies, MHC antigens, and complement, as well as abnormalities of phagocytes. A report on immunodeficiencies published in 1995 by the World Health Organization listed forty-five primary immunodeficiencies, all classical inborn errors, and a further thirty-five associated with other disorders—chromosome anomalies, metabolic errors, and the like (8). No one supposes this to be the end of it; given the number and variety of unit steps in the whole apparatus of defense, many more such inborn errors should emerge.

What has been discovered so far are the most profound deficiencies, all infrequent, easily perceived as inborn errors, and readily distinguished from normal. As expected, there is variation within each, but many are lethal early in life and all exact a significant price in reduced life expectancy and curtailment of reproduction. So these monogenic immunodeficiencies represent the upper reaches of a gradient of selective effect that must decline through lesser degrees of susceptibility to resistance.

This continuity has been demonstrated repeatedly. For example, for some people infection with *Haemophilus influenza* is familial; they have a quantitative variation—not a deficiency—in their immune response. There is also evidence of multigenic control in the magnitude of response to vaccines. Further testimony for continuity is given in an investigation into the causes of death of people separated from their biological parents very early in life (9). When a biological parent died of infection at or before age seventy, the relative risk of dying of the same cause for their children was increased fivefold. That is, the correlation in cause of death was between the biologically related but separated persons, not the adopted child and foster parent. There was no conventional immunodeficiency here, only enhanced susceptibility.

In a more recent paper, it was reported that the probability that patients hospitalized for pneumococcal pneumonia would be readmitted for the same disease was more than five times that of other patients to be readmitted for their particular illnesses (10). Evidently there are people especially susceptible to the pneumococcus. And why not? Each of us must have a unique set of molecules pertaining to responses to all sorts of infection, and what we know of mutation tells us that where there are devastating inborn errors, there are also lesser grades of deviation (11). That the potential for such differences lurks in our gene pool was demonstrated by Biozzi et al., who, after fifteen generations of selection, succeeded in breeding strains of mice that were high and low responders to a specific antigen (12). That these less well-defined susceptibilities will soon be given molecular identity is attested by the work of Skamene and others, who, by linkage analysis, have discovered genes contributing as a part of multifactorial systems to both susceptibility and resistance to a variety of organisms (13).

What about genetic variations in microorganisms? Inborn errors of neurospora and E. coli played prominent parts in defining what genes are and what they do, but such handicapped organisms are not likely to go far in the business of infection. On the other hand, a mutation leading to an advantage might make itself known. For example, a variant was discovered in a strain of meningococcus that produced localized epidemics of meningitis in England and Wales (14). This strain was found to differ from others in a single base substitution in a gene that specifies the outer membrane protein of the meningococcus. Evidently, this point mutation gave this strain a sufficient advantage to account for most of the cases of meningitis in the affected areas. The nature of the advantage was not reported, but it has been proposed that the glycoproteins of the meningococcal surface so resemble their human congeners as to allow access to human cells without immunological interference.

Such mimicry, attained by microbial mutation and selection, is one of many mechanisms that evolved to facilitate microbial careers. Others include the ability of trypanosomes to change surface proteins at intervals that coincide with the time required for an immune response; they stay just ahead of the immune system, creating in the affected patient a sort of immunological incompetence. Other organisms are able to set up housekeeping inside the phagocytes that are meant to kill them, while still others, notably schistosomes, hijack the surface proteins of the cells of their victims and so pass as self (15–18). Indeed, so ingenious are the means "devised" by microbes to preserve themselves and to fulfill their "plans" that we tend to see them as resourceful, crafty foes, endowing them with human attributes, when, in fact, they are at the mercy of chance. They engage in the most wasteful enterprises, in which billions of organisms die because lacking the wherewithal to find conditions favorable for reproduction, while a single organism, one out of those billions, is endowed with a mutant protein that, quite by chance, conforms as a ligand to the structure of a human "receptor" to make its way to a safe haven where reproduction can occur.

Such encounters, lacking purpose or strategic aim, are simply the kind of jostling that goes on in an ecology in which the survival of species depends upon their ability to adapt to and to reshape an environment in their own interest. These microbial mutational adaptations that fulfill both of these functions represent a microbial logic complementary to that of human congruence and disease. For example, microbial mutants that make unit steps of human homeostasis into points of vulnerability validate the idea of the unitary step as the central feature of human disease. Further, nothing demonstrates more clearly the unity of life than, on the one hand, the capacity of microorganisms to mimic human structures and, on the other, the human ability to specify antibodies to microbial antigens.

All this seems to suggest that infections are no less exemplary of unity and continuity than other diseases, or perhaps even of a classification based on vulnerability of unit steps of homeostasis. That is, infections might be classified according to their avenues of access or transmission, or the means they use to evade or engage the immune system. Clinical expressions must be linked to these qualities.

Finally, how do we characterize infections? Certainly in the general estimation they are diseases of environmental origin; without the microorganisms there is no disease. And it is to changing the environment, to ridding society of its nether millstone, that public health and preventive medicine are dedicated. Public health authorities are also engaged, to the limit of their capacities, in the amelioration of the effects of the upper millstone. They do this by clarifying the role of deprivation and want in creating conditions favorable for the growth and transmission of pathogenic organisms and for depressing human resistance, to their depredations. And we have seen some genuine successes in these actions in the improvement of housing and nutrition; the mortality from infections had dropped significantly long before the introduction of antibiotics. In addition, immunization has become widespread, and public health planning has scored a smashing triumph in the eradication of smallpox. So, clearly, infections are environmental diseases. But an equally compelling case can be made for infections as genetic disorders; there are inborn errors of the defense system and there is a selective gradient that runs continuously from inevitable disease to resistance, a range of variability observed in all disorders associated with variant genes.

So what is the answer to the question? In fact, infections cannot legitimately be called "environmental" only, nor are they solely genetic. They are neither and they are both. In an African population where civil war, hunger, and fear prevail, infections of many kinds are rife and genetic variation is of little significance in differentiating who has disease. But in a suburban U.S. population where life-threatening infections are less frequent anyway, immunodeficiency, or individual vulnerability, is more likely to come to mind. It is not clear that the incidence of immunodeficiency or susceptibility is rising; rather, such vulnerability is more prominent as the frequency of infections declines; a case can be made for a rising heritability. So we can say that the either-or position—genetic or environmental—is a nonstarter. It is an exercise in typological thinking. The population thinker, in contrast, visualizes populations as assemblies of organisms—people, in this case—each with an individual, and relative, readiness to receive or reject the advances of microorganisms; the specificity of infections resides in the degree of the compatibility of the relevant elements of human homeostasis with those of the infecting organism. In analyzing a population we may take the historical path of an analysis of heritability, or we may focus sharply on the molecular characteristics of individual encounters between man and microbe. Clearly the future belongs to the latter, but not, we should hope, at the expense of the former. The state of populations, their genetic composition, their social, economic, and cultural properties, and the dynamism of relationships among the contending organisms are as critical for prevention as the molecular identity of the immunological competence of each of the individuals of which the populations are composed. We have always to keep in mind that it is the remote causes, genetic and cultural, that determine the proximate causes in pathogenicity.

As for the educators who stress the humanities in medical education, infections as disruptive influences in both societies and individual lives have been repeatedly chronicled. I was brought up on DeKruif's *The Microbe Hunters* and Zinsser's *Rats, Lice and History.* More recent accounts are McNeill's *The Human Condition,* already cited, as well as his *Plagues and Peoples.* Crosby's *Ecological Imperialism* is still another. No doubt there are others, but these books describe the struggles between human beings and organisms that pursue their careers unseen by their victims, but not unnoticed. They also expose the paradox revealed in McNeill's metaphor of the millstones. Even today there is still in the world an unconscious cooperation between oppressors who are natural enemies. That is, we struggle mightily and expensively to create antibiotics and vaccines while responding less vigorously to the challenge inherent in the inverse relationship between SES and infections, even in the developing nations.

VII
An Analysis of Disease
in Three Time Frames

This part is devoted to observing how the synthesis of genetic and medical thought expressed in genetic medicine can shape the thinking of the agents of the medical enterprise—mainly in education, but in practice, too. Questions include "Does such a synthesis provide an infrastructure of ideas that helps us to understand why human beings get sick at all, which of us is likely to do so, when in the lifetime, and at what risk to permanent injury or life expectancy? And does that infrastructure serve as a context within which to grasp the meaning of causes, the origins of pathogenesis, and rationales for treatment, as well as to account for the hazards and harmonies of the articulation of open systems with their surroundings?"

These questions will be answered in reference to the three time frames. First, a study of a single disease, type I diabetes, illustrates how the logic illuminates the principles of (a) the nominalist definition of disease; (b) individuality and population thinking; (c) heterogeneity; (d) the unity of disease, its continuity, and the gradient of selective effect; and (e) the interrelationships of proximate and remote causes. Although the expression of every disease is necessarily forged on the anvil of all three time frames, the description of this disorder emphasizes events of the moment.

A second example emphasizes the dynamism of disease and its relationship to the developmental matrix, to the events of the lifetime. The genes, present from conception, specify products whose competences as unit steps in hierarchies of homeostatic integrations are tested across development and as long as life endures. Pathogenesis may be accumulative over many years, may require the completion of several separate steps, may be held in abeyance by homeostatic compensation, or may follow the course of all three together, emerging as overt disease only after some developmental change or as a result of aging. Given the continuity of expression of disease, it is possible that some, or even many, human beings express modified or subclinical forms of chronic disorders. Some are destined to come to fruition while others are held below the threshold of attention by homeostatic compensation, perhaps waxing and waning according to variations in the kind, intensity, and duration of provocations, so that the number of such individuals should vary directly with chronological age. In later life, overt expression is likely to represent only a fraction of the vulnerable. How many octogenarians, dying of whatever cause, are shown to be free of atherosclerosis? And prostatic carcinoma is a frequent incidental finding at autopsy among old men.

A third analysis embraces the context of phylogeny within which the destiny of our species has been shaped. It embraces also cultural evolution, the means whereby the human species has facilitated its own adaptation, the better to succeed in phylogeny. This atmosphere of genetic-cultural harmony, however instrumental in the success of the species, supports incongruities for individuals that circumstances may raise to overt disease. So there is a tension between medicine, the champion of the individual, and a social organization that, although presumed to exist for the public good, may be inimical to some of its individual elements.

And finally, there is an analysis of disease in all three time frames at once, constituting a point of view in which genetic medicine is seen to represent a synthesis of the logic of disease with the metaphor of the machine. Above all, the analysis reveals the paradox between the longitudinal direction of life and the cross-sectional practice of medicine.

25

The Moment

Type 1 Diabetes

Diagnosis of disease follows the assembly of historical information, signs, symptoms, and laboratory data, so as to name a disease that experience tells us responds to a particular treatment. When a disease is not well understood, many cases are investigated to discover its cause, describe its properties, and identify risk factors in the form of experiences and qualities that characterize susceptibility. In these too often typological exercises the qualities described are those of the disease, and it is assumed that any individual patient will resemble, although variably, the average or common character.

How does the logic help in this practical pursuit of diagnosis—in this case in the description of individuals with type I diabetes? The aim is to discern not only that a person has diabetes, but the character of his or her particular version of it.

Type I diabetes, while commonly perceived to be the property of endocrinologists, is familiar to physicians of all specialties. The disease engenders complications that engage the attention of ophthalmologists, cardiologists, nephrologists, neurologists, dermatologists, orthopedists, and others, too, and since its victims survive—some to old age—the disease may add to the hazards of whatever other disorders may come the patient's way. It is not a common disease, nor is it rare. The incidence for children under seventeen years of age varies worldwide between 5 and 35 per 100,000. Age at onset varies from infancy to adulthood—sometimes in persons above forty or even fifty years of age; there is a principal peak at puberty and a smaller one around five years. So it is a transitional disorder, resembling in cases of early onset the infrequency, severity, and biochemical detail of the classical inborn errors of infancy and childhood, while in cases of later onset that are milder and more tractable, it resembles the multifactorial disorders of adult life. We should expect, therefore, a continuity of many characteristics along the axis of age at onset, which stands in here for the gradient of selective effect. The cases with earliest and latest onset should be the easiest to differentiate and perhaps the easiest to make predictions about, but specificity and sensitivity of characteristics deteriorate

Table 7 **Factors Involved in Type I Diabetes**

Genes	Development	Environment
HLA, DR3, DR4	Age	Infection
Many others	Maternal age	Season
	Sex of affected parent	Geography
		Year
		Human milk

as we approach the middle of this distribution, so there is practical use in individual assessments.

Table 7 lists the elements that enter the analysis in the familiar three columns. The list is incomplete; for example, that of the genes is subject to constant revision as new linkages are added and the genes and their specificities are exposed (1,2). Analyses commonly take the form of characterizing populations of cases in regard to each of these qualities, with calculations that indicate their risk to the population or to an abstract, representative diabetic. But population thinking requires that we know how each individual fares in regard to all the factors, and that is the direction more recent analyses are taking.

Consider first the genes. The best understood are those of the MHC, which represent, for this disease, the "main genes"—all others seem less directly implicated in risk and at present are perceived as modifiers (1,2). There is also heterogeneity and variable risk within the MHC alleles. Patients who are heterozygotes for the genotype $\frac{D2A1 * 0501 \quad DQB1*0201}{DQA1*0301 \quad DQB1*0302}$,

once designated DR3/DR4, top the list, while numerous others are of intermediate risk. Still others, including DQA1*0102 and DQB1*0602, once designated DR2, are seldom found in diabetes and so are presumed to be protective, acting to ameliorate the malign effects of others (3). How this gradient of risk within the MHC relates to differences in pathogenesis remains obscure.

The insulin gene, 3'INS, contains in its 3' noncoding region a tandem repeat whose number is polymorphic in the population (1,2). There is evidence that it augments the risk when found in association with MHC alleles, but its role in pathogenesis is unknown. Other genes contributing to the phenotype are so far known only as linkage associations. Currently about ten are known.

Next are factors of the environment. Infection is presumed to be a first step in a chain of events leading to an autoimmune disorder; anti-insulin and other antibodies attest to an autoimmune process and appear also in relatives, some of whom later develop the disease. That more new cases turn up in winter than summer is also cited in favor of the infectious origin, as is variation in incidence from year to year (4). But no one knows why the worldwide incidence is increasing or why the frequency among immigrants compares more favorably with their new place of living than with that whence they came (5).

One experience that has attracted attention is early exposure to cow's milk (6). Evidence is indirect but is increasingly compelling as the association is confirmed again and again. First, antibodies to cow's milk proteins are found in the blood of young diabetics. Second, when the feeding histories of diabetics were compared with those of nondiabetics, babies fed cow's milk were consistently overrepresented among the diabetics. Third, in Scandinavian countries, correlation was demonstrated between the incidence of diabetes and rates of cow's milk feeding, and in an Italian study there was an inverse relationship between the incidence of breastfeeding and that of type I diabetes. Clearly, there is here a nexus of causes—genetic and cultural, proximate and remote. But the issue is not yet decided. Some studies do not find the association. That is to be expected given that each population is likely to differ in representation of individuals to whom cow's milk is injurious. That is, it is unlikely that everyone is equally susceptible to injury by cow's milk protein.

Among developmental factors are age at onset, maternal age at birth, sex of the affected parent, and weight gain early in life (7,8). When fathers are affected, a surplus of DR4 alleles are transmitted (9).

How are these properties assorted to account for expression in individual diabetics? The answer will require prospective studies. One such study involved several thousand newborn babies, among whom more than 2 percent had the high-risk genotypes and a further 20 percent had the moderate-risk versions (10). We know that only a fraction of these high-risk babies will ever have diabetes, so the individuality of the disease will be exposed by following them, preferably for as long as forty years. This is a very forward-looking study, exemplary of what must be done for many diseases in which genes are perceived to be risks. Such prospective observations are the only way we will ever know the risks for populations or for individuals. The latter aim is promoted by observing arrays of genes and other elements in both affected and unaffected individuals at risk, with arrangement according to probability of disease and its severity. The circumstances surrounding the advent of, or escape from, the disease in individuals would then be laid before us in detail.

Other studies of diabetes have revealed a profound effect of age; for example, the high-risk genotypes and high antibody titers are concentrated in diabetics with the earliest onset (11). Further, the earlier the onset, the higher is the familial recurrence rate and the greater the MZ twin concordance—and the greater the probability of having been raised on cow's milk (6,12,13). Conversely, breastfed babies who became diabetic did so at a later age. In contrast, in a population of 190 patients with type I diabetes with onset at over twenty years of age, 16 percent were reported to lack any of the high-risk alleles, to be less severely affected, and to have low levels of antibody and few affected relatives (14). The authors suggested etiologic heterogeneity by way of explanation and cited these patients as evidence of the need for individual analysis of cases.

Winter onset is also associated with severe disease and with the high-risk genotypes, but it is unclear whether winter-onset cases are also of early onset (4,5). If not, when the disease has onset in the winter in the very young, is it worse than when onset in such patients occurs in the summer? Other associations are still unexplored: for example, we don't know the particulars of the diabetes of patients born to elderly mothers, only that there are more of them (15). Also, if breastfeeding reduces the incidence of diabetes, what besides early onset characterizes patients who get the disease despite such feeding? And if the incidence is rising, are the patients observed in the years with higher frequency in some way different? Is the heritability changing? And why is the frequency so high in Scandinavian countries as opposed to, say, South America or Japan? In time it should be possible to correlate all these risk factors with particular constellations of genes, at which point the disorder will doubtless be seen to be an indivisible continuum along an axis, perhaps of age at onset, but with humps in the distribution that constitute syndromes of variable frequency.

In its focus on the particular set of variables possessed by each of many individuals, such analyses go beyond epidemiology which characterizes populations. Each different combination of such variables must be expressed in a unique version of the disease. Subtle differences in constellations of qualities may have little impact on the treatment, which may be equally appropriate for some or many of the versions. But is it not likely that those characteristics we all admire in superior clinicians derive from their intuitive perception of just such subtleties? And clearly their careful adjustment of treatment to the apparent need of each patient represents a response to individuality, an expression of what we all applaud as the "art" of medicine. Intuition has been all but replaced by technology, and in one sense, no one can fail to be pleased by that. But is it not likely that a mentality that is most comfortable with the representation of each case as a unique example, a mentality informed by the nominalist view of disease, is also more likely to see that that unique assembly of informative facts is made possible only by the individuality of the patient? Such a perception of the humanity of the sick is unlikely when the patient is viewed as a broken machine.

Physicians who have been treating type I diabetics over the years have recognized the individuality of each patient; this is a disease in which failure to do so can be disastrous. So it is careful observation, appeal to intuition, and attention to individual detail that have distinguished the management of this disease since the advent of insulin. It is only now that the sources of that individuality are being exposed. Will such revelations improve the treatment? Certainly, but they will do so because the new treatments will be seen to suit the special properties of each patient: the diabetes of Jane Jones will be distinguished from that of John Smith. Failure to attend to the social identity of patients is one aspect of the dissatisfaction expressed by the critics of medical education. Perhaps that recognition of the individuality of disease, an individuality compounded of both biological and social qualities, will go some way to re-establish that interest?

26

The Lifetime

Some readers may recall a cartoon map of the United States that appeared in the *New Yorker* years ago. Drawn by Saul Steinberg, it was a satirical view of the nation, an expression of the narcissism of the East. At least half the map consisted of New York City and a further 30 percent of a much-distorted eastern seaboard. The remainder was a bizarre rendering of all the rest of the country, very little of it west of the Mississippi.

Although hardly the cartoonist's intent, the drawing might serve as a metaphor for a similarly distorted notion of how disease affects the human species. The conventional wisdom about the lifetime distribution of human diseases shows the same provincial preoccupation with the obvious: what is obvious to New Yorkers is New York, what medical people know is that the main burden of disease falls upon adults, especially old people. But it is a distortion that reflects the machine mentality that is stirred only by something clearly broken and in need of fixing. And why not? The physician's business is with living patients who have complaints that lead to a diagnosis and treatment.

Although representative of disease after birth, this traditional view is not inclusive of the whole lifetime. It omits a period that, however brief, embraces the genesis, not only of the patients who suffer disease after birth, but of both their diseases and the human individuality that make them various. So genetic medicine begins with the zygote, whose individuality is strongly genetic, and is guided by the logic already outlined: the genetically variable unit step of homeostasis, the gradient of selective effect, the unity and continuity of disease, and so on. The gradient of selective effect begins at conception, where genetic individuality is at a maximum, and declines through life to the centenarian whose individuality has been so much shaped by decades of experiences. But outcomes of the experiences of each life are always constrained by the way gene products internalized those experiences and wove them into the fabric of individuality, a fabric that derives its distinctive character from modification of trajectories established early in life. Some of that fabric is likely to represent incongruence.

Figure 4 (chapter 22) shows age-defined mortality rates that confirm the conventional emphasis on the latter part of life. But elsewhere in this book the mayhem of intrauterine life was exposed, and it was revealed that the conventional distribution of human disease and mortality is no more an accurate depiction of reality than is Steinberg's cartoon map of the United States. The difference between the two distributions of disease is that the conventional one embraces only that which comes to the doctor's attention, while the alternative includes diseases that affect conceptuses, embryos, and fetuses that never make an appearance in daily life and that are not easily recognized as human beings. But they have human genes and soon become open systems with homeostatic apparatuses, and the principle of the continuity of disease, based on the idea of incongruity between a genetically specified homeostasis and the environment, requires that fertilized ova and embryos be deemed a part of the continuum. One is reminded here of Garrod's concept of the continuity of chemical individuality: the inborn errors he observed were merely the visible range of a vast continuum of chemical variety that was, in his time, invisible and unknowable.

Now, keeping in mind that the child is father of the man and that our days are bound each to each in a historical process, each day's homeostatic competences must reflect the variety of the elements of the genotype, including those genes whose presence will be known only in later life, and the products of such genes must participate, each in its own way, in the trajectory taken by the integrated whole. If so, then the seeds of disease, sown at conception, may germinate very early, even in utero. No doubt some genes of early development turn off, but only after imposing their individual stamp, while others await a time of action—at birth, say, or at adolescence. If some of those that turned off early or came on late are variants, those that turn on subsequently enter a system already shaped by development, and they may enhance the unfavorable direction of these prior variants, or they may negate their effects. If the former, a vulnerability may arise that can respond to conditions that lead, perhaps through other vulnerabilities, to later disease. The point is that because the genes that specify the unit steps of homeostasis that constitute points of vulnerability—and that lead, under appropriate conditions, to overt disease—are present from the beginning and are in action before—even long before—the advent of disease, they must be seen as taking part in the orientation taken by development, biasing it, each in its own special way. So variants, present from the start, germinate the soil, preparing it for experiences that will find it favorable, early or late, as life, ontogeny, and aging unfold.

Gestation, not ordinarily a major element in the medical curriculum, fills less than 1 percent of an eighty-five–year lifetime, the first two years perhaps 3 percent, and the bulk of development—say fifteen years—17 percent, and yet these early times overshadow all the rest. The metaphor of a relay race may be useful here, a race toward a goal of, say, eighty-five years. In such a race the team performance depends upon that of each runner, and we know that in this race, the last runner is the weakest. So the others must present the last with a substantial lead. To that end, the first runner should be the most fleet, the most reliable, the better to pass an early advantage down the line. No doubt there would be intense competition (selection) for this first position. Many would be called, few chosen, because the performance of the first runner is critical to the whole. Of course, some modest hitch in the effort of the first may be made up by the exertions of the second and third, but should the second fail also, the whole burden is laid on the third. That is, the earlier the failure, the less likely will there be any advantage to pass on to the last, and least, runner.

So it is in these early developmental phases that the human individual we know and recognize comes into being. We cannot neglect the influence of the original stamp upon the rest of life, no matter how much plasticity and adaptability are built into the design. Indeed, the mechanisms of plasticity, themselves mediated by gene products, must be subject to variation and vulnerability as well as to the proviso just cited. Reduced plasticity is to be expected in old age, but its lack early in life must reduce the capacity to seize options—which, in turn, must foreclose others.

Clearly, selection acts to reduce unwanted variants; hence the losses in utero and the many hundreds (thousands?) of single-gene disorders known today. But continuity and the selective gradient require that, in our thinking about medicine and in teaching, we integrate these developmental periods into our concept of the human lifetime and that we recognize that mutants that escape early selection lead to vulnerability, potential disease, and possibly handicap. Now, having fixed in our minds that all of us, right now, today, regardless of age, and in ways both straightforward and convoluted, reflect our early lives—not only those of adolescence, childhood, or infancy, but that of gestation, too—how do we translate this into action in medical thinking and teaching? There are two ways: (a) in the description of early expressions of pathogenesis that emerge as disease later in life, and (b) in observing the special vulnerabilities of life's developmental phases.

Early Expressions

Tests of the hypothesis that events early in life influence later disease have only lately become possible. Much of the relevant thinking has been laid out in the sections on homeostasis, especially that on development. Adult life is an outcome of early life as a result of adaptation and change constrained by the genotype and proceeding day by day to form individual matrixes within which the events of later days are influenced by those of the past. And because each step in this progression will be influenced, not only by the original impetus, but by all the conditions prevailing in the evolving matrix, predictions based on

Analysis of Disease in Three Time Frames

that which set the process in motion are sure to be uncertain; we are reminded of the ambiguity of the locution "genes for."

Despite these complexities there is a movement, now gathering momentum, to test the proposition outlined above: that conditions in early life set in motion events that lead to later vulnerability and disease (1,2). The methods employed are mainly epidemiological and include correlations between (a) qualities expressed early in postnatal life and those of later years; (b) low birth weight and disease late in life; and (c) infant and later mortality in the same areas of poverty. The question here is, "Does high infant mortality suggest conditions that have impaired growth in utero with reflections on the whole of life?"

Correlations, Early and Late

Lucas concludes that malnutrition, both in utero and after birth, programs developmental events (3). That is, the fetus and infant monitor the nutritional environment and adapt metabolism appropriately. Then, since the processes of growth are set for the energy available and since this happens during rapid developmental change, the results of the adaptation may be permanent. Some of Lucas's work in comparing the development of premature infants fed cow's milk as opposed to human milk has already been reviewed (see chapter 8). In other work, the influence of the genes is revealed. Feeding cow's milk to premature babies heightened the incidence of later asthmatic attacks, but only when there was a family history of allergy (3).

Type II Diabetes

Several investigators have found significant correlations between low birth weight and type II diabetes associated with insulin resistance in patients fifty to sixty years old (4–6). The role of the intrauterine environment is further suggested by observation among Pima Indians of a five-times higher incidence of NIDDM at age twenty to twenty-five years among the offspring of mothers who were diabetic during pregnancy than among those of prediabetic women (4). The latter were known to have a genetic predisposition since they developed the disease later, so an intrauterine influence in addition to the genetic impulse was suggested. Other postnatal qualities, including urban living, education of both parents and subject, childhood activity, and obesity, have been shown to be correlated with NIDDM in adult life (7).

Hypertension

Once again, as in NIDDM, a significant correlation between hypertension in adult life and low birth weight has been observed—and, in addition, between hypertension and placental enlargement (8,9). In one study the relationship was particularly pronounced when the adults were obese (9). Edwards et al.'s explanation for the intrauterine growth retardation is overexposure of the fetus to active glucocorticoid as a result of reduced activity of hydroxysteroid dehydrogenase, an enzyme that inactivates glucocorticoid (10). He postulates that the glucocorticoid, which is known to affect vascular tone, affects the growth of the fetal vasculature, with effects on blood pressure throughout life. Lever and Harrap, in an article entitled "Essential Hypertension: A Disorder of Growth with Origins in Childhood," suggest two phases in the establishment of high blood pressure (11). One is in early life, where there is excessive vascular growth, and this is followed by other mechanisms that cause the elevated pressure to persist.

So, different events and mechanisms working at different times of life may be required to bring the adult patient to the doctor, whether with asymptomatic hypertension or with stroke. To experience all of these events and mechanisms may mean serious trouble; to omit the first, expressed in early life, may mean none at all.

Atherosclerosis

Investigations into relationships between events in early life and ischemic heart disease have been pursued most vigorously by Barker and co-workers (1). They have demonstrated (a) correlations of low birth weight and enlarged placenta with mortality due to heart attack later in life; (b) an inverse correlation between mortality from coronary artery disease and weight at one year of age; and (c) an inverse correlation between weight at one year and serum fibrinogen levels in adult life. So they contend that there is an association between growth in early life and premature mortality due to heart attack.

The reader may protest that the evidence for all of these conditions is insubstantial and indirect and, indeed, cogently argued reservations of the sort have been expressed (12). But the position is a familiar one: a new idea runs counter to conventional thought and, because not yet thoroughly tested, is spurned. Fair enough. The advocates of these early origins of diseases that characterize later life have much to do to validate their assertions. Especially do they need to describe the intrauterine events that contribute to fetal retardation and to examine these experiences of early life prospectively and in the context of family histories. It is known, for example, that the lipid risk factors for atherosclerosis vary in infancy and childhood in accord with family history, but nothing is known about uterine growth and family history for any of these diseases. The report of the Pima Indians and the heightened rate of diabetes in the offspring of diabetic mothers made no mention of birth weight.

In summary, this work has a strong appeal in its compatibility with the logic of disease being developed in this book. If the child is father of the man in health, does it not follow that such influences exist also in disease?

Development as a Remote Cause of Disease

The infant offspring of an antelope must be ready within minutes to run with the herd, lest it be consumed by predators, and to this end, its central nervous system is sufficiently mature at birth. Not so with human babies, who must experience years of maturation before attaining the same competence, and it is to neotonous development with its prolonged juvenility that we owe the adaptability and plasticity of our nervous systems and our special cognitive qualities. But prolonged development does not mean that a fully competent brain is merely taking its time working out the intricacies of behavior; rather, it means that the formation of structure and the integration of physiology have still a long way to go in postnatal life, and an incomplete nervous system is a vulnerable one. Indeed, the human newborn is, in comparison with that of other primates, still a fetus, with the necessity at birth of assuming responsibility for its own metabolism. Human babies are helped over the initial phases of maturation by products of the human breast, which, standing in for the placenta, acts as an essential element in the infant's homeostasis. It is this physiological immaturity that, when combined with that of the structure and function of the brain, constitutes the infant's vulnerability to the intrusion of experiences for which it is unready. So, neoteny, however inestimable its advantage in the formation of our cognitive lives, has its darker side as a remote cause of disease.

Disorders of Neotonous Development

Several disorders of early life are a consequence of such immaturity. One example is phenylketonuria in which phenylalanine or a metabolic product become toxic to the immature brain. Were the human brain as far along as that of the animal that runs at birth, PKU might be merely a harmless metabolic variant. Other examples are (a) lead poisoning, which in childhood damages the brain but in adult life produces peripheral neuritis; (b) cretinism, which again disrupts brain development, as opposed to hyperthyroidism later in life that does no such harm to the brain; and (c) kernicterus, a condition of brain damage in newborn babies due to an excess of bilirubin that has not yet been detoxified because time is required for the induction of the enzyme glucuronyltransferase. So there is a trade-off: unparalleled opportunities for variety and flexibility for the majority against risks of developmental damage for a minority.

Osteoporosis

A particularly instructive example of lifetime impact is in variations in homeostasis of bone that lead to fractures in old people. The state of bone at any moment is a result of a balance between bone formation and destruction that is influenced by stresses, nutrition, and hormones, including vitamin D, parathyroid, and sex hormones. All of the cellular mechanisms—including absorption and excretion of calcium, the synthesis, secretion, and degradation of hormones, and the processes of bone formation and destruction—are mediated by protein products of genes susceptible to mutation. These include the hormones themselves as well as the transcription factors they influence, many growth factors, some specialized morphogenetic bone proteins, as well as the vitamin D receptor that regulates calcitonin and whose polymorphisms are thought to be predictors of bone density (13). So it can be no surprise that the heritability of the attainment of bone mass is high—for example, mother-daughter correlations for measures of bone mass are high. When the mother had suffered fractures, her daughters' measures of bone mass were likely to be below normal. The implication of this heritability is that osteoporosis and fracture can be familial (14).

Most of the genetic variation is expressed in the attainment of peak bone mass, while most of the variation expressed in the loss of bone is associated with experiences (15). Both encompass a great deal of individual variation. Peak bone mass is reached in early adult life, and twin studies show the heritability to be high. In males, bone mass is influenced by testosterone, so that boys with delayed puberty or hypogonadism attain a lesser peak (16).

Bone mass is then maintained until an indeterminate time when, with great individual variability, it begins a very slow descent, hastened in women by the loss of estrogen at the menopause. Much of the individual variation has to do with poor nutrition, lack of exercise, alcohol, smoking, and other influences, all modified by the variable ways people age. Smoking is of particular interest since it is often a teenage habit indulged at the very moment of a spurt in bone mass, a spurt of much import to the teenager, who may pay for this indulgence in later years, since sufferers of fractures and collapsed vertebrae in late life are those whose peak bone mass was below par to begin with. What seems of so little moment at teen age is anything but thirty to fifty years later. The question here is how to teach the teenage smoker that her days are bound each to each in fidelity to genetic obligations that, together with her own set of experiences (over which she has some control), specify a trajectory that can lead either to illness and debility or to a healthy old age. Teenagers are notoriously resistant to constraint, but one wonders how many have a visceral grasp of the continuity of their physiological lives or that what we do early in life may decide our health as old people.

The moral of the story is plain. An elderly grandmother who has shrunk a few inches or had a fracture is a signal to her daughters and granddaughters to look to their own bones and to think of exercise as a useful preventive, and perhaps to consider estrogen after the menopause as a measure necessary to preserve a bone mass that might have little margin for loss. Similarly, a grandson whose puberty was delayed might see salvation in exercise and add this to a dozen reasons for not smoking.

The limitation of medical practice that is engaged only when a patient is already sick is nowhere so starkly evident as in these impacts of early life on later disease. First, disease is likely to be a family matter—even when only one person is affected, others may be liable—and second, as molecular pathogenesis is exposed and as we learn how particular experiences interact with the products of specific genotypes over the lifetime, medical education and practice can hardly fail to accept the primacy of prevention.

CONCLUSION

In this chapter I have tried to show that there is a limbo between health and disease, a transitional zone wherein overt expression hangs in the balance. The thinking I have outlined here puts it that our diseases are in us and of us. They are as expressive of us as the characteristic features of our faces, wherein we recognize one another not because one has a face and another does not, but because of the arrangement, shapes, sizes, colors, and contours of the features thereof, features that identify us both early in life and late. So the physician needs to know the biology, not only of Homo sapiens, but in some significant degree that of individuals with names and social security numbers who are representative of the species. In so doing, the doctor's gaze is shifted away from each patient's approximation to an abstract stereotype to the reality of one person's expressions of disease. It is the qualities of each metaphorical child—the qualities of inheritance, of experience, and of maturation—that determine whether the metaphorical man will have disease at all, which ones, when in life, which among all possible forms it will take, whether and in what degree treatment will succeed, and whether by some judicious intervention it can be prevented. Such a construction of disease attains the humane goal of putting the doctor right into the context of a patient's life, there to observe how one set of days bound each to each have brought a singular human being to a particular present state. Surely this sense of the unity and continuity of one's own life is uppermost in the minds of any of us when we consult a doctor. Isn't it up to the doctor to match that concern?

Biology and Social History, and a Vision of Disease in Three Time Frames

The history of the present illness given by a sick patient is a product of the history of the patient's development and maturation as well as his participation in phylogeny. It is the latter that provides the genes that make his homeostatic apparatus both human and representative of all life, impose upon it constraints that we cannot transgress, and provide the means to create, through development, the individuality that colors all aspects of our lives. And it is the remote causes that makes the experience of disease a personal one. But it has not only a biological dimension, it embraces culture, too. Human existence must have a culture of some kind no matter how primitive, and our ancestral primates and hominids adapted to it, with selection eliminating the incongruent while adding that which facilitated adaptation. So our phylogenetic history leaves us adaptable, more capable of creating environments in which to thrive than any other organism. But that flexibility is based in part on homeostatic elements that have been successful in all life forms and that we transcend at our peril. However ingenious the creations that enable human beings to master the environment, human diversity will leave some individuals vulnerable. Accordingly, some disease is a consequence of incongruence of experience with processes representative of the remote past, some with processes characteristic only of human beings, and both are a consequence of incongruences of individual homeostasis with individual experiences of the environment, natural and contrived.

Biological history is slow, measured in hundreds of millions of years. Social and cultural history are more likely to be reckoned in generations and seem now to be measured in decades—or less. The asynchrony of these two histories has significant human consequences. Human ingenuity has added social adaptation to biological evolution, enabling us to broaden our experiences of the planet and even to give ourselves social definition as people with names, identities, attainments, and many other characteristics, definitions that transcend, but do not defy, biology. At least, when we do the latter, as in our "conquest" of space, it is at no small physiological cost.

In the developed nations, cultural and social history has brought adjustments in housing, nutrition, education, and medicine that have reduced sickness and mortality and doubled the average life expectancy, with significant and unanticipated changes in our demography: for example, no one foresaw that today the oldest old—eighty-five years and up—would be the fastest growing segment of the population (1). At the same time this evolutionary asynchrony gives origin to much of our disease. Examples are (a) unintended ecological disruptions that lead to incongruence and disease—fouling of the atmosphere, a damaged ozone layer, desertification of arable land, pollution of the seas, and misuse of drugs; and (b) Iatrogenic disease, which is by no means unknown—drugs said to be sovereign for a particular disease prove to be intolerable for some individuals. But nowhere is the clash more evident than in the disorders associated with the habits and modes of living observed in the developed nations. The excesses and deficiencies of the present overtax the resilience of a homeostasis designed for the past.

These are conditions of the environment that we know and understand. But behind that knowledge, there lurks the question of how much of the whole of disease is accountable to these rather straightforward proximate causes that act on genetically vulnerable substrates. Are there not more complex interactions, too? In the last chapter, we saw that there are. Phylogeny and the conditions of the moment (genes and experiences) conspire to create a developmental matrix within which such interactions occur. Latency of disease is a property of the matrix, so diseases must have a far longer history than we know. But we need such knowledge if prevention is to matter. We need to understand vulnerabilities as outcomes of developmental trajectories.

So, what should we be looking for? For example, how many vulnerabilities are outcomes of the directions taken by developmental trajectories under the influence of events early in development? We know that outstanding performance in adult life is often associated with precocity early in life; there are no end of photographs of Tiger Woods, the celebrity golfer of the moment, whacking away at the ball at age five. So if early training is a prescription for later proficiency, why not for disease as well? If we are ever to surmount such circumlocutions as "gene-environment interaction" or to explain heritability coefficients of 0.5, we will have to come more realistically to grips with what they mean.

Much is being made of the Human Genome Project, and rightly so, but let us be clear: that effort will uncover an effusion of proximate causes that will illuminate pathogenesis and, perhaps, lead to specific treatments. Of course, it should lead to prevention, too, but if this is to happen, we must know what needs changing—qualities and events that may be lost in the mist of long-forgotten development. The Genome Project will certainly be extended to discover the influences of the genes it exposes on development and aging. But genetic individuality is only part of the story. We need a companion effort to discover the conditions within which the gene-specified variant proteins direct home-ostasis into channels that predispose to disease later in life. Again we are in the house that Jack built.

Objection might be raised on the grounds that we could never observe the lives of individuals closely enough to detect such differences and, if we could, the data would be so dense as to defy interpretation. Of course, they would be dense and complicated, but the study would be systematized to start with. As for complexity, we are told that 50,000 to 100,000 genes are going to be de-scribed, after which their protein products and the latter's functions are to be discovered, too. So new ways of handling data are being devised. The point is that the organization that is making the Genome Project successful might be adapted to the study of the relation of development and maturation to disease. Let us remember that until we approach the "environment," including devel-opment, systematically, we shall be left with heritability coefficients. They do tell us something important, but they say that we must look for the genes and beyond the genes to whatever it is that creates the conditions within which the genes' products fail in their duties. So heritabilities are worthwhile, but very unfulfilling—a shredded wheat biscuit as opposed to a feast. Perhaps heri-tabilities are like classical Greek figures, separated heads, limbless trunks, and the like. They have beauty in themselves and suggest the lives they represent, but they are a long way from the intentions of the artist.

Just as the Genome Project has called upon the varied expertness of many biologists, so must an intensive study of the origins of disease in individuals in the experiences of development call upon more than physicians. Again we per-ceive the virtues of the representatives of those other disciplines that have dealt themselves a hand in medicine. Anthropologists should have much to offer; habits and qualities of development must differ markedly among populations, and so does the incidence of disease. Epidemiologists, geneticists, statisticians, and demographers, as well as psychologists, sociologists, historians, and, of course, physicians, perhaps mainly pediatricians, could all contribute were there some concerted effort to find the conditions of the developmental matrix that raise vulnerabilities to disease. To omit these factors just when the genet-ic elements are the object of such perfervid zeal is to seem to be accepting the genetic determinism that we all reject.

A VISION OF DISEASE IN THE THREE TIME SCALES

In this analysis of disease at the three levels of history, genetic thinking and the metaphor of the machine come together to provide a coherent context for medical thinking that embraces education, practice, and public health. It is a context of three levels in which the first is embraced within the second and both within the third, like a set of fitted boxes, and there is an uninterrupted continuity of thought as one moves from one box to the next. In the innermost box is diagnosis and treatment of a particular patient, whose genetic and developmental individuality is incongruent with experience. But the individuality of the patient cannot be clearly perceived apart from the second box; indeed, individuality is defined only in comparison of one to others. So individuality is first tested in the family, which must come to be the primary focus of the physician—primary because it is in the family setting that individuality takes shape, where the most significant developmental events occur, including the inheritance of genes, the most explosive growth and maturation, the beginning of acculturation, and the origin of the developmental trajectories that differentiate individuals. Sibs share parental genes, parental culture, and household experiences. These are all sources of within-family likeness in vulnerability, and since different families are likely to vary in constellations of both genes and experiences, a better sense of the future for any individual is more likely to derive from observations of a whole family than from any single person.

The third box includes the elements of which incongruence is made, the wherewithal the species uses to get on with its business of living and reproduction: mutation, recombination, genetic polymorphism, and the composition of the gene pool, as well as the cultural and social attributes that characterize and differentiate ethnic groups and larger communities. These are remote causes that tell us why human beings must suffer disease at all and how incongruities arise.

The continuities in going from one box to the next are obvious. The first starts from the present—the patient in box 1—and goes, by way of the lifetime of development and aging within the influence of the family (box 2), to biological and cultural history (box 3). Second, in passing from the first box to the third, kinship is diluted; relatives share peculiarities of both genes and experiences and so, in progressively lesser degree, do members of ethnic groups and larger communities. But the diversity within such groups is greater than that between them; in the end, our humanness transcends our ethnic or other differentiation. So at the basis of ideas about disease that include genetic variation there is always a powerful constraint. Remote causes, inherent in evolution, lead to disease but also constrain its forms.

In a third continuity there is a progression of forms of management. Treatment in the form of medication or surgery is focused sharply on individual patients (box 1). Prevention is most easily perceived and executed in families of individuals who share genes and habits (box 2), and preventive medicine and public health are most comfortably embraced in box 3, among the remote causes.

A fourth continuity is critical for medical teaching, where a tension exists between education and practical training. Education was defined in the introduction as disposing principles and ideas, their relationships, how they evolved, and how they inform practical training. The latter is defined as teaching how to care for patients and includes diagnosis and management, which is rote learning unless taught in the context of ideas. Practice (box 1) taught unclothed in the ideas of boxes 2 and 3 risks limiting the doctor-patient encounter to technology. Perhaps it is a lack of reconciliation between education and practice that has so stirred those critics of medical education whose view it is that failure to observe the patient's social integration—and biological, too, they might have added—leads to omission of ethical and humanistic dimensions essential for good management. Confirmation of the critics' contention is given by Kunitz, who observed that the physicians most attentive to patients' values and sensibilities were family practitioners and pediatricians—that is, those whose mission includes the family (box 2) as a primary concern (2). So unity of ideas and practice is most naturally attained in the context of the family, wherein development and the experiences of the lifetime are also most readily comprehended.

Such continuities flow naturally from the different ideas expressed in the three boxes, and I believe some such medicine of ideas was in Garrod's mind when he sat down to write *Inborn Factors in Disease*. The idea of the inborn error, limited at its inception to alkaptonuria, soon took in three more variants, and today there are hundreds, and while it is unlikely that anyone could, or would want to, recite from memory the whole list of their names, all medical students should be comfortable with the concept and perceive how central it is in our thinking today. Logic took Garrod's thinking from the inborn error to chemical individuality which, transcending individuals, can be seen to characterize species, too. From there it was only a short step to the perception that chemical individuality is the wherewithal for selection, which defines our evolutionary advantages as well as the disadvantages that may constitute disease.

What Garrod lacked to test his ideas was the rich detail of today's cell and molecular biology. This we have, and we are seeing how seemingly trivial changes in chemical individuality can be translated into devastating disease. In doing so we observe new mechanisms and generalizations that Garrod could not even have imagined, but rather than leading to significant departures from his original principles, these novelties give them new meaning, lending coherence and logic to explanations of disease.

VIII
The Logic and Modern Medicine

It remains in this final section of the book to consider whether and how the thinking of genetic medicine as it has been defined here provides a context in which to deal with the problems of medicine outlined in chapter 3, as well as with the concerns of those disciplines that have asserted their interests (see chapter 1). No one denies that the evidence of human genetic variation has had a signal influence on our understanding of pathogenesis of disease or that those insights are going to be deepened as the products of the Genome Project flow into medicine. The question is how the information, new and old, is to be used. So the first chapter in this section is devoted to how the fruits of the Genome Project are likely to affect medicine. There will be a spate of information about human gene loci as well as about the homeostatic elements their occupants specify. Such information will be useful to those studying the physiological impact on both congruence and incongruence of allelic variation at these loci. But how will such information be perceived within the logic of disease? And, particularly, how is it likely to affect medical education?

The second chapter poses the question of how the logic can help in integrating the ideas of human biology and medicine with those of cultures and societies, particularly how the logic might influence medical education to reestablish the primacy of the individual patient in medical care, and in so doing, how it might lead to emphasis on prevention and public health. If there is objection to medicine entering more prominently into how we carry on our social lives in both communities and larger societies, one can only say that any aspect of society that commands so imposing a fraction of the gross national product has already entered that sphere and has already affected social life to a degree comparable with education, the church, or defense.

A further question is, what is it in genetic medicine that will accommodate, even advance, the cause of at least some of those nonmedical disciplines? A case could be made that the people they embrace are not "outsiders" at all, that we are all in the same boat and that our problems of health will be solved only by a concerted effort to cultivate and impose a public will. The medical pro-

Table 8 **A Logic of Disease**

Qualtiy	Genetic Medicine	Body as Machine
Concept of disease	Nominalist	Essentialist
Classes	Individual	That of the class
Causes	Complex, multiple, both proximate and remote	Simple, single, proximate
Heterogeneity of cause	Expected until shown not to exist	Opposed until shown to exist
Time	Disease in three time scales	Present illness, past history
Mentality	Populational	Typological
Variability	Both intrinsic and extrinsic, extensive	Extrinsic, small
Relationship to selection	Strong, disease is a consequence of necessity for variation	Weak, disease is due to origins outside the body, apart from "genetic" disease
Familiarity	Expected in most disease, family included in diagnosis	Ignored, or recognized in "genetic" disease
Frequency of disease	Inverse relationship with selective gradient	Depends upon frequency of outside cause or of gene in "genetic" disorder
Incidence	Depends upon frequency and distribution of both genes and experiences	Depends upon frequency and distribution of cause
Age at onset	Depends on postion in selective gradient and developmental matrix	Depends upon when in the lifetime the cause acts
Classification of disease	Systematic	Pragmatic
Prevention	Natural, inherent in the nature of the causes, takes form of protection of the vulnerable	Awaits onset of disease
Doctor–patient relationship	Necessary, opportunity for sympathy is reinforced	Depends on temperament of doctor
Social attitudes	Includes relationship between physiological, developmental, genetic, and social homeostasis	None—what has society to do with medicine?—doctor's social attitudes are personal
Therapy	Directed to remote as well as proximate causes	Directed to proximate causes
Ultimate outcomes	Uncertain	Disease-free society

fession would then be in a kind of executive position, using expert knowledge to carry on the public's business.

The question for the final chapter is whether genetic medicine provides a basis for a medical education capable of implanting new ideas in the minds of medical students. No new curriculum is needed, nor necessarily need there be a change in anyone's precious hours; it is simply a matter of teaching the existing curriculum from a new point of view.

To refresh the reader's memory and to lay out the elements of the logic of genetic medicine in comparison to that of the machine mentality, Table 8 is included here. The table provides the context in which to recount the ideas and issues of the final three chapters.

28

The Human Genome Project

Out of the crooked timber of humanity, no straight thing was ever made.
—Isaiah Berlin, *The Crooked Timber of Humanity*

This line, which originated with Kant, was cited by Isaiah Berlin in an essay called "The Pursuit of the Ideal." It was his belief that human diversity stands in the way of the conformity required to attain an ideal society. One person's Eden is another's prison, and the latter is unlikely to accept willingly the coercion of the former. The uses of the crooked timber have to be adapted to it rather than it to them.

Berlin argued the case cogently by examining the limitations of the social utopias proposed in the Enlightenment, in the romantic movement in Germany, and in the tyrannies of the recent past. Always the different paths toward the ideal failed to cohere; whoever went one way could not go the other. Although Berlin argued on cultural grounds, the lesson is that if the human timber is to be fashioned into something, it must be done in accord with its qualities, both inherent and cultural, and the most prominent of these is diversity. So if, for example, we want a disease-free society, we are likely to find the road blocked by human variety. What will wipe out disease for some will harm others, and to adapt the means to those others may fail the some. Furthermore, there will always be those who reject whatever is proposed, perhaps on the grounds of belief in an alternative or because of fear, failure to understand, or just indifference. The ambiguity of technological success is one of the properties that attracted the interest of representatives of those other disciplines listed in the introduction who are not willing to leave medicine wholly to the doctors.

Berlin's slogan was applied to politics, but when fitted to medical aspirations, its virtue lies in its denial of typology and its appeal to population thinking. It seems to attest to the limitations of the machine mentality and to affirm the logic of disease: utopian proposals for medicine will have to pass the test of human diversity and therefore may be beyond our grasp. But this is hardly a prescription for pessimism; now is the time for us to test our grasp against the reach of the Human Genome Project.

Nature encourages diversity, and on the path to new states of congruence, much incongruence is generated. It is the job of medicine so to change conditions as to make congruent that which is incongruent, and the essence of our investigative mission is to define how nearly we can attain so desirable an end. So we must understand the nature of the crooked timber, its tolerance for manipulation, and the extent to which we must adapt our ends to its intransigence. And the human timber is not all that has limits: all of the elements of Darwin's bank demand adaptation to them as well. We have the advantage of nature in our capacity to adjust the environment, but nature has the advantage of us in eons of refinement of homeostatic adaptations, not only within single organisms but between them—and within and between species as well. We meddle with its complexity at our peril.

Thus far in medicine we have been pragmatic, doing what we can and being remarkably successful, too, but such success is usually defined in comparison to the diseased state rather than to health. We are pleased with outcomes that, when compared to being sick, are tolerable but are a good deal less than the health the patient once enjoyed. We are pleased with our progress but salways aim for more. Now we are going to have the benefits of the Human Genome Project, and speculation about the quality and extent of those benefits is accompanied by predictions of unintended hazards. The apposite title of a recently published book is *Why Things Bite Back: Technology and the Revenge of Unintended Consequences* (1); another is *Worse Than the Disease: Pitfalls of Medical Progress* (2).

THE GENOME PROJECT

A cardinal question raised by medical thinkers, as well as by those others who have asserted an interest, is how is medicine to adapt to an increasingly technological future? Most of our attention at the moment goes to the changes in practice that are being forced by an enterprise that, although exploitive of both profession and patients, styles itself as "free." Medicine's other side—its ideas and intellectual content—is also under siege, this time by the arrival of genetics; the prospect of a genetic medicine is no less threatening to complacency than is managed care.

Novelty in medical thinking leads to reworking of medical education. The influence of the medical genetics enterprise is one source of impetus toward what seems inevitable. Another is the promise of exposure to scrutiny of the whole of the human genetic apparatus, a natural outcome of a reductionist molecular biology, even a logical fulfillment of Garrod's postulate of chemical individuality.

The Human Genome Project has been argued and advanced in large part by nonmedical biologists, and the field has attracted the attention of ethicists, philosophers, lawyers, and others nonmedical (3,4). Successful outcomes of the promises of the project will be enthusiastically received by physicians, too; indeed, prototypical attainments already have been. But given the variation in where we are all coming from, a great deal of exchange and compromise is required. This coming together of diverse viewpoints has been going on for some time and is built into the fabric of the project in the form of the Joint Working Group on Ethical, Legal and Social Issues (ELSI), so information is already in some degree "out there," and seeping into the consciousness of whomever gets involved with relevant patients. Problems arise in the context of genetics in medical education, too, but because physicians will necessarily appreciate the information that accrues to the project according to the context in which they think and work, a comparison of the vision of the Genome Project in the context of the machine mentality as opposed to that of the synthetic alternative may be useful.

Outcomes of the Human Genome Project

First, it must be said that the project is an extraordinary undertaking, a marvel of technology that grows more wondrous as it matures (4). Its impact and meaning will take decades to unfold. For medicine, most of the predictions of outcomes have been in the engineering vein of the machine mentality—typological and in the main restricted to proximate causes, diagnosis, and the technology of treatment and prevention, and if we reach anything like what is proposed, we shall have advanced a good deal. But from the standpoint of genetic medicine, all the other predicted insights into biology are of no less moment to medicine than to biology. Simply to expose the whole of the human genome and then to be able to go on to discover the relationship of each gene to its product and that of the latter to its homeostatic home lays a groundwork for understanding disease in the three time scales. Such an information bank may be tapped to fill gaps in our knowledge that exist because what we know already was gathered in studies with necessarily limited goals. With the whole list, together with those of such other organisms as *C. elegans,* drosophila, and the mouse, we will be able at last to discover the denominators required for quantitative estimates of many genetic properties and probabilities. Some of these follow.

Polymorphism

Harris and Lewontin set out to discover the extent of genetic variation in human beings and drosophila. As the Human Genome Project proceeds, additional studies should give us answers to questions they asked without the wherewithal to answer them, but answers are needed if we are to understand disease. We might learn the following:

(a) How many loci fulfill the definition for polymorphism of Harris and Lewontin?

(b) What is the frequency of polymorphism according to the structure and function of protein products? So far we know most about loci specifying soluble enzyme proteins which seem to be more frequently polymorphic than those of other kinds of proteins, but the information is far from sufficient for a definitive answer. Such differentiations are worth making because the polymorphic loci represent a reservoir of alleles most likely to turn up in association with common diseases.

(c) What is the extent of heterozygote advantage? We still do not know whether heterosis is of any significance in human biology or, if it is, whether it varies according to the qualities of the molecules the genes specify. It will also be of interest to know how many and what kinds of unit steps of homeostasis are likely to show clinical expression in people who are heterozygous for mutants that in homozygotes produce a severe disease.

(d) Are conserved loci likely to be polymorphic? We might suppose them not to be on the grounds that they represent steps in homeostasis that tolerate little variation. Alternatively, they might turn up frequently in disease for the same reason.

The Range of Human Disease

Similarly, there may be answers to questions of the possible range of human disease.

(a) Is there at least one allele at every locus, whether frequent or rare, that is associated with disease? Or are some loci, whether possessed of polymorphic variants or not, rarely or never to be found in disease? And if so, what distinguishes each group?

(b) Is there something characteristic about disease expression depending upon the type of gene product that is variable? Do enzyme deficiencies differ from disorders due to variant receptors, neurotransmitters, transcription factors, structural proteins, and so on?

(c) How many diseases engage only one major variant, no doubt with modifiers? How many with two or more alleles of discretely salient effect, and how many are a product of several genes, none more prominent than others? Given the continuity of phenotypes, the number of diseases would be expected to decline and the heterogeneity and frequency to rise as the number of genes engaged increases.

(d) Might we be able to fit variants into a gradient of selective effect? Obviously it could not be a "great chain" of alleles since the effects of so many variants are provisional, contingent, and promoting disease in one person and not another in response to the variable effects of other genes, development, and experiences. But it might be possible to classify them in a continuous chain as always associated with disease, often, occasionally, rarely, or never.

(e) In time it will be possible to characterize the whole range of disease. Then all diseases will be described in relation to the specificity of the unit steps involved, their number and quality, as well as the kinds of variants responsible. New relationships between diseases will be divulged, so that whatever varicose veins have in common with hyperthyroidism and both with hyperbilirubinemia of the newborn will be made apparent. Given the genes and their products, computer programs should be capable of discovering relationships not immediately apparent. For example, (1) some alleles will appear in several disorders while others will be confined to only one; (2) the specificity of unit steps of homeostasis may confer similarities in signs and symptoms of disease across organ systems; and (3) if the relationship of proximate cause to description of disease can be clarified and the origins of the proximate in remote causes can be exposed, then disease, the emergent phenotype, may become more nearly scrutable, and to the degree that these relationships are exposed, possibilities for treatment and prevention might be maximized.

(f) How many diseases are there of the homeostasis of chromosome organization? There are many proteins engaged in packaging of chromosomes and in the maneuvers of mitosis and meiosis. Deficiencies of these could be disastrous. Would such defects be expressed in failure of cell division or in the many forms of chromosome anomaly?

(g) Are there implications for aging? How many variants of the machinery of transcription and repair lead to excessive somatic mutation? Are some loci more susceptible than others to mutants that promote aging processes? Will the hypothesis that genes have positive effects early in life but contribute to aging late in life turn out to have validity? Insights into aging should be a principle benefit of the Human Genome Project.

(h) Finally, will we be able to base a definition of disease and health on the presence or absence of particular alleles? To me, the answer is "No," because disease is always contingent upon the actions of specific proteins in the contexts of development and experience. So genes alone do not determine disease, and the increasing contingency of the actions of their protein products as we descend the selective gradient make those phenotypes increasingly uncertain. So, too, is the definition of normality unsure. While we may agree that at the two ends of the gradient of selective effect outliers promote undoubted disease at one end and health at the other, in the broad middle range, one person's normal is another's abnormal. We have known this for sometime already, but not with the precision that the Genome Project will give us.

Development

Diseases of development are among the most baneful of human afflictions, so insights into genes that influence the developmental phases of life must be an important goal. For example, how many loci are reserved exclusively for embryogenesis, subsiding into silence after their duties are done? How many others are reserved for fetal life, and how many and what loci turn on at birth and adolescence? Are there any relationships between the genes of early life and those of aging? And are there mutations of the genes of embryogenesis that result in their being reactivated later in life to cause disease? Shall we at last know the details of those pre- and postimplantation intrauterine losses?

Classification

We have seen that the elaboration of a classification of diseases according to vulnerability of unit steps of homeostasis has been handicapped by the gaps in our knowledge. Certainly a signal benefit of the Human Genome Project must be to show the way to a definitive classification dependent upon the proteins that constitute the unit steps of homeostasis. And perhaps as a corollary to classification there may come a resolution of the tangled semantics of human genetics. If we know all the genes and all of their products and how all of the unit steps are integrated into increasingly complex integrons, we may well need a language of physiology, some would say a language of complexity, rather than that of the phenotype (drosophila) or of the gene (molecular biology). What that language will be is unclear; physiology up to now has been indifferent to genetics. But new thinking about complexity is advancing rapidly, so the new language will surely differ from the locutions of either drosophila or molecular genetics (5).

Finally, it is plain that the Genome Project, in exposing so many genes with their undoubted association with disease, however contingent, however direct or indirect, must deal a fatal blow to the essentialist concept of disease, even while establishing the nominalist vulnerability of the genetically specified homeostasis as the only tenable view.

Treatment

Much is made of new kinds of therapy based on knowledge of the variant proteins that are at the root of disease. Nothing could be more natural than gene therapy, which derives from the engineering principle that is the operating arm of the machine mentality (6). And who can doubt that there will be some brilliant successes? Technology will be devised, ingenious ways of "thinking around" all sorts of obstacles will be invented, and diseases will be cured as absolutely as if by surgery. So far, efforts are directed to disorders that are invariable consequences of variants at one locus. Moving further down the selective gradient, however, the crooked timber will begin to show itself in variability in expression, modifying genes, differences in provocative experiences, and the like. At some point in the continuum further attempts will be profligate of resources and, in any case, it will be impossible to determine which individual might benefit and in what degree. But what of that? Hardly any physician who has attended the tribulations of human beings has expectations of perfection, so we will look forward to those successes, however many or few they may be.

Prevention

Finally, will the outcomes of the Genome Project lead to new ways of thinking about prevention? When the extent of polymorphism and heterogeneity are laid bare and as the range of disease in both causes and expression is grasped, a new depth of meaning of the crooked timber of humanity will be disclosed. We will be given more than glimpses of the influence of genetic variation on homeostatic products, and as we observe the further variation induced by the particularities of the environment experienced by each separate open system, the concept of individuality will take on a concrete meaning. Then prospects for prevention may become more realistic. Estimates of probabilities for developing diseases, originally based on population frequencies, may be made more nearly appropriate for individuals; we may be able to understand how the genetic and developmental context in which a particular variant exists could be such as to bring on its expression early in life, late in life, or not at all.

But still, in the end it may be that the assignment of a particular probability for an individual to have or escape a disease may elude us. We shall be testing the tolerance of the crooked timber of humanity. It is an exciting prospect, but one unlikely to go as far as we might wish until something is done in a concerted way to discover the complementary conditions of incongruence that predispose to disease. The need for such a project, equivalent to that of the genome, was raised in chapter 27.

THE PROJECT AND MEDICAL THINKING

It cannot be denied that genetics has changed medical discourse even while not much altering medical thought. Molecular biology permeates diagnosis and treatment, and does so comfortably within the purview of the machine mentality. But now, even while enriching the armamentaria for further diagnostic and therapeutic triumphs in making possible the exposure of the variety inherent in the collective human genome and in fostering population thinking and the kind of biology it entails, the Human Genome Project promises to change medical thinking as well.

It is not clear that significant change in medical thought was in the minds of those who proposed the project. Rather, it was perceived as "a natural extension of the current themes of biology as a whole" (7). The technology was ready or envisioned, interest was high, and because the DNA was perceived as "the most fundamental property of the body" (7), a successful completion of the job could not fail to alter medical thinking. Indeed, one of the project's originators pronounced its successful completion as a biological holy grail (7). This is a felicitous metaphor, embracing both the romance of a quest for something ultimate and the recognition that the attainment may not be exactly what is envisioned. After all, historians of the early centuries of the Christian era have found that, although emblematic of the religion of the time, the Holy Grail was never clearly defined as to what it was, how many of them there were, or where it (or they) resided, and those who are said to have seen it (or them), themselves shrouded in myth, were said to have been blinded by its effulgence and so could not describe what they saw (8).

As plans for the project moved forward, there seems not to have been much medical contribution to the design. It was largely under the direction of biologists not primarily engaged in medical pursuits (3). But that is entirely compatible with the medical thinking of the time. From the 1950s, when genetics began to be much noticed in medicine, its impact was perceived primarily in diagnosis, but in the 1970s, screening and antenatal diagnosis gained prominence and medical genetics came to be taken seriously as a career. In the meantime, as microbial genetics flourished and the manipulation of genes in viruses and bacteria became an everyday event, biologists, extrapolating their experiences to human beings, evinced concern about manipulation of human genes to enhance or otherwise influence human qualities and even to develop methods such as cloning of people to serve the evil purposes of ruthless dictators (9).

Table 9 lists books published between 1962 and 1974 (9)—well before the Genome Project was proposed—reporting symposia at which the future uses of genetics in human populations was the issue (10–19). Their apocalyptic titles give clues to the intensity of concern for man's future in the face of what, at the time, seemed limitless possibilities to meddle in the quality and direction of human biology. The table also shows that medical representation at these meetings was in a minority, and yet where were such manipulations to take place? The physicians who attended these exercises tended to draw attention to diagnostic uses, potential treatments including gene therapy, and antenatal diagnosis and abortion. And they found the eugenic fears and the possibilities for misuse of the new knowledge improbable and unconvincing.

Time passed without the fears of the biologists being realized and with it came all the new developments that culminated in the Human Genome Project (3). Now gene manipulation is used in the elucidation of development and cell biology in drosophila, *C. elegans,* mice, and other organisms. What has been happening is the discovery of the genes that specify the unit steps of home-

Table 9 Books Reporting Symposia on Eugenics and Human Evolution

Title (ref. no.)	Participants		
	Nonmedical	Medical	Total
Evolution and Man's Progress (10)	9	0	9
The Control of Human Heredity and Evolution (11)	7	1	8
Biology and the Future of Man (12)	7	1	8
The Future of Man (13)	19	7	26
Genetics and the Future of Man (14)	7	0	7
Who Shall Live (15)	6	0	6
Changing Mores of Biomedical Research (16)	7	3	10
Genetic Engineering (17)	6	2	8
The New Genetics and the Future of Man (18)	9	3	12
Ethical Issues in Human Genetics (19)	16	19	35
Total (%)	93 (72.1)	36 (27.9)	129 (100.0)

Childs, B. Galton, Garrod and clinical medicine. Reproduced by permission of *Yale Journal of Biology and Medicine* 46: 297–313, 1973.

ostasis and that, when discovered in drosophila or the mouse, can be shown to have human homologies that are often the seat of human disease. So the most important initial impact on medicine of the Genome Project will be the discovery of genes that specify those unit steps. Such homeostatic units constitute the central theme of medicine, the chief focus of pathogenesis whence come descriptions of disease and the target of therapeutic and, one hopes, preventive exercises.

So why is the Genome Project not an object of keen attention in medicine? Why is it not the subject of editorials in medical journals, addresses of retiring presidents of medical societies, named lectures, and symposia at medical meetings? Why is it not of great interest to the American Medical Association and the academies and colleges that look to the interests of practitioners? It is not that medicine shies away from big projects. Most of the institutes of the National Institutes of Health are named for diseases that are expected to be the object of the research they support. And in the 1970s a war on cancer was declared and supported by the president of the United States. So it cannot be that big projects or big money are inhibiting.

One reason for medical inertia might be that medical attention is still riveted on phenotypes, while that of the adherents of the Genome Project is on genotypes. Medicine proceeds traditionally in an analysis from the top down, while the rewards of the Genome Project will flow from the bottom up. Medical attention is stimulated by sick people; the Genome Project expects to expose loci whose variants produce diseases yet undescribed. Perhaps medicine does not yet perceive the unit step of homeostasis as the interface between phenotype and genotype, the product of the latter and the source of the former, and the point of union of the physician and the biologist. So it is again a difference in mentality, but a difference that the outcomes of the Human Genome Project will certainly resolve, and soon.

The Project and Humanity

It is sometimes said that the list of genes will be an account of our humanity (7), and in a limited sense, this observation is true. Because the avowed purpose of the project is a catalogue of all gene loci, together with everything else in the genome, it is possible to see its aim, in a typological context, as a search at once for proximate causes of disease and for the wherewithal for the function of the brain in cognition and behavior. In that sense the project will produce a flat and two-dimensional blueprint of humanity's essence. But in population thinking, humanity has no essence. It is above all variable in its emergent properties, products of (a) development, itself contingent upon both the variability of the genes and the interactions of their products with variable experiences, and (b) the variety inherent in the gene pool, a consequence of selection and randomness. So whatever humanity is, its meaning cannot reside exclusively in a genome that represents possibilities and limits, but not predictions. Rather, humanity resides in the diversity exemplified in open systems, whether intact or diseased, adapting as best they can to the diversity of the environment. Humanity resides in the qualities of the crooked timber.

29

The Medical-Genetic Synthesis and Society

We have become increasingly aware that even the internal logic of formal thought can be shaped by social needs and assumptions; the domain of seemingly value free inquiry grows ever smaller. We have become aware as well that specific institutional structures mediate the relationship between men of learning and the society that supports them. In sum, we have become conscious of the need to integrate knowledge into a more general understanding of organizational and attitudinal trends.

—Charles Rosenberg, "Toward an Ecology of Knowledge" (1)

Rosenberg is a leader among those medical historians who no longer write only of medical personalities and events but who pay more attention to social conditions that influence how medicine is carried on (2). When applied to medicine, his statement says that the thinking that informs the institutions of medical teaching and action can be influenced by the requirements of the society medicine serves. Perhaps today we are seeing some consequences of medicine's failure to make concessions to the society that supports it. Certainly such a perception was reflected in the conclusions reached by those committees of concerned educators. So the question for this chapter is, can genetic medicine help to reshape the institutions through which knowledge flows from medicine to society?

In the past, medicine enjoyed an unassailable authority over the knowledge that informed medical teaching and complete autonomy in its use (3). So it is not surprising that, uninfluenced by any but its own interpretation of "social needs and assumptions" and apparently isolated from any but its own institutions, medicine turned inward to validate its authority in technology and reductionist explanations of disease, and it did seem for a while that nothing could interfere with medicine's own vision of progress. But since new technology and knowledge are likely to expose the crooked timber, we began in the 1960s to hear with increasing urgency from those interested parties who think that medicine is too important to leave to the doctors. They have added themselves to previously established "institutions that mediate" the connection of medicine to society.

The machine mentality, best adapted to times of authority and autonomy, has not the resiliency to accommodate in ways that best serve both medicine and its constituents. What the machine mentality lacks, and one reason why commerce has moved in on medicine as if it were an appropriate object for its interest, is recognition that diagnosis and treatment are not the whole of the doctor-patient relationship. If they did constitute the whole of the transaction, then the encounter would, indeed, have the quality of the sale of a commodity. But if the doctor is acting as the agent of something that transcends the immediacy of the meeting, if the sale and purchase of medical expertness have a social purpose that goes beyond the visit of the moment, then medicine has a public domain that cannot be treated as something to be sold by the pound or the hour.

In fact, medicine has always had a pastoral mission. There has always existed a bond between doctor and patient that includes for the former a concern for the social and emotional effects of disease on the latter, and if this side of medicine is at the moment somewhat attenuated, we need to seek ways to amend it. Equally, disease has always exerted a profound social impact in families, communities, and national economies. Patients may lose income, with serious repercussions in families. Business losses in productivity due to the illness of workers are computed annually, and the threat of disease to communities is the responsibility of such agencies as the Food and Drug Administration, the Centers for Disease Control, and state and city health departments. These latter perceive their role as preventive and apart from therapeutic medicine, and in their concept of populations, they are embraced comfortably within the machine mentality.

So it seems that where the individual, the private person with a name, a social security number, and a unique genetic and developmental identity, is not paramount, as in public health, or wherever the reductive approach to pathogenesis is emphasized to the neglect of individuality, the machine mentality prevails. Indeed, the visibility of the patient as a person seems to vary inversely with the degree of adherence to the machine mentality. So, some modifications of the institutions that mediate the flow of knowledge to the society that supports them are needed. Here the word *institution* is taken to include traditions or established points of view as opposed to formally constituted bodies.

MODIFICATIONS OF CURRENT INSTITUTIONS

What modifications? Some are inherent in the logic of disease.

All Disease Has a Social Component

If human open systems are congruent with experiences of the physical and social environment, and if disease is a consequence of incongruence stemming from variably adaptive unit steps of homeostasis, then every disease has a social component that cannot be denied, but is ignored when thinking stops at proximate causes. Proximate causes are outcomes of remote causes, and it is the latter that make a case of disease into a particular person suffering the consequences of his or her uniquely incongruent physiology. Remote causes are of no interest to the machine mentality that concentrates on proximate causes in an essentialist framework of disease. But the population thinker is driven to the nominalist interpretation of disease in which the uniqueness of the sick individual, the heterogeneity of genes and experiences, the continuity of disease from lethal to none discernible, and the dynamic quality of disease in which heritability changes, are all evidence of the rule of remote causes.

One provisional answer, then, to the question of modified institutions might be an acknowledgment that disease is a social phenomenon that has both proximate and remote causes, that concatenations of proximate causes are a consequence of both biological and social conditions, and that solutions must be in part social and so must include representation from elements of society. In the evolution of the public position on tobacco, for example, medicine's role was dominated at first by exhortations to stop smoking lest one or other of the numerous dire outcomes befall, and no doubt lives were saved. But such advice absolves medicine of further responsibility by transferring it to the smoker. For many years the sale of this substance, so incongruent with human physiology as to put vulnerable people at risk for a disease of nearly every organ system in the body, was socially acceptable. But gradually a consensus has formed to move toward limiting that sale. The first step in attaining such a consensus is a general acceptance of the social origin of disease, to be dealt with not only by medicine, as it is conventionally defined, but also by medicine in concert with agencies of the society whose health is threatened by its own organization.

This kind of consensus is needed if we are to go beyond tobacco to search for experiences of life that are specific to other complex disorders. And medicine, through its various organizations, must be a prominent partner in such ventures. How such agreement is to be attained is unclear. It is likely to engage a different cast of characters in each disorder, and the crooked timber will ensure that agreements are not easily reached. But the first step is clear: it is general acceptance of the social nature of disease. After all, we are each an independent open system, dependent upon the environment for sustenance.

The Primacy of Prevention

A second institutional modification flows naturally from the first. Here change is compelled by the discovery, at exponential rates, of homeostatic variants that constitute genetic vulnerabilities. Some of these may provide points for the design of treatment, but many will act as markers of risk. And no doubt the provocative experiences that raise such susceptibilities to overt disease are woven into the fabric of ordinary experiences. So again there is a necessity for consensus about how to deal, both as a society and as individuals, with the discovery in ourselves of genetic differences that can lead to disease or even to premature death.

A part of the debate—that having to do with "genetic" disease—has been going on for more than twenty years. Ethicists, sociologists, theologians, lawyers, educators in health and biology, philosophers, geneticists, and a variety of representatives of the public, including disease-related family support groups of which there are now above a hundred, have in meetings, symposia, books, pamphlets, and handouts generated a good deal of heat and no little light. Questions of privacy, confidentiality, legal and civil rights, insurance, education, and whether or not in whom, by whom, and when and where testing for vulnerabilities is to be done, are all objects of intense scrutiny (4).

What are the concerns expressed by these observers of today's medicine? They are fears of an imperious technology, of genetic determinism, and of loss of individual autonomy and identity. The observers fear that indiscriminate exposure of genetic vulnerability will have social consequences in the form, say, of cancellation of insurance or the loss of jobs, or that the lack of any preventive appropriate for some traits will impose an unrelievable sense of doom. The observers fear laws that require testing for susceptibility or that do not protect the exposed citizen, and they fear labeling of people according to traits rather than by the aggregate of qualities that constitute a unique human being. They fear a new eugenics based on knowledge of the genes, not of normality, but of disease.

Table 10 shows the variety and extent of these concerns. It is a list, not necessarily exhaustive, of books published in the 1990s on the subject of social consequences of genetic knowledge. A small minority were written by physicians, and some report the transactions of symposia that included physicians among the participants. But most are the product of nonmedical observers— biologists, ethicists, philosophers, sociologists, historians, lawyers, and others who wish to make public their uneasiness about the uses of genetic knowledge. In contrast to those of thirty years ago (see Table 9 in the preceding chapter on the Human Genome Project), the titles are less foreboding, certainly more realistic and representative of concerns that are shared by all, medical people no less than others. Indeed, the books and their contents represent the start of rapprochement, of progress in drawing together people who perceive common ground whereon some realistic understanding is possible. There is a long way to go, but in embracing the whole range of concerns, even including disapproval of almost all uses of genetic knowledge in medicine, the books represent the beginning of discourse, the first requisite for understanding.

Table 10   Recent Books on the Social Consequences of Genetic Knowledge

1. Suzuki, K., and P. Knudtson. *Genetics: The Clash between the New Genetics and Human Values.* Cambridge: Harvard University Press, 1990.
2. Wingerson, L. *Mapping Our Genes.* New York: Plume, 1990.
3. Davis, B. D. (ed.). *The Genetic Revolution.* Baltimore: Johns Hopkins University Press.
4. Keveles, D. J., and L. Hood. *The Code of Codes: Scientific and Social Issues in the Human Genome Project.* Cambridge: Harvard University Press, 1992.
5. Hubbard, R., and E. Wald. *Exploring the Gene Myth.* Boston: Beacon, 1995.
6. Jones, S. *The Language of the Genes: Biology and the Evolutionary Future.* New York: HarperCollins, 1993.
7. Andrews, L. B., J. E. Fullarton, N. A. Holtzman, and A. G. Motulsky. *Assessing Genetic Risks: Implications for Health and Social Policy.* Washington, DC: National Academy of Sciences Press, 1994.
8. Neel, J. V. *Physician to the Gene Pool.* New York: Wiley, 1994.
9. Duster, T., and K. Garrett. *Cultural Perspectives on Biological Knowledge.* Norwood, NJ: Ablex, 1984.
10. Drlica, K. A. *Double-Edged Sword: The Promises and Risks of the Genetic Revolution.* Reading, MA: Addison-Wesley, 1994.
11. Weir, R. F., S. C. Laurence, and E. Fales. *Genes and Human Self-Knowledge: Historical and Philosophical Reflections on Modern Genetics.* Iowa City: University of Iowa Press, 1994.
12. Weatherall, D. *Science and the Quiet Art.* New York: Norton, 1995.
13. Russo, E., and D. Cove. *Genetic Engineering: Dreams and Nightmares.* New York: W. H. Freeman, 1995.
14. Jones, S. *In the Blood: God, Genes and Destiny.* New York: Penguin, 1995.
15. Nelkin, D., and M. S. Lindee. *The DNA Mystique: The Gene as a Cultural Icon.* New York: W. H. Freeman, 1995.
16. Kelear, E. F. *Refiguring Life: Metaphors of Twentieth-Century Biology.* New York: Columbia University Press, 1995.
17. Cranor, C. (ed.). *Are Genes Us? The Social Consequences of the New Genetics.* New Brunswick, NJ: Rutgers University Press, 1995.
18. Rollin, B. E. *The Frankenstein Syndrome: Ethical and Social Issues in the Genetic Engineering of Animals.* New York: Cambridge University Press, 1995.
19. Bodmer, W., and R. McKie. *The Book of Man.* New York: Scribner's, 1995.
20. Nathan, D. G. *Genes, Blood and Courage* Cambridge: Harvard University Press, 1995.
21. Cook-Degan, R. M. *The Gene Wars: Science, Politics and the Human Genome.* New York: Norton, 1995.
22. Aldridge, S. *The Thread of Life: The Story of Genes and Genetic Engineering.* New York: Cambridge University Press, 1996.
23. Kitcher, P. T*he Lives to Come: The Genetic Revolution and Human Possibilities.* New York: Simon & Schuster, 1996.

Education

Changes in a third institution or tradition are required to mediate this alignment of medicine with society: that of educating the public in what genetics in medicine means in their lives. Some would say that the educational mission is well on its way; books, magazines, newspapers, television, even the comic strips—all refer to the genes and their works. But the references to genetics are typological, in the essentialist tradition of disease, and strongly determinist. Nelkin and Lindee have surveyed this literature and its language and testify again and again to the curse of "genes for," a usage that, in seeming to say it all, stifles further thought (5). In addition, they demonstrate that such locutions as "genes for" criminal behavior, or even for happiness, are often uncritically accepted as equivalent to "genes for" hemophilia, say, or for cystic fibrosis, as if there were lurking somewhere in the genotype of each of us a gene or genes that determine whether we are happy or sad.

But the usage "genes for," when appropriately employed, is actually based on empirical observation and is merely a shorthand expression of complex suppositions and realities. No doubt medicine is in part responsible for this misunderstanding, since in informal conversation and press conferences such shorthand acknowledgments of gene-phenotype relationships are usually employed. But if the fruits of the Genome Project are to fit rationally into the pursuit of standard medical aims, and if people are to have the wisdom to be engaged responsibly in the preservation of their health, they must have the intellectual wherewithal to receive whatever the purveyors of the "news" offer, some sort of context within which to sort it out and to see it for what it is.

Progress in this vein is being made in primary and secondary education, where the principles of biology are taught in a human context (6). Further, recognizing the inaccessible volume of the available information in biology, emphasis is given to (a) building a conceptual framework within which to sort it out, (b) exposing students to its personal and social implications, and (c) understanding its nature and how its principles flow from those of evolution and natural selection. The most enlightened of such educators ask not "What should the students know?" but "How can we best prepare their minds for what, in time, they will come to know?"

Does medicine have a role in public education? History makes clear that it does: the American Heart Association, the American Cancer Society, and the March of Dimes, among others, are all very active in informing the public about their diseases, and genetics has necessarily entered in. And both biologists and physicians engage in occasional teaching, usually in schools where their own children are students. But the emphasis in these efforts is on spreading information to the general, less so to the individual.

Medical genetics has taken a different tack, offering information about specific diseases to affected patients and their families in the form of genetic counseling in connection with testing for genetic risk factors. The counselors' mission is educational and fits readily into medicine's social domain. Their teaching, advice, and support of families suddenly made aware of vulnerabilities and diseases deriving from the patient's unique genetic constitution are an essential part of medical care. Although the information and knowledge are not inherently incomprehensible, the public mind has not yet the understanding to receive it, so the counselor's job is one of iteration until something is perceived to be lodged. The value of this function is measured by the necessity for knowledge to make informed decisions about further reproduction, for informing other relatives, and for deciding on the path to take in future medical care. Counseling is also integral to the establishment of a new and unanticipated vision of life in the future of families who must care for afflicted children or themselves endure the uncertainty of constraint by genetic probabilities. And it is a measure of societal ignorance that medical insurers decline to pay for it.

So there is a new medical mission to be filled, a gap made apparent by a nominalist view of disease wherein the genetic and developmental individuality of each patient requires unique care, a part of which is to assist in the attainment of an intellectual grasp. Medicine's role in filling this gap remains undefined. Perhaps a more formal effort on the part of medical schools and universities would help.

Medicine and Society

Relations with individuals is the essence of medical practice, but what are medicine's points of contact with society as embodied in the homeostasis of social organizations and cultures? They are county, state, and national medical societies, specialist colleges and associations, and the numerous disease-related organizations. It is through these bodies that medicine speaks to the public. But what of a future when there is a general consensus on the social component of disease? Will medicine become activist? There is the example of the Physicians for the Prevention of Nuclear War, and physicians, individually and as agents of their organizations, have lobbied, often successfully, for legislation in the public interest; for example, pediatricians of the American Academy of Pediatrics have appeared before legislative bodies advocating safety in infant beds, toys, bottle tops, seat belts, and the like. But if all disease has a social component, is there not a need for something more concerted, something more representative of a general aim of medicine to find the provocations in the environment, to prevent disease—indeed, to advocate the institution of such measures as to push the heritability of disease toward 1.0? Were something of the sort to emerge it would surely be informal, a sort of entente of like-thinking groups, each with its special identity to preserve and advance within the common purpose. The crooked timber might preclude anything formal.

The common currency of such an entente should be ideas that exert centripetal forces toward unity, ideas that inform a philosophy to which all elements can subscribe. The synthesis of medical and genetic ideas offered here is one source of such ideas. But where, in general, are such thoughts likely to be generated? Medical schools, of course—but where in the medical school system of departments? Possibly in new departments of medicine and society, or more likely of medical philosophy, or perhaps it is a role for departments of history of medicine. Historians of science have perceived the fertility for their work of the last fifty to seventy-five years of genetics, but what medicine has taken from, or contributed to, that history has received less attention. Other possible sources of ideas are the schools of public health that are oriented to distributions of disease and prevention. They have departments of environmental medicine, health policy, population dynamics, and epidemiology that are already oriented to social roles. These departments have not been pioneers in weaving genetics into their thinking, but the fruits of the Genome Project and the principle of disease as a social phenomenon make such a shift inevitable.

No doubt the form of any such common understanding is unpredictable, but to the degree that the generation of ideas is its purpose, it must be a true university function, ramifying beyond the medical school into anthropology, sociology, economics, and philosophy, including ethics—all those disciplines described at the beginning of the book that perceive a stake in medicine—and beyond them into other aspects of the humanities as well. If we are to take seriously the proposition that our genotype participates in any way in our "humanity" or, more realistically, in the integrated homeostasis which those genes specify, we had better see whether we can reconcile variations in protein-mediated steps of development and metabolism with the ideas of poets and novelists who describe humanity in other terms. Or with the thoughts of philosophers of medicine, who, in addition to their contributions to the ethics of new ventures into genetics, will be interested in the social meaning of our new and extensive knowledge of genetic variation in disease and health.

It might be said that such a common understanding is at hand, exemplified in the courses on medicine and society or medicine and the humanities in the new curricula and in the participation of representatives of the other disciplines in these courses. And that is true. But it is true because medicine has reacted to the urgency of its observers. What is needed is not a reactive but a creative incorporation of some of the ideas of the other disciplines into the thinking of medicine, the active creation by medical thinkers of a philosophy that provides a bridge between human biology and medicine on one side and human culture on the other, to the benefit of both individuals and communities. Certainly medical schools as the principal repositories of knowledge of human biology have an obligation to provide such ideas in the setting of their universities and thereby to fulfill a true university function. In a re-evaluation of universities, Jaroslav Pelikan justifies the university status of professional schools, including those of medicine, by their "tradition of critical philosophical reflection," and adds that the university is the "only possible setting in which such reflection on a profession . . . can be carried on in a full intellectual context" (7).

As it is now, such "critical philosophical reflection" is a peripheral occupation, without influence on how medicine is carried on. But if given support, it could result in the embodiment of thought from which a new medical rationale—broader, more encompassing than the present—might be composed. And such a structure of ideas should inform medical education, still another institution in need of modification.

30

A Basis for Medical Education

Rather it views the construction of a framework of knowledge, ways of thinking about human beings in health and disease, as an essential component of an effective program of general medical education. . . . Such a philosophical framework for medicine should include at least three dimensions. First, it should recognize human beings as living organisms both closely related chemically and physically to all living organisms and also remarkably diverse, as revealed by modern molecular and cell biology. Second, the framework should view humans as members of society. Third, physicians must view their patients not only as living organisms and members of society but also as unique individuals.

—D. C. Tosteson, S. James Adelstein, and Susan T. Carver,
New Pathways to Medical Education

The above reveals the motor that drove the reforms in medical education at Harvard. It suggests that underlying the empiricism of medical knowledge and practice there is a system of thought and ideas, a philosophy that embraces the principle of the molecular and biochemical unity of all organisms, the social nature of human beings, and the uniqueness of the individual. *Philosophy* is not a word that comes often or easily to the mind of the physician. And yet doctors are aware that medical and biological investigators are seeking "the most general facts and principles of reality and of human nature and behavior." These words are enclosed in quotation marks because they appear in *Webster's* dictionary as a definition of *philosophy*.

In the past, philosophers of medicine, who tend to observe rather than to practice medicine, were handicapped because we lacked the kind of understanding of physiology and disease we have today, so that, although the ethical side of philosophy has had a thorough exposure in medicine, the epistemological side may have been less developed (1). But the flood of molecular facts and the promise, through the yield of the Human Genome Project, of insights into our "humanity" have stimulated interest, and we may anticipate some brisk exchanges between physicians, perhaps especially medical educators, and philosophers of science and medicine.

The epigraph to this chapter also reveals some of the ideas that constitute a framework of knowledge, ideas that resemble those of the logic outlined in this book. So this final chapter will be devoted to how the synthesis of medical and genetic thinking outlined in previous chapters can help in the construction of such a framework or infrastructure for medical education.

A framework is constructed of ideas that articulate well together to form a basis from which flow other ideas, related but perhaps of more restricted or special application. It might be argued that no such framework could have any permanence, that medicine changes overnight, a result of new technology and the flood of knowledge it generates. But, in fact, the framework is independent of contemporary events in the conduct of medicine. No one doubts that medicine is in flux, but if disease in human beings stems from incongruities between the unit steps of our homeostatic identities and our experiences, then the changes in disease and medicine must be attributed to the latter since our homeostasis is as old as our species. If AIDS is a new disease, it is because its virus evolved to become pathogenic, not because of some new human susceptibility; some fraction of humanity has been vulnerable to the HIV since long before the virus took its present form. And if atherosclerosis is in some parts of the world a disease of the twentieth century, it is because of a culture of dietary and other habits that is incongruent with an ancient homeostasis. So the logic presented here is as suitable for the twenty-first century as for the twentieth.

Further evidence of the structural durability of the logic, as well as its principal virtue, is how its parts flow predictably from its most central principles. For example, if it is agreed that mutations generated at meiosis are a source of adaptive variability, that such mutations are translated into variant proteins acting as unit steps of homeostasis, and that incongruence of such variants with provocative experiences creates proximate causes that promote disease, then we may say that disease is a consequence of both the necessity of a species for a reservoir of variability and the action of selection against the phenotypes of nonadapting variants. That is, both disease and nature's response to it flow from the processes of evolution, as do all other aspects of the logic, thus:

1. Disease must be described in the historical context of the three time scales because variant unit steps of homeostasis arise in the course of phylogeny, become a part of a unique individual homeostasis in ontogeny, and, depending upon their position in a selective gradient, exert their effects directly or as traits vulnerable to provocative experiences.

2. The specificity of disease as to cell type and organ system and the genetic het-

erogeneity that affects phenotypic variation are attributable to the randomness of mutation.

3. Age at onset and frequency of disease, as well as severity of phenotype, are properties of the gradient, while relationships between variant unit steps and the presence, kind, duration, and intensity of provocative experiences that determine whether disease ensues are expressed in variable coefficients of heritability.

4. The specificity of individuals affected is associated with remote causes of disease, such as the distribution of variants in populations and the matings of their possessors, whether random or assortative.

5. The selective gradient is continuous, varying from phenotypes associated with genes of lethal effect both early and late to those arising in all degrees of contingency. The discovery of so many genes that represent varying degrees of contingency imposes major adjustments in medical intervention that include abortion of affected fetuses, gene manipulations, targeting of variant homeostatic steps for medication or immunological treatments, and avoidance of provocations. The aim of all of these is intervention before the onset of disease, which by definition is prevention, a purpose that has been honored more in the breach than in the observance of it, simply because means to attain it were so seldom at hand.

This is a context, a framework, an infrastructure, that offers an expanded populational perspective as opposed to a narrow typology. It creates a necessity to conjure with remote causes no less than proximate if prevention is to have its due, to adhere to a flexible and embracing nominalist concept of disease as opposed to the limiting essentialist version, and to class each individual as a genetic and developmental experiment whose experience with disease will reflect one particular phylogenetic and developmental past.

A further virtue of the logic, another prediction stemming from evolution and natural selection, is its independence of species limits. The lesson of phylogeny is that since all of life shares, in the DNA, a common basis subject in all species to mutations that are reflected in homeostatic proteins that are, across species, similar or nearly identical, the mechanisms of disease are of general application. The reader will recall how Beadle and Tatum created inborn errors in Neurospora in the work that established a relationship between genes and proteins. Those were nutritional diseases that represent no less a burden to us than to Neurospora, and we suffer the same fate unless raised on a "complete" medium.

What is it about the logic that fills existing needs in medical education, or that supplies something not yet recognized as a need? To begin, there is that dissatisfaction with the status quo expressed by medical educators during the past twenty years or so. Although many have alluded to frameworks and infrastructures, few have offered much guidance, although some—Harvard's effort is an example—are seriously looking for ways to accommodate to the expanding information. Because so much of the latter is molecular and genetic and because the word is getting around that people are differentially susceptible to disease, efforts to supply such a framework are very much apropos.

A second concern expressed by many of the critics is for coherence: medicine is so fractionated and the new information is so copious as to be nearly impossible to assimilate. Here, too, the logic is responsive, supplying generalizations that accommodate all disease. For example, in the genetic analysis of complex disorders, the first genes to be found usually account for only a small fraction of all cases. But that is to be expected: genes highest in the selective gradient are the most assertive, both early in life and in the most severe phenotypic effect. Or, it might be said that in youthful populations heritability is high.

A third want, often expressed, is that of a satisfactory way of expressing the symbiosis of medicine and society, a condition to which we may be blind when we focus narrowly on proximate causes. Some of these proximate causes are a part of the culture, but there is in addition the larger range of remote causes both biological and cultural whence the proximate derive and which provide the particularity of each case.

A fourth need is for attention to the intellectual disjunction between the preclinical and the clinical years (2). The preclinical teaching fulfills the definition of education: it is abstract and general. But the clinical teaching is largely training, the application of the general to the specific. Teaching in the clinical years is around cases that are specific in both disease and individuality. Other contrasts are book learning versus hands on experience, health versus disease, and congruence versus incongruence.

Perhaps the most formidable hurdle is pedagogic. In the past, medical education began with anatomy, both gross and microscopic, in which individuals more or less like the student were dissected, the various organ systems were identified, and their cells were examined. This was followed by physiology and biochemistry—that is, the integrated human body came first, the reductionist sciences second. But today, the preclinical teaching proceeds from reduction to integration, from the molecular biology of the cell to anatomy, to physiology by way of biochemistry, and thence to pathology or pathophysiology. This bottom-up approach is in contrast to the top-down stance of the clinical teaching, in which the student-physician proceeds from the history to the physical examination to the laboratory, which is the real interface between the two sides of the street.

But is it an interface, or does it represent a wall, something to surmount? Students do experience dissonance at this point in their education, some a great deal, but they see that the earlier experience is intended to teach them about health and the latter about disease, and being talented people they adjust. And that is education of a sort. But this year or so, during which a switch is made from preclinical to clinical, from generalizations about biology to disease in individual human beings, may be a critical period in the ontogeny of the physician akin to other critical periods in human development: if fulfilled in a timely way, all is well, but if not, catch-up may be imperfect. Accordingly, it would be worthwhile to find some way to ease the transition, to make it more in keeping with the principles of human biology and therefore anticipated by the student. No doubt this can be achieved, but only in cooperation with teachers who are willing to make some changes in their approach.

The point is that the generalizations of the preclinical teaching are not compatible with the individuality of the diseased patient, especially given the limited grasp of that individuality imposed by the typology of the machine mentality. Perhaps there is an assumption that if you know congruence, you will know incongruence; the latter is simply the former gone wrong, and a knowledge of normal homeostasis is all it takes to grasp how disease can harrow it up. But such an assumption can do nothing to close the transitional gap. For that, other knowledge is required; the student needs to know (a) that congruence was attained through the phylogeny of the unit steps of homeostasis and their integration through development, and (b) how these processes account for the uniqueness of genotypes, the uniqueness of developmental trajectories, and the singularity of people who are uniquely adapted to experiences of the environment. They should also know that disease is a consequence of an evolutionary imperative and that it is experienced differentially according to unique susceptibilities to provocation from within or without in association with remote causes expressed in an evolving culture, and that the consequent disease is experienced uniquely.

The injection of such ideas may seem as much a transgression of the domain of the preclinical scientists as it is of the machine mentality of the clinicians. The days of physician teachers of basic sciences are long gone. Now the role is filled by biologists strongly committed to investigation and graduate teaching, as well as to educating medical students. But if medicine is to be based on a biological and social infrastructure that informs the pursuit of medical missions, why should not those who introduce students of medicine to their field share the ideas that compose that foundation? The basic scientists might say that they do just that, but some significant differences between biologists and physicians in approach and solutions to problems, were reviewed in chapter 6. Resolution of those differences could go a long way to answering the questions of the critics of medical education.

Some medical schools require a return to basic science in the clinical years. After experiences with patients, the students can see a relevance not apparent before. But I suggest that the understanding of the basic sciences both before and after the clinical experiences would be much enriched if taught on both sides of the street in the context of some framework of ideas held in common. Under present conditions it would be no surprise were the biologists to perceive teaching medical students as peripheral to their principal interests. And why not? The students have already made decisions that orient them away from those interests. Further, the present teaching of basic science translates easily into the machine mentality in clinical medicine. So why does not a remedy for most of the complaints of the critics lie in a logic that bases the aims of medicine on biological principles that are inclusive, going beyond cell biology, molecular genetics, biochemistry, and physiology to evolution and natural selection and, above all, to population biology, variation, and individuality? Such an expanded foundation would go a long way to enhancing a community of interests between pre- and postclinical teachers, and it could hardly harm biologists whose education must have included such ideas, perhaps forgotten in the excitement of today's reductionist fever.

Biologists often say that they are pleased when the outcomes of their work include benefits to human beings, and this interface is overtly acknowledged in the mix of names appended to papers reporting the molecular details of diseases as well as in the choice of names of such journals as *Nature Genetics* and *Nature Medicine,* where a journal devoted to all science has perceived the common ground between biology and medicine and has created journals to accommodate it. Presumably this perception is a general one and, if so, an additional way for preclinical scientists to serve humanity is to give medical education a foundation of biology that goes beyond the molecular details to say more about where the molecules come from, how as unit steps they became integrated into the physiological homeostasis of species, and how disease in all species is an inevitable product of the mechanisms for change. Indeed, the student should come to the clinical years ready to distinguish the Oslerian question from those of Garrod. The former asks, "What disease does this patient have and how do I treat it?" while the latter ask, "What disease does this particular human being have, in what way does this patient differ from others among whom he lives, and what can I do to restore this person's unique orientation to the environment?" Without an appropriate foundation the student sees only the Oslerian as relevant, overlooking the far more profound grasp of human variation and individuality of the Garrodian. They are questions that, although including the Oslerian appeal to the molecular details of disease, go beyond them to the unique biological and social particularity of one human being in distress.

In ending this chapter I cite some remarks made by Joshua Lederberg in 1990 at a symposium on cancer in a medical school setting, that of Mount Sinai, in New York. After reviewing the development of the reductionist approach to disease with appropriate approbation, he ended his talk as follows:

My fear is that in the great excitement of this new wave of knowledge, we may lose some of the convergence, the feel for the organism, the natural historical context, the excitement and provocations that come from clinical observations which, in my view, will be necessary not only to further clinically important needs but even to give us the most important revolutionary findings within biology itself (3).

This convergence, feel for the organism, and historical context are cardinal features of the genetic medicine described in this book, which represents not a curriculum, but a way of thinking useful in the design of curricular change. Curricular changes always depend upon individuals to whom education is a matter of first importance. My hope is that some such people will find the ideas in this book congenial and that they will use them, adding to or altering them to suit the climate of each school. Changes in neither thinking nor curricula are likely overnight. It will be an evolutionary process—trial and error, descent with modification, continuity and change. But evolution is what the book is about.

Notes

PREFACE

1. Wright, S. Genetics, the gene and the hierarchy of biological sciences. In *Proceedings of the Tenth International Congress of Genetics*. Toronto: University of Toronto Press, 1958.

2. Temkin, O. The historiography of ideas in medicine. In E. Clarke (ed.). *Modern Methods in the History of Medicine*. London: Ashlane Press, 1971.

3. Brandt, A. M. Emerging themes in the history of medicine. *Milbank Quarterly* 69: 199–214, 1991.

CHAPTER 1: INTRODUCTION

There is a voluminous literature on how various disciplines mesh with medicine; for example, the Welch Medical Library carries more than 250 volumes on medical ethics and philosophy alone. Books listed here are representative of their subjects. Others are cited where appropriate in subsequent chapters.

1. Kleinman, A. *Patients and Healers in the Context of Culture*. San Francisco: University of California Press, 1980.

2. Weiss, K. M. *Genetic Variation and Human Disease*. New York: Cambridge University Press, 1993.

3. Hahn, R. A. *Sickness and Healing: An Anthropological Perspective*. New Haven, CT: Yale University Press, 1995.

4. Fein, R. *Medical Care, Medical Costs*. Cambridge, MA: Harvard University Press, 1986.

5. Schramm, C. J. *Health Care and Its Costs*. New York: Norton, 1987.

6. Ginsberg, E. *The Medical Triangle: Physicians, Politics and the Public*. Cambridge, MA: Harvard University Press, 1990.

7. Callahan, D. *What Kind of Life: The Limits of Medical Progress*. New York: Simon and Schuster, 1990.

8. Rothman, D. J. *Strangers at the Bedside*. New York: Basic Books, 1991.

9. Jonson, A. R., M. Siegler, and W. J. Winslade. *Clinical Ethics*. 4th ed. New York: McGraw-Hill, 1998.

10. Milunsky, A., and G. J. Annas. *Genetics and the Law*. Vols. I–III. Boston: Plenum, 1976–1984.

11. Stevens, R. *American Medicine and the Public Interest*. New Haven, CT: Yale University Press, 1971.

12. Starr, P. *The Social Transformation of American Medicine.* New York: Basic Books, 1982.

13. Arney, W. R., and B. J. Bergen. *Medicine and the Management of Living.* Chicago: University of Chicago Press, 1984.

14. Dutton, D. *Worse than the Disease: Pitfalls of Medical Progress.* Cambridge: Cambridge University Press, 1988.

15. Stevens, R. *In Sickness and in Wealth.* New York: Basic Books, 1989.

16. Nelkin, D., and J. Tancredi. *Dangerous Diagnostics: The Social Power of Biological Information.* Chicago: University of Chicago Press, 1994.

17. Hunter, K. M. A science of individuals: Medicine and uncertainty. *Hospital Practice* 27: 183–218, 15 May 1992.

18. King, L. S. *Medical Thinking: A Historical Preface.* Princeton, NJ: Princeton University Press, 1982.

19. Ludmerer, K. M. *Learning to Heal: The Development of American Medical Education.* New York: Basic Books, 1985.

20. Rosenberg, C. E. *The Care of Strangers: The Rise of America's Hospital System.* New York: Basic Books, 1987.

21. Rosenberg, C. E. *Explaining Epidemics and Other Studies in the History of Medicine.* Cambridge: Cambridge University Press, 1992.

22. Rosenberg, C. E., and J. Golden (eds.). *Framing Disease: Studies in Cultural History.* New Brunswick, NJ: Rutgers University Press, 1992.

23. Murphy, E.A. *The Logic of Medicine.* Baltimore, MD: Johns Hopkins University Press, 1976.

24. Pellegrino, E. D., and D.C. Thomasma. *A Philosophical Basis of Medical Practice.* New York: Oxford University Press, 1981.

25. Reznek, L. *The Nature of Disease.* London: Routledge and Keegan Paul, 1987.

26. Kitcher, P. *The Lives to Come: The Genetic Revolution and Human Possibilities.* New York: Simon and Schuster, 1996.

CHAPTER 2: INBORN ERRORS AND CHEMICAL INDIVIDUALITY

1. Scriver, C., A. L. Beaudet, W. S. Sly, and D. Valle (eds.). *The Metabolic and Molecular Bases of Inherited Disease.* 7th ed. New York: McGraw-Hill, 1995.

2. Childs, B. *The Metabolic and Molecular Bases of Inherited Disease,* 6th edition [review]. *American Journal of Human Genetics* 46: 848–851, 1990.

3. Stanbury, J. B., J. B. Wyngaarden, and D. S. Fredrickson (eds.). *The Metabolic Basis of Inherited Disease.* New York: McGraw-Hill, 1960.

4. Garrod, A. E. *Inborn Errors of Metabolism.* Oxford: Oxford University Press, 1909.

5. Carter, B., T. H. Beaty, G. D. Steinberg, B. Childs, and P. C. Walsh. Mendelian inheritance of familial prostate cancer. *Proceedings of the National Academy of Sciences* 89: 3367–3371, 1992.

6. Sanda, M. G., T. H. Beaty, R. E. Stutzman, B. Childs, and P. C. Walsh. Genetic susceptibility of benign prostatic hyperplasia. *Journal of Urology* 152: 115–119, 1994.

7. Bearn, A. G. *Archibald Garrod and the Individuality of Man.* Oxford: Oxford University Press, 1993.

8. Garrod, A. E. The incidence of alkaptonuria: A study in chemical individuality. *Lancet* ii: 1616–1620, 1902.

9. Scriver, C. R., and B. Childs (eds.). *Garrod's Inborn Factors in Disease*. Oxford: Oxford University Press, 1989.

10. Fruton, J. S. *Molecules and Life*. New York: Wiley, 1972.

11. Cushing, H. *The Life of Sir William Osler*. Vols. I, II. Oxford: Oxford University Press, 1926.

12. Bryan, C. S. What is the Oslerian tradition? *Annals of Internal Medicine* 120: 682–687, 1994.

13. Stone, M. J. The wisdom of Sir William Osler. *American Journal of Cardiology* 75: 269–276, 1995.

14. Osler, W. *The Principles and Practice of Medicine*. New York: Appleton, 1892.

15. Osler, W. The natural method of teaching the subject of medicine. *Journal of the American Medical Association* 36: 1673–1679, 1901.

16. Osler, W. On the need of a radical reform in our methods of teaching medical students. *Medical News* 82: 49–53, 1904.

17. Osler, W. Teaching and thinking. An address given at McGill Medical School, October 1894. In J. P. McGovern and C. G. Roland (eds.). *The Collected Essays of Sir William Osler*. Vol. 2. Birmingham, UK: Classics of Medicine Library, 1985.

CHAPTER 3: THE TRANSITION FROM OSLERIAN TO GARRODIAN MEDICINE

1. Christakis, N. A. The similarity and frequency of proposals to reform U. S. medical education. *Journal of the American Medical Association* 274: 706–711, 1995.

2. Powles, J. On the limitations of modern medicine. *Science, Medicine and Man* 1: 1–30, 1973.

3. McKeown, T. *The Role of Medicine*. London: Nuffield Trust, 1976.

4. Freymann, J. G. The origins of disease orientation in American medical education. *Preventive Medicine* 10: 663–673, 1981.

5. McKeown, T. *The Origins of Human Disease*. Oxford: Basil Blackwell, 1988.

6. Foss, L. The challenge to biomedicine. *Journal of Medicine and Philosophy* 14: 165–191, 1989.

7. Thomas, L. The future impact of science and technology on medicine. *Bioscience* 24: 99–105, 1974.

8. Seldin, D. W. The boundaries of medicine. *Transactions of the Association of American Physicians* 94: 75–86, 1981.

9. Harvey, A. M., R. J. Johns, V. A. McKusick, A. H. Owens, and R. S. Ross. *The Principles and Practice of Medicine*. 22nd ed. New York: Appleton Century Crofts, 1988.

10. Kevles, D., L. and Hood (eds.). *The Code of Codes*. Cambridge, MA: Harvard University Press, 1992.

11. Reiser, S. J. *Medicine and the Reign of Technology*. New York: Cambridge University Press, 1978.

12. Greaves, D. What is medicine: Towards a philosophical approach. *Journal of Medical Ethics* 5: 29–32, 1979.

13. Council on Medical Education, American Medical Association House of

Delegates. Future directions for medical education. *Journal of the American Medical Association* 248: 3225–3239, 1982.

14. Muller, S., and J. A. D. Coope. Physicians for the twenty-first century. Report of the project panel on the general professional education of the physician and college preparation for medicine. *Journal of Medical Education* 59, suppl.: 1–200, 1984.

15. Odegard, C. E. *Dear Doctor. A Personal Letter to a Physician*. Menlo Park, CA: Henry J. Kaiser Family Foundation, 1986.

16. Rothstein, W. G. *American Medical Schools and the Practice of Medicine*. New York: Oxford University Press, 1987.

17. White, K. L. *The Task of Medicine*. Menlo Park, CA: Henry J. Kaiser Family Foundation, 1988.

18. Schroeder, S. A., J. S. Zones, and J. A. Showstack. Academic medicine as a public trust. *Journal of the American Medical Association* 262: 803–826, 1989.

19. Colloton, J. W. Academic medicine's changing covenant with society. *Academic Medicine* 64: 55–60, 1989.

20. Cantor, J. C., A. B. Cohen, D. E. Barker, A. L. Shuster, and R. C. Reynolds. Medical educators' views on medical education reform. *Journal of the American Medical Association* 265: 1002–1006, 1991.

21. Jonas, H. S., S. I. Etzel, and B. Barzansky. Educational programs in U.S. medical schools. *Journal of the American Medical Association* 266: 913–920, 1991.

22. Marston, R. Q., and R. M. Jones. *Medical Education in Transition*. Princeton, NJ: Robert Wood Johnson Foundation, 1992.

23. Lowry, S. *Medical Education*. London: BMJ Publishing Group, 1993.

24. Reiser, S. J. Technology and the use of the senses in twentieth-century medicine. In W. E. Bynum and R. Porter (eds). *Medicine and the Five Senses*. New York: Cambridge University Press, 1993.

25. Greer, D. S., K. N. Bhak, and B. M. Zenker. Comments on the AAMC policy statement recommending strategies for increasing the production of generalist physicians. *Academic Medicine* 69: 245–259, 1994.

26. Feinstein, A. R. Twentieth century paradigms that threaten both scientific and humane medicine in the twenty-first century. *Journal of Clinical Epidemiology* 49: 615–617, 1996.

27. Weatherall, D. *Science and the Quiet Art*. New York: Norton, 1995.

28. Gunderman, R. B. Rethinking our basic concepts of health and disease. *Academic Medicine* 70: 676–683, 1995.

29. Cassell, E. J. The body of the future. In D. Leder (ed.). *The Body in Medical Thought and Practice*. Boston: Kluwer, 1992.

30. McDermott, W. General medical care: Identification and analysis of alternative approaches. *Bulletin of the Johns Hopkins Hospital* 135: 292–321, 1974.

31. Rosenberg, C. E. *The Care of Strangers: The Rise of America's Hospital System*. New York: Basic Books, 1987.

32. Silver, G. A. Social medicine and social policy. *Yale Journal of Biology and Medicine* 57: 851–864, 1984.

33. McKeown, T., and C. R. Lowe. *An Introduction to Social Medicine*. Oxford: Blackwell, 1966.

34. Engel, G. L. The need for a new medical model. *Science* 196: 129–136, 1977.

35. Engel, G. L. The clinical application of the biopsychosocial model. *American Journal of Psychiatry* 137: 535–544, 1980.

36. Moore-West, M., M. Regan-Smith, A. Dietrich, and D. O. Kollisch. Innovations in medical education. In H. C. Hendrie and C. Lloyd (eds.). *Educating Competent and Humane Physicians*. Bloomington, IN: Indiana University Press, 1990.

37. Tosteson, D. C. New pathways in general medical education. *New England Journal of Medicine* 322: 234–238, 1990.

38. Reiser, S. J. The era of the patient: Using the experience of illness in shaping the mission of health care. *Journal of the American Medical Association* 269: 1012–1017, 1993.

39. Freymann, J. G. The public's health care paradigm is shifting. *Journal of General Internal Medicine* 4: 313–319, 1989.

40. Woodward, A. Public health has no place in undergraduate medical education. *Journal of Public Health Medicine* 16: 389–392, 1994.

41. White, K. L., and J. E. Connelly. The medical school's mission and the population's health. *Annals of Internal Medicine* 115: 968–972, 1991.

42. Bondurant, S. Health care reform continues: Themes for academic medicine. *Academic Medicine* 70: 93–97, 1995.

43. Reiser, S. J. The coming resurgence of the generalist in medicine. *Pharos* 58: 8–11, 1995.

44. Lee, P. R. Health system reform and the generalist physician. *Academic Medicine* 70: 510–513, 1995.

45. Ebert, R. H. Medical education at the peak of the era of experimental medicine. *Daedalus* 115: 55–81, 1986.

46. Garrod, A. E. The incidence of alkaptonuria: A study in chemical individuality. *Lancet* ii: 1616–1620, 1902.

47. Scriver, C. R., and B. Childs (eds.). *Garrod's Inborn Factors in Disease*. Oxford: Oxford University Press, 1989.

Chapter 4: Individuality and Causes

1. Gregorian, V. A place elsewhere: Reading in the age of the computer. *Bulletin of the American Academy of Arts and Sciences* 49: 54–64, 1996.

2. Mayr, E. *The Growth of Biological Thought*. Cambridge, MA: Harvard University Press, 1982.

3. Scriver, C. R., and B. Childs (eds.). *Garrod's Inborn Factors in Disease*. Oxford: Oxford University Press, 1989.

4. Winkelstein, J. A., and B. Childs. Genetically determined variation in the immune system: Implications for host defense. *Pediatric Infectious Disease Journal* 8: 531–534, 1989.

5. Childs, B. Public attitudes toward the handicapped. In A. Milunsky and G. J. Annas (eds.). *Genetics and the Law*. Vol. II. New York: Plenum Press, 1979.

6. Susser, M. What is a cause and how do we know one? A grammar for pragmatic epidemiology. *American Journal of Epidemiology* 133: 635–648, 1991.

7. Renton, A. Epidemiology and causation: A realist view. *Journal of Epidemiology and Community Health* 48: 4–10, 1994.

8. Mayr, E. Cause and effect in biology. In *Toward a New Philosophy of Biology.* Cambridge, MA: Harvard University Press, 1988.

CHAPTER 5: DEFINITIONS OF DISEASE

1. Temkin, O. The scientific approach to disease: Specific entity and individual sickness. In A. C. Crombie (ed.). *Scientific Change.* New York: Basic Books, 1963.

2. King, L. S. What is disease? *Philosophy of Science* 21: 193–203, 1954.

3. Galdston, I. *The Meaning of Social Medicine.* Cambridge, MA: Harvard University Press, 1954.

4. Sheldon, A. Toward a general theory of disease and medical care. *Science, Medicine and Man* 1: 237–262, 1974.

5. Engelhardt, H. T. Explanatory models in medicine: Facts, theories, and values. *Texas Reports on Biology and Medicine* 32: 225–239, 1974.

6. Copeland, D. D. Concepts of disease and diagnosis. *Perspectives in Biology and Medicine* 20: 528–538, 1977.

7. Risse, G. Epidemics and medicine: The influence of disease on medical thought and practice. *Bulletin of the History of Medicine* 53: 505–519, 1979.

8. Toon, P. D. Defining diseases. *Journal of Medical Ethics* 7: 197–201, 1981.

9. Kunitz, S. J. The historical roots and ideological functions of disease concepts in three primary care specialities. *Bulletin of the History of Medicine* 57: 412–432, 1983.

10. Scriver, C. R. An evolutionary view of disease in man. *Proceedings of the Royal Society* 220: 273–298, 1984.

11. Gillick, M. R. Common sense models of health and disease. *New England Journal of Medicine* 313: 700–703, 1985.

12. Cassell, E. J. Ideas in conflict: The rise and fall (and rise and fall) of new views of disease. *Daedalus* 115: 19–42, 1986.

13. Engelhardt, H. T. Clinical complaints and the ens morbus. *Journal of Medicine and Philosophy* 11: 207–214, 1986.

14. Merskey, H. Variable meanings for the definition of disease. *Journal of Medicine and Philosophy* 11: 215–232, 1986.

15. Nordenfeldt, L. Health and disease: Two philosophical perspectives. *Journal of Epidemiology and Community Health* 41: 281–284, 1986.

16. Rosenberg, C. E. Disease and social order in America: Perceptions and expectations. *Milbank Quarterly* 64, suppl. 1: 34–48, 1986.

17. Reznek, L. *The Nature of Disease.* London: Routledge and Kegan Paul, 1987.

18. Toombs, S. K. The meaning of illness. *Journal of Medicine and Philosophy* 12: 219–240, 1987.

19. Rosenberg, C. E. Disease in history. Frames and framers. *Milbank Quarterly* 67, suppl. 1: 1–15, 1989.

20. Rosenberg, C. E., and J. Golden (eds.). *Framing Disease: Studies in Cultural History.* New Brunswick, NJ: Rutgers University Press, 1992.

21. Fox, R. The medicalization and demedicalization of American society. *Daedalus* 106: 9–22, 1977.

22. Cohen, H. The evolution of the concept of disease. *Proceedings of the Royal Society of Medicine* 48: 159–169, 1955.

23. Anonymous. The concept of disease. *British Medical Journal* 2: 751–752, 1979.

24. Campbell, E. J. M., J. G. Scadding, and R. S. Roberts. The concept of disease. *British Medical Journal* 2: 757–762, 1979.

25. King, L. S. *Medical Thinking: A Historical Preface.* Princeton: Princeton University Press, 1982.

26. Seldin, D. W. The boundaries of medicine. *Transactions of the Association of American Physicians* 94: 75–86, 1981.

PART II: A LOGIC OF DISEASE: INTRODUCTION

1. Greaves, D. What is medicine: Towards a philosophical approach. *Journal of Medical Ethics* 5: 29–32, 1979.

2. Alberts, B., D. Bray, J. Lewis, M. Raff, K. Roberts, and J. D. Watson. *Molecular Biology of the Cell.* 1st ed. New York: Garland, 1983.

CHAPTER 6: BIOLOGY AND MEDICINE

1. Maynard Smith, J. H. *Problems of Biology.* Oxford, UK: Oxford University Press, 1986.

2. Weatherall, D. *Science and the Quiet Art.* New York: Norton, 1995.

3. Medawar, P. B. *The Art of the Soluble.* London: Methuen, 1967.

4. Delbrêck, M. A physicist looks at biology. In J. Cairns, G. S. Stout, and J. D. Watson (eds.). *Phage and the Origins of Molecular Biology.* Cold Spring Harbor, NY: Cold Spring Harbor Laboratory of Quantitative Biology, 1966.

5. Jacob, F. *The Logic of Life.* New York: Pantheon, 1973.

6. Bury, J. B. *The Idea of Progress: An Inquiry into Its Origin and Growth.* New York: Dover, 1955.

7. Lovejoy, A. O. *The Great Chain of Being.* Cambridge, MA: Harvard University Press, 1936.

8. Ayala, F. J. The concept of biological progress. In F. J. Ayala and J. Dobzhansky (eds.). *Studies in the Philosophy of Biology: Reduction and Related Problems.* Berkeley, CA: University of California Press, 1974.

9. Bonner, J. T. *The Evolution of Complexity.* Princeton, NJ: Princeton University Press, 1988.

10. Fries, J. F. Aging, natural death and the compression of mortality. *New England Journal of Medicine* 303: 130–135, 1980.

11. Thomas, L. The deacon's masterpiece. In *The Medusa and the Snail.* New York: Viking, 1979.

12. Fries, J. F., and L. M. Crapo. *Vitality and Aging.* New York: Freeman, 1981.

CHAPTER 7: A SYNTHESIS

1. Beadle, G. W. The genetic control of biochemical reactions. *Harvey Lectures,* Series XL, 1944–1945.

2. Mayr, E., and W. B. Provine. *The Evolutionary Synthesis. Perspectives on the Unification of Biology.* Cambridge, MA: Harvard University Press, 1980.

3. Smocovitis, V. B. Unifying biology: The evolutionary synthesis and evolutionary biology. *Journal of the History of Biology* 25: 1–65, 1992.

4. Harwood, J. Metaphysical foundations of the evolutionary synthesis: A historiographical note. *Journal of the History of Biology* 27: 2–20, 1944.

5. Holton, G. Analysis and synthesis as methodological themata. In G. Holton. *The Scientific Imagination.* Cambridge, UK: Cambridge University Press, 1978.

6. Muller, H. J. Progress and prospects in human genetics. *American Journal of Human Genetics* 1: 1–18, 1949.

Chapter 8: Lessons from Phylogeny

1. Williams, G. C., and R. M. Nesse. The dawn of Darwinian medicine. *Quantitative Review of Biology* 66: 1–22, 1991.

2. Nesse, R. M., and G. C. Williams. *Why We Get Sick.* New York: Times Books, 1994.

3. Gould, S. J., and R. C. Lewontin. The spandrels of San Marcos and the Panglossian paradigm. *Proceedings of the Royal Society,* Series B, 205: 581–598, 1979.

4. Lewontin, R. C. Gene, organism and environment. In D. S. Bendall (ed.). *Evolution from Molecules to Men.* Cambridge, UK: Cambridge University Press, 1985.

5. Doll, R., and A. B. Hill. Smoking and carcinoma of the lung. *British Medical Journal* 2: 739-748, 1950.

6. Ochsner, A., and M. DeBakey. Carcinoma of the lung. *Archives of Surgery* 42: 209–258, 1941.

7. Peto, R., A. D. Lopez, J. Boreham, M. Thun, and C. Heath. Mortality from tobacco in developed countries. *Lancet* 339: 1268–1278, 1992.

8. Dugdale, A. E. Evolution and infant feeding. *Lancet* i: 670–673, 1986.

9. Palloni, A., and M. Tienda. The effects of breast feeding and pace of childbearing on mortality at early ages. *Demography* 23: 31–66, 1986.

10. Thapa, S., R. V. Short, and M. Potts. Breast feeding, birth spacing and their effects on child survival. *Nature* 335: 679–682, 1988.

11. Oski, F. A. Infant nutrition, physical growth, breastfeeding, and general nutrition. *Current Opinion in Pediatrics* 5: 385–388, 1993.

12. Lucas, A., R. Morely, T. J. Cole, G. Lister, and C. Leeson-Payne. Breast milk and subsequent intelligence quotient in children born pre-term. *Lancet* i: 261–264, 1992.

13. Menkes, J. H. Early feeding history of children with learning disorders. *Developmental Medicine and Child Neurology* 19: 169–171, 1977.

14. Rodgers, B. Feeding in infancy and later ability and attainment: A longitudinal study. *Developmental Medicine and Child Neurology* 20: 421–426, 1978.

15. Makrides, M., M. Neumann, K. Simmer, J. Pater, and R. Gobson. Are long-chain polyunsaturated fatty acids essential nutrients in infancy? *Lancet* 345: 1463–1468, 1995.

16. Karjalainen, J., J. M. Martin, M. Knop, J. Ilonen, B. Robinson, E. Savilahti, H.

K. Akerblow, and H. Dosh. A bovine albumin peptide as a possible trigger of insulin-dependent diabetes mellitus. *New England Journal of Medicine* 327: 302–307, 1992.

17. Newberg, D. S., S. Ashkenazc, and T. G. Clearly. Human milk contains the *Shiga* toxin and *Shiga*-like toxin receptor glycolipid Gb3. *Journal of Infectious Disease* 166: 832–836, 1992.

18. Yolken, R. H., J. A. Peterson, S. L. Vonderfecht, E. T. Fouts, K. Midthun, and D. S. Newburg. Human milk mucin inhibits rotavirus replication and prevents experimental gastroenteritis. *Journal of Clinical Investigation* 90: 1984–1991, 1992.

19. Pabst, H. F., and D. W. Spady. Effect of breast feeding on antibody response to conjugate vaccine. *Lancet* ii: 269–270, 1990.

20. Eaton, S. B., M. Shostak, and M. Konner. *The Paleolithic Prescription*. New York: Harper & Row, 1980.

21. King, M. C., and A. C. Wilson. Evolution at two levels: Molecular similarities and biological differences between humans and chimpanzees. *Science* 188: 106–116, 1975.

22. Neel, J. V. *Physician to the Gene Pool*. New York: Wiley, 1994.

23. Gardner, L. I., E. A. MacLachlan, W. Pick, M. L. Terry, and A. M. Butler. Etiologic factors in tetany of newly born infants. *Pediatrics* 5: 228–239, 1950.

24. Zuelzer, W. W., and F. N. Ogden. Megaloblastic anemia in infancy: A common syndrome responding specifically to folic acid therapy. *American Journal of Diseases of Children* 71: 211–243, 1946.

25. Bessey, O. A., D. J. D. Adam, and A. Hansen. Intake of vitamin B6 and infantile convulsions. *Pediatrics* 20: 33–44, 1957.

26. Scriver, C. R. Vitamin B6 dependency and infantile convulsions. *Pediatrics* 26: 62–74, 1960.

PART IV: ADAPTIVE FLEXIBILITY: INTRODUCTION

1. Lederberg, J. The genetics of human nature. *Social Research* 40: 375–406, 1978.

2. Waddington, C. H. *The Strategy of the Genes*. London: Allen and Unwin, 1957.

3. Burke, P. *The French Historical Revolution*. Stanford, CA: Stanford University Press, 1990.

4. Braudel, F. *The Mediterranean and the Mediterranean World in the Age of Philip II*. Vol. 1. New York: Harper & Row, 1972.

5. Milstein, C. Antibodies: A paradigm for the biology of molecular recognition. *Proceedings of the Royal Society*, Series B, 239: 1–16, 1990.

CHAPTER 9: PHYSIOLOGICAL HOMEOSTASIS

1. Holmes, F. L. Claude Bernard: The *milieu intérieure*, and regulatory physiology. *History of Philosophy of the Life Sciences* 8: 3–25, 1986.

2. Bernard, C. *Lectures on the Phenomena of Life*. Springfield IL: C. C. Thomas, 1974.

3. Cannon, W. B. Biographical memoir of Lawrence Joseph Henderson. *National Academy of Sciences Biographical Memoirs* 23: 31–58, 1943.

4. Parascandola, J. Organismic and holistic concepts in the thought of L. J. Henderson. *Journal of the History of Biology* 4: 63–113, 1971.

5. Henderson, L. J. The practice of medicine as applied sociology. *Transactions of Association of American Physicians* 51: 8–22, 1936.

6. Russett, C. E. *The Concept of Equilibrium in American Social Thought.* New Haven, CT: Yale University Press, 1966.

7. Cannon, W. B. *The Wisdom of the Body.* Cambridge, MA: Harvard University Press, 1939.

8. Allen, G. E. *Life Science in the Twentieth Century.* New York: Wiley, 1975.

9. Murphy, E. A., and R. E. Pyeritz. Homeostasis VII: A conspectus. *American Journal of Medical Genetics* 24: 735–751, 1986.

10. Toulmin, S. Concepts of function and mechanism in medicine and medical science. In H. T. Engelhardt and S. F. Spicker (eds.). *Evaluation and Explanation in the Biomedical Sciences.* Dordrecht, Netherlands: Reidel, 1975.

11. Loomis, W. F., and P. W. Sternberg. Genetic networks. *Science* 269: 649, 1965.

12. Dawkins, R. *The Selfish Gene.* Oxford, UK: Oxford University Press, 1976.

13. Alberts, B., D. Bray, J. Lewis, M. Raff, K. Roberts, and J. D. Watson. *Molecular Biology of the Cell.* 3rd ed. New York: Garland, 1994.

14. Jacob, F. *The Logic of Life.* New York: Pantheon, 1973.

15. Schmidt-Nielsen, K. *Scaling: Why Is Animal Size So Important?* New York: Cambridge University Press, 1984.

16. Moore-Ede, M. C., F. M. Sulzmare, and C. A. Fuller. *The Clocks That Time Us.* Cambridge, MA: Harvard University Press, 1982.

17. Edmunds, L. N., Jr. *Cellular and Molecular Bases of Biological Clocks.* New York: Springer-Verlag, 1988.

18. Dunlap, J. C. Genetic analysis of circadian clocks. *Annual Review of Physiology* 55: 683–728, 1993.

19. Barinaga, M. New clues found to circadian clocks—including mammals. *Science* 276: 1030–1031, 1997.

20. Muller, J. E., G. H. Tofler, and P. H. Stone. Circadian variation and triggers of onset of acute cardiovascular disease. *Circulation* 79: 733–743, 1989.

21. Pepine, C. J. Circadian variations in myocardial ischemia. *Journal of the American Medical Association* 265: 386–390, 1991.

22. Henderson, L. J. Acidosis. *Science* 46: 73–83, 1917.

CHAPTER 10: GENETIC HOMEOSTASIS

1. Scriver, C. R., and B. Childs (eds.). *Garrod's Inborn Factors in Disease.* New York: Oxford University Press, 1989.

2. Dubos, R. *Mirage of Health.* New York: Harper, 1959.

3. Dubos, R. *Man Adapting.* New Haven, CT: Yale University Press, 1965.

4. Dubos, R. *A God Within.* New York: Scribners, 1972.

5. Dobzhansky, J. *Mankind Evolving.* New Haven, CT: Yale University Press, 1962.

6. Dobzhansky, T. *Genetic Diversity and Human Equality.* New York: Basic, 1973.

7. Darlington, C. D. *The Evolution of Man and Society.* New York: Simon and Schuster, 1969.

8. Neel, J. V. *Physician to the Gene Pool.* New York: Wiley, 1994.

9. Wolstenholme, G. *Man and His Future.* Boston: Little, Brown, 1963.

10. Fisher, R. A. *The Genetical Theory of Natural Selection.* 2nd ed. New York: Dover, 1958.

11. Provine, W. H. *Sewall Wright and Evolutionary Biology.* Chicago: University of Chicago Press, 1986.

12. Haldane, J. B. S. *Causes of Evolution.* London: Longmans, Green, 1932.

13. Hoffman, A. A., and P. A. Parsons. *Evolutionary Genetics and Environmental Stress.* New York: Oxford University Press, 1991.

14. King, M. C., and A. C. Wilson. Evolution at two levels: Molecular similarities and biological differences between humans and chimpanzees. *Science* 188: 106–116, 1975.

15. Crow, J. Muller, Dobzhansky and overdominance. *Journal of the History of Biology* 20: 351–380, 1987.

16. Avise, J. C. *Molecular Markers, Natural History and Evolution.* New York: Chapman and Hall, 1994.

17. Dobzhansky, T. A review of some fundamental concepts and problems of population genetics. *Quantitative Biology* 20: 1–15, 1955.

18. Muller, H. G. Our load of mutations. *American Journal of Human Genetics* 2: 111–176, 1949.

19. Harris, H. *The Principles of Human Biochemical Genetics.* 3rd ed. New York: Elsevier, 1980.

20. Lewontin, R. C. *The Genetic Basis of Evolutionary Change.* New York: Columbia University Press, 1974.

21. Kimura, M. *The Neutral Theory of Molecular Evolution.* Cambridge, UK: Cambridge University Press, 1983.

22. Milton, J. B. Enzyme heterozygosity, metabolism and developmental stability. *Genetika* 89: 47–65, 1933.

23. Vogel, F. Clinical consequences of heterogeneity for autosomal recessive diseases. *Clinical Genetics* 25: 381–415, 1984.

24. Kacser, H., and J. A. Burns. The molecular basis of dominance. *Genetics* 97: 639–666, 1981.

25. Lewontin, R. C. Population genetics. *Annual Review of Genetics* 19: 81–102, 1985.

Chapter 11: Developmental Homeostasis

1. Monod, J. *Chance and Necessity.* New York: Knopf, 1971.

2. Hoffman, A. A., and P. A. Parsons. *Evolutionary Genetics and Environmental Stress.* New York: Oxford University Press, 1991.

3. Ruddle, F. H., J. L. Bartels, K. L. Bentley, C. Kappen, M. J. Murtha, and J. Pendleton. Evolution of Hox genes. *Annual Review of Genetics* 28: 423–442, 1994.

4. Jacob, F. Evolution and tinkering. *Science* 196: 1161–1165, 1977.

5. King, M. C., and A. Wilson. Evolution at two levels: Molecular similarities and biological differences between humans and chimpanzees. *Science* 188: 106–116, 1975.

6. Gould, S. J. *Ontogeny and Phylogeny.* Cambridge, MA: Harvard University Press, 1977.

7. Stent, G. S. Strengths and weaknesses of the genetic approach to the development of the nervous system. In W. M. Cowan (ed.). *Studies in Developmental Neurobiology.* New York: Oxford University Press, 1981.

8. Waddington, C. H. *The Strategy of the Genes.* London: Allen & Unwin, 1957.

9. Scarr, S., and A. McCartney. How people make their own environments: A theory of genotype-environment effects. *Child Development* 54: 424–435, 1983.

10. Hill, J. A. Immunological mechanisms of pregnancy maintenance and failure: A critique of theories and therapy. *American Journal of Reproductive Immunology* 5: 331–334, 1989.

11. Efstradiatis, A. Parental imprinting of autosomal mammalian genes. *Current Opinion in Genetics and Development* 4: 265–280, 1994.

12. Sapienza, C., and J. G. Hall. Genetic imprinting in human disease. In C. R. Scriver, A. L. Beaudet, W. S. Sly, and D. Valle (eds.). *The Metabolic and Molecular Bases of Human Disease.* 7th ed. New York: McGraw-Hill, 1995.

13. Shock, N. Systems integration. In C. E. Finch and E. T. Schneider (eds.). *Handbook of the Biology of Aging.* New York: Van Nostrand, Reinhold, 1977.

14. Shock, N. Longitudinal studies of aging in humans. In C. E. Finch and E. T. Schneider (eds.), *Handbook of the Biology of Aging.* 2nd ed. New York: Van Nostrand, Reinhold, 1985.

15. Williams, G. C. Pleiotrophy, natural selection and the evolution of senescence. *Evolution* 11: 398–411, 1957.

16. Kirkwood, T. B. L. The nature and causes of aging. In *Research and the Aging Population.* Ciba Foundation Symposium No. 134. Chichester, UK: Wiley, 1988.

17. Albin, R. L. Antagonistic pleiotropy, mutation accumulation, and human genetic disease. *Genetica* 91: 279–286, 1993.

18. Martin, G. M., S. N. Austad, and T. E. Johnson. Genetic analysis of ageing: Role of oxidative damage and environmental stresses. *Nature Genetics* 13: 25–34, 1996.

19. Rowe, J. W., and R. L. Kahn. Human aging: Visual and successful. *Science* 237: 143–149, 1987.

20. Finch, C. E. *Longevity, Senescence and the Genome.* Chicago: University of Chicago Press, 1990.

21. Rose, M. R. *Evolutionary Biology of Aging.* Oxford, UK: Oxford University Press, 1991.

22. Rose, M. R., and C. E. Finch. The Janiform genetics of aging. *Genetica* 91: 3–10, 1993.

23. Martin, G. M. Abrotrophic gene action in Homo sapiens: Potential mechanisms and significance for the pathobiology of aging. *Genetica* 91: 265–277, 1993.

24. Jarwinski, S. M. Longevity, genes and aging. *Science* 273: 54–58, 1966.

CHAPTER 12: SOCIOCULTURAL HOMEOSTASIS

1. Parascandola, J. Organismic concepts in the thought of L. J. Henderson. *Journal of the History of Biology* 4: 63–113, 1971

2. Lewontin, R. C. The analysis of variance and the analysis of causes. *American Journal of Human Genetics* 26: 400–411, 1974.

3. Dobzhansky, T. *Mankind Evolving*. New Haven, CT: Yale University Press, 1962.

4. Schama, S. *Landscape and Memory*. New York: Knopf, 1995.

5. Lewontin, R. C. Gene, organism and environment. In D. S. Bendall (ed.). *Evolution from Molecules to Men*. Cambridge, UK: Cambridge University Press, 1983.

6. Thompson, J. N. *The Coevolutionary Process*. Chicago: University of Chicago Press, 1994.

7. Collins, J. P. Evolutionary ecology and the use of natural selection in ecology theory. *Journal of the History of Biology* 19: 257–288, 1983.

8. Hoffman, A. A., C. M. Sgro, and S. H. Lawler. Ecological population genetics: The interface between genes and the environment. *Annual Review of Genetics* 29: 349–370, 1995.

9. Lovelock, J. *The Ages of Gaia*. New York: Norton, 1988.

10. Cavalli-Sforza, L. L., and M. W. Feldman. *Cultural Transmission and Evolution: A Quantitative Approach*. Princeton, NJ: Princeton University Press, 1981.

11. Boyd, R., and P. J. Richerson. *Culture and the Evolutionary Process*. Chicago: University of Chicago Press, 1985.

12. Durham, W. H. *Coevolution*. Stanford, CA: Stanford University Press, 1991.

13. Ammerman, A. J., and L. L. Cavalli-Sforza. *The Neolithic Transition and the Genetics of Populations in Europe*. Princeton, NJ: Princeton University Press, 1984.

14. Cavalli-Sforza, L. L., and F. Cavalli-Sforza. *The Great Human Diasporas*. New York: Addison-Wesley, 1995.

15. Flatz, G. The genetic polymorphism of intestinal lactase activity in adult humans. In C. R. Scriver, A. L. Beaudet, W. S. Sly, and D. Valle (eds.). *The Metabolic and Molecular Bases of Inherited Disease*. 7th ed. New York: McGraw-Hill, 1995.

16. Sigerist, H. *Civilization and Disease*. Chicago: University of Chicago Press, 1943.

Chapter 13: Homeostatic Interactions

1. Childs, B. Nephrogenic diabetes insipidus. *Archives of Pediatric and Adolescent Medicine* 149: 181–186, 1995.

2. Waring, A. J., L. Kajdi, and V. Tappan. A congenital defect of water metabolism. *American Journal of Diseases of Children* 69: 323–324, 1945.

3. Williams, R. H., and C. Henry. Nephrogenic diabetes insipidus: transmitted by females and appearing during infancy in males. *Annals of Internal Medicine* 27: 84–95, 1947.

4. Bode, H. H., and J. D. Crawford. Nephrogenic diabetes insipidus in North America: The Hopewell hypothesis. *New England Journal of Medicine* 280: 750–754, 1969.

5. Toulmin, S. Knowledge and art in the practice of medicine: Clinical judgement and historical reconstruction. In C. Delkescamp-Hayes and M. A. G. Cutter (eds.). *Science, Technology and the Art of Medicine*. Amsterdam: Kluwer Academic Publishers, 1993.

PART V: DESCENT WITH MODIFICATION: INTRODUCTION

1. Alberts, B., D. Bray, J. Lewis, M. Raff, K. Roberts, and J. D. Watson. *Molecular Biology of the Cell.* 3rd ed. New York: Garland, 1994.

CHAPTER 14: WHAT IS A GENE?

1. Watson, J. D., N. H. Hopkins, J. W. Roberts, J. A. Steitz, and A. M. Weiner. *Molecular Biology of the Gene.* 4th ed. Menlo Park, CA: Benjamin-Cummings, 1987.

2. Darnell, J., H. Lodish, and D. Baltimore. *Molecular Cell Biology.* 2nd ed. New York: W. H. Freeman, 1990.

3. Alberts, B., D. Bray, J. Lewis, M. Raff, K. Roberts, and J. D. Watson. *Molecular Biology of the Cell.* New York: Garland, 1989.

4. Berg, P., and M. Singer. *Dealing with Genes: The Language of Heredity.* Mill Valley, CA: University Science Books, 1992.

5. Olby, R. C. Mendel no Mendelian. *History of Science* 17: 53–72, 1974.

6. Callender, L. A. Gregor Mendel: An opponent of descent with modification. *History of Science* 26: 42–75, 1988.

7. Lewontin, R. C. *The Genetic Basis of Evolutionary Change.* New York: Columbia University Press, 1974.

8. Frogatt, P., and N. C. Nevin. The "Law of Ancestral Heredity" and the Mendelian-ancestrian controversy in England, 1889–1906. *Journal of Medical Genetics* 8: 1–24, 1971.

9. Fisher, R. A. The correlation between relatives on the suppositions of Mendelian inheritance. *Transactions of the Royal Society, Edinburgh* 52: 321–341, 1918.

10. Norton, B., and E. S. Pearson. A note on the background to, and refereeing of, R. A. Fisher's 1918 paper "On the suppositions of Mendelian inheritance." *Notes and Records, Royal Society London* 30–31: 151–155, 1975–1977.

11. Falk, R. The gene in search of an identity. *Human Genetics* 68: 195–204, 1984.

12. Carlson, E. A. *The Gene: A Critical History.* Los Angeles: University of California Press, 1966.

13. Portin, P. The concept of the gene: Short history and present status. *Quarterly Review of Biology* 68: 173–223, 1993.

14. Provine, W. B. *The Origins of Theoretical Population Genetics.* Chicago: University of Chicago Press, 1971.

15. Lewis, E. B. Clusters of master control genes regulate the development of higher organisms. *Journal of the American Medical Association* 267: 1524–1531, 1992.

16. Fedoroff, N. Maize transposable elements. *Perspectives in Biology and Medicine* 35: 2–19, 1991.

17. Morgan, T. H. The relations of genetics to physiology and medicine. *Scientific Monthly* 41: 5–18, 1935.

18. Wright, S. Color inheritance in mammals. *Journal of Heredity* 8: 224–235, 1917.

19. Wright, S. The physiology of the gene. *Physiological Review* 21: 487–527, 1941.

20. Beadle, G. W. Genes and chemical reactions in neurospora. *Science* 129: 1715–1719, 1959.

21. Horowitz, N. Fifty years ago: The neurospora revolution. *Genetics* 127: 631–635, 1991.

22. Delbrück, M. Discussion. *Cold Spring Harbor Symposium Quantitative Biology* 11: 22–23, 1946.

23. Olby, R. *The Path to the Double Helix.* Seattle, WA: University of Washington Press, 1974.

24. Scott-Moncrieff, R. The classical period in chemical genetics. Recollections of Muriel Wheldale Onslow, R. and G. Robinson and J. B. S. Haldane. *Notes and Records, Royal Society London* 36–37: 125–154, 1981–1983.

25. Bearn, A. G. *Archibald Garrod and the Individuality of Man.* Oxford, UK: Oxford University Press, 1993.

26. Neel, J. V. The detection of the genetic carriers of hereditary disease. *American Journal of Human Genetics* 1: 19–36, 1949.

27. Childs, B. *The Metabolic and Molecular Bases of Inherited Disease,* 6th edition [review]. *American Journal of Human Genetics* 46: 848–851, 1990.

28. Muller, H. J. The gene. *Proceedings of the Royal Society, London* 134: 1–37, 1947.

29. Stent, G. S. That was the molecular biology that was. *Science* 160: 390–395, 1968.

30. Avery, O. T., C. M. MacLeod, and M. McCarty. Studies on the chemical nature of the substance inducing transformation of pueumococcal types. *Journal of Experimental Medicine* 79: 137–158, 1944.

31. Lederberg, J. What the double helix (1953) has meant for basic biomedical science. *Journal of the American Medical Association* 269: 1981–1985, 1993.

32. Delbrück, M. A physicist looks at biology. In J. Cairns, G. S. Stout, and J. D. Watson (eds.). *Phage and the Origins of Molecular Biology.* Cold Spring Harbor, NY: Cold Spring Harbor Laboratory Press, 1966.

33. Hershey, A. D., and M. Chase. Independent functions of viral protein and nucleic acid in growth of bacteriophage. *Journal of General Physiology* 36: 39–56, 1952.

34. Benzer, S. Genetic fine structure. *Harvey Lectures* 56: 1–21, 1960–1961.

35. Lederberg, J. Genetic recombination in bacteria: A discovery account. *Annual Review of Genetics* 21: 23–46, 1987.

36. Yanofsky, C. Gene structure and protein structure. *Harvey Lectures* 61: 145–167, 1965–1966.

37. Jacob, F., and J. Monod. Genetic regulatory mechanisms in the synthesis of proteins. *Journal of Molecular Biology* 3: 318–356, 1961.

38. Berget, S. M., C. Moore, and P. A. Sharp. Spliced segments at the 5' terminus of advenoviur 2 late mRNA. *Proceedings of the National Academy of Sciences* 74: 3171–3175, 1977.

39. Kellum, R., and P. Schedl. A position-effect assay for boundaries of higher order chromosomal domains. *Cell* 64: 941–950, 1991.

40. Dorit, R. L., and W. Gilbert. The limited universe of exons. *Current Opinion in Genetics and Development* 1: 464–469, 1991.

41. Hobbs, H. H., D. W. Russell, M. S. Brown, and I. L. Goldstein. The LDL re-

ceptor locus and familial hypercholesterolemia: Mutational analysis of a membrane protein. *Annual Review of Genetics* 24: 133–170, 1990.

42. Dietz, H., J. M. Saraiva, R. E. Pyeritz, G. R. Cutting, and C. A. Francomano. Clustering of fibrillin (FBN1) missense mutations in Marfan syndrome patients of cysteine residues in EGF-like domains. *Human Mutation* 1: 336–374, 1992.

43. Furie, B., and B. C. Furie. The molecular basis of blood coagulation. *Cell* 53: 505–518, 1988.

44. Fogle, T. Are genes units of inheritance? *Biology and Philosophy* 5: 349–371, 1990.

45. Robbins, R. Representing genomic maps in a relational database. In S. Suhai (ed.). *Computational Methods in Genome Research.* New York: Plenum, 1993.

46. Viskochil, D., R. Cawthorn, P. O'Connell, G. Xu, J. Stevens, M. Culver, J. Carey, and R. White. The gene encoding the oligodendrocyte-myelin glycoproteins is embedded within the neurofibromatosis type 1 gene. *Molecular and Cellular Biology* 11: 906–912, 1991.

47. Douglass, J., O. Civelli, and E. Herbert. Polyprotein gene expression: Generation of diversity of neuroendocrine peptides. *Annual Review of Biochemistry* 53: 665–715, 1984.

48. Wakil, S. J. Fatty acid synthase, a proficient multifunctional enzyme. *Biochemistry* 28: 4523–4530, 1989.

49. Padgett, R. A., G. M. Wahl, and G. R. Stark. Structure of the gene for C.A.D., the multifunctional protein that initiates U.M.P. synthesis in N-(phosphonacetyl) L-aspartate-resistant hamster cells. *Molecular and Cellular Biology* 2: 293–301, 1982.

50. Smith, C. W. J., J. G. Patton, and B. Nadal-Ginard. Alternative splicing in the control of gene expression. *Annual Review of Genetics* 23: 527–577, 1989.

51. Redman, J. B., R. G. Fenwick, F. Ying-Hui, A. Pizzuti, and C. T. Caskey. Relationship between parental trinucleotide GCT repeat length and severity of myotonic dystrophy in offspring. *Journal of the American Medical Association* 269: 1960–1965, 1993.

52. Bhattacharyya, M. K., A. M. Smith, T. H. N. Ellis, C. Hedley, and C. Martin. The wrinkled-seed character of pea described by Mendel is caused by a transposon-like insertion in a gene encoding starch-branching enzyme. *Cell* 60: 115–122, 1990.

53. Caskey, C. T. Molecular medicine: A spin-off from the helix. *Journal of the American Medical Association* 269: 1986–1992, 1993.

CHAPTER 15: THE PATHS OF GENE ACTION

1. Keller, E. F. Language and science. In E. F. Keller. *Refiguring Life.* New York: Columbia University Press, 1995.

2. Yates, F. E. Self-organizing systems. In C. A. R. Boyd and D. Noble (eds.). *The Logic of Life.* Oxford, UK: Oxford University Press, 1993.

CHAPTER 16: WHATEVER IS, IS VARIABLE

1. Wilson, A. C., S. S. Carlson, and T. J. White. Biochemical evolution. *Annual Review of Biochemistry* 46: 573–639, 1977.

2. Ohno, S. *Evolution by Gene Duplication.* New York: Springer-Verlag, 1970.

3. Bodmer, W. F. The William Allen Memorial Award Address: Gene clusters, genome organization and complex phenotypes. *American Journal of Human Genetics* 33: 664–682, 1981.

4. Cleaver, J. E., and K. H. Kraemer. *Xeroderma pigmentosum* and Cockayue syndrome. In C. R. Scriver, A. L. Beaudet, W. S. Sly, and D. Valle. (eds.). *The Metabolic and Molecular Bases of Inherited Disease.* 7th ed. New York: McGraw-Hill, 1995.

5. Cooper, D. N., M. Krawczak, and S. E. Antonarakis. The nature and mechanisms of human gene mutation. In C. R. Scriver, A. L. Beaudet, W. S. Sly, and D. Valle. (eds.). *The Metabolic and Molecular Bases of Inherited Disease.* 7th ed. New York: McGraw-Hill, 1995.

CHAPTER 17: THE SEMANTICS OF GENETICS

1. Kohler, R. E. *Lords of the Fly: Drosophila Genetics and the Experimental Life.* Chicago: University of Chicago Press, 1994.

2. Wilkie, A. O. M. The molecular basis of dominance. *Journal of Medical Genetics* 31: 89–98, 1994.

3. Stern, C. *Human Genetics.* New York: Freeman, 1949, 1960 (2nd ed.), 1973 (3rd ed.).

4. Limoges, C. Errare humanum est: Do genetic errors have a future? In C. Cranor (ed.). *Are Genes Us?* New Brunswick, NJ: Rutgers University Press, 1994.

5. Schrödinger, E. *What Is Life?* Cambridge, UK: Cambridge University Press, 1967.

CHAPTER 18: CLASSIFICATION OF DISEASE

1. Kunitz, S. J. Classification in medicine. In R. C. Manlitz, and D. E. Long (eds.). *Grand Rounds: One Hundred Years of Internal Medicine.* Philadelphia: University of Pennsylvania Press, 1988.

2. Faber, K. *Nosography: The Evolution of Clinical Medicine in Modern Times.* New York: Hoeber, 1930.

3. King, L. S. *Medical Thinking.* Princeton, NJ: Princeton University Press, 1982.

4. *International Classification of Disease.* 10th revision. Geneva: WHO, 1992.

5. Holton, G. *The Scientific Imagination.* Cambridge, UK: Cambridge University Press, 1978.

6. Brusilow, S. W., and A. L. Horwich. Urea cycle enzymes. In C. R. Scriver, A. L. Beaudet, W. S. Sly, and D. Valle (eds.). *The Metabolic and Molecular Bases of Inherited Disease.* 7th ed. New York: McGraw-Hill, 1995.

7. Tanaka, K. R., and D. E. Paglia. Pyruvatekinase and other enzymopathies of the erythrocyte. In C. R. Scriver, A. L. Beaudet, W. S. Sly, and D. Valle (eds.). *The Metabolic and Molecular Bases of Inherited Disease.* 7th ed. New York: McGraw-Hill, 1995.

8. Scriver, C. R., A. L. Beaudet, W. S. Sly, and D. Valle (eds.). *The Metabolic and Molecular Bases of Inherited Disease.* 7th ed. New York: McGraw-Hill, 1995.

CHAPTER 19: THE DIPLOID STATE

1. Delbrück, M. A physicist looks at biology. In J. Cairns, G. Stout, and J. D. Watson (eds.). *Phage and the Origins of Molecular Biology.* Expanded ed. Cold Spring Harbor, NY: Cold Spring Harbor Press, 1992.

2. Lederberg, J. Genetic recombination in bacteria: A discovery account. *Annual Review of Genetics* 21: 23–46, 1987.

3. Provine, W. B. *Sewall Wright and Evolutionary Biology.* Chicago: University of Chicago Press, 1986.

4. Provine, W. B. *The Origins of Theoretical Population Genetics.* Chicago: University of Chicago Press, 1971.

5. Brusilow, S. W., and A. L. Horwitch. Urea cycle enzymes. In C. R. Scriver, A. L. Beaudet, W. S. Sly, and D. Valle (eds.). *The Metabolic and Molecular Bases of Inherited Disease.* 7th ed. New York: McGraw-Hill, 1995.

6. Ostrer, H. *Non-Mendelian Genetics in Humans.* New York: Oxford University Press, 1998.

CHAPTER 20: GENE FREQUENCY

1. Provine, W. B. *Sewall Wright and Evolutionary Biology.* Chicago: University of Chicago Press, 1986.

2. Wright, S. Physiological aspects of genetics. *Physiological Reviews* 5: 75–106, 1945.

3. Blumberg, B. *Genetic Polymorphisms and Geographic Variations in Disease.* New York: Grune & Stratton, 1961.

4. Goldschmidt, E. (ed.). *The Genetics of Migrant and Isolate Populations.* Baltimore, MD: Williams & Wilkins, 1963.

5. Rothschild, H.R. (ed.). *Biocultural Aspects of Disease.* New York: Academic, 1981.

6. Ramot, B. *Genetic Polymorphisms and Disease in Man.* New York: Academic, 1974.

7. Jacobs, P., and T. J. Hassold. Chromosome abnormalities: Origins and etiology in abortions and live births. In F. Vogel and K. Sperling (eds.), *Proceedings of the Seventh International Congress on Human Genetics.* Berlin: Springer-Verlag, 1986.

CHAPTER 21: HETEROGENEITY

1. Woolf, V. On not knowing Greek. In *The Common Reader.* 1st series. New York: Harcourt Brace, 1984.

2. Haldane, J. B. S. *New Paths in Genetics.* London: Allen & Unwin, 1941.

3. Harris, H. *The Principles of Human Biochemical Genetics.* New York: Elsevier, 1980.

4. Harris, H., U. Mittwoch, E. B. Robson, and F. L. Warren. Phenotypes and genotypes in cystinuria. *Annals of Human Genetics* 20: 57–91, 1955.

5. Luzzato, L., and A. Mehta. Glucose-6-phosphate deficiency. In C. R. Scriver, A. L. Beaudet, W. S. Sly, and D. Valle. (eds.). *The Metabolic and Molecular Bases of Inherited Disease.* 7th ed. New York: McGraw-Hill, 1995.

6. Multifactorial inheritance: A special issue. *Trends in Genetics* 11: 463–524, 1995.

7. Falconer, D. S. The inheritance of liability to certain diseases estimated from the incidence among relatives. *Annals of Human Genetics* 29: 51–71, 1965.

8. Weissman, S. M. Genetic basis for common polymorphic disease. *Proceedings of the National Academy of Sciences* 92: 8543–8545, 1995.

9. Lifton, R. P. Genetic determinants of human hypertension. *Proceedings of the National Academy of Sciences* 92: 8545–8551, 1995.

10. Schellenberg, G. D. Genetic dissection of Alzheimer disease, a heterogeneous disorder. *Proceedings of the National Academy of Sciences* 92: 8552–8559, 1995.

11. Todd, J. A. Genetic analysis of type I diabetes using whole genome approaches. *Proceedings of the National Academy of Sciences* 92: 8560–8565, 1995.

12. Kinzler, K. W., and B. Vogelstein. Colorectal tumors. In C. R. Scriver, A. L. Beaudet, W. S. Sly, and D. Valle. (eds.). *The Metabolic and Molecular Bases of Inherited Disease.* 7th ed. New York: McGraw-Hill, 1995.

13. Murphy, E. A. Genetics in hypertension. *Circulation Research* 32, suppl. 1: 129–137, 1973.

14. Humphries, S. E., Y. Shu, P. Talmud, L. Bara, L. Wilhelmsen, and L. Tiret. European atherosclerosis study: Genotype at the fibrogen locus (G-455-A Æ gene) is associated with differences in fibrogen levels. *Atherosclerosis, Thrombosis and Vascular Biology* 15: 96–104, 1995.

15. Pfeffer, M. ACE inhibition in acute myocardial infarction. *New England Journal of Medicine* 332: 118–120, 1995.

CHAPTER 22: UNITY AND CONTINUITY OF DISEASE

1. Costa, T., C. R. Scriver, and B. Childs. The effect of mendelian disease on human health. *American Journal of Medical Genetics* 21: 231–242, 1985.

2. Hayes, A., T. Costa, C. R. Scriver, and B. Childs. The effect of mendelian disease on human health. II: Response to treatment. *American Journal of Medical Genetics* 21: 243–255, 1985.

3. Treacy, E., B. Childs, and C. R. Scriver. Response to treatment in hereditary metabolic disease: 1993 survey and 10-year comparison. *American Journal of Human Genetics* 56: 359–367, 1995.

4. Bassett, D. E., Jr., M. S. Boguski, F. Spencer, R. Reeves, M. Goebl, and P. Hieter. Comparative genomics, genome cross referencing and XREFdb. *Trends in Genetics* 11: 322–373, 1995.

5. Childs, B. Age at onset and causes of disease. *Perspectives in Biology and Medicine* 29: 437–460, 1986.

6. Johnston, C., D. A. Pybe, A. G. Cudworth, and E. Wolf. HLA-DR typing in identical twins with insulin-dependent diabetes. *British Medical Journal* 286: 253–255, 1983.

7. Marmot, M. G., M. J. Shipley, and G. Rose. Inequalities in death-specific explanations of a general pattern. *Lancet* I: 1003–1006, 1984.

8. Weissman, M., P. Wikmaratne, and K. R. Merikangas. Onset of major depression in early adulthood. *Archives of General Psychiatry* 41: 1136–1143, 1984.

9. Pulver, A. E., and K. Y. Liang. Estimating effects of proband characteristics on familial risk, II. *Genetic Epidemiology* 8: 339–350, 1991.

10. Taylor, S. I. Diabetes mellitus. In C. R. Scriver, A. L. Beaudet, W. S. Sly, and D. Valle (eds.). *The Metabolic and Molecular Bases of Inherited Disease.* 7th ed. New York: McGraw-Hill, 1995.

11. Lifton, R. P. Genetic determinants of human hypertension. *Proceedings of the National Academy of Sciences* 92: 8545–8551, 1995.

12. Couch, F., and B. L. Webe. Breast cancer. In B. Vogelstein and K. W. Kinzler (eds.). *The Genetic Basis of Human Cancer.* New York: McGraw-Hill, 1998.

13. Carter, B. S., T. H. Beaty, G. D. Steinberg, B. Childs, and P. C. Walsh. Mendelian inheritance of familial prostate cancer. *Proceedings of the National Academy of Sciences* 89: 3367–3371, 1992.

14. Kinzler, K. W., and B. Vogelstein, B. Colorectal tumors. In C. R. Scriver, A. L. Beaudet, W. S. Sly, and D. Valle (eds.). *The Metabolic and Molecular Bases of Inherited Disease.* 7th ed. New York: McGraw-Hill, 1995.

15. Sanda, M. G., T. H. Beaty, R. E. Stutzman, B. Childs, and P. C. Walsh. Genetic susceptibility of benign prostatic hyperplasia. *Journal of Urology* 152: 115–119, 1994.

16. Rubinstein, D. C., D. E. Barton, B. C. C. Davidson, and M. A. Ferguson-Smith. Analysis of the Huntington gene. *Human Molecular Genetics* 2: 1713–1715, 1993.

17. Wenger, N. Coronary disease in women. *Annual Review of Medicine* 36: 285–294, 1985.

18. Knudson, A. G. Mutation and cancer: Statistical study of retinoblastoma. *Proceedings of the National Academy of Sciences* 68: 820–824, 1971.

CHAPTER 23: HERITABILITY

1. McInerney, J. D. Why biological literacy matters. *Quarterly Review of Biology* 71: 81–96, 1996.

2. Lewontin, R. C. The analysis of variance and the analysis of causes. *American Journal of Human Genetics* 26: 400–411, 1974.

3. Zimmet, P. Type 2 (non-insulin-dependent) diabetes: An epidemiologic overview. *Diabetologia* 22: 399–411, 1982.

4. Terrenato, L., M. F. Gravina, A. San Martini, and L. Ulizzi. Natural selection associated with birth weight. III. Changes over the last twenty years. *Annals of Human Genetics* 45: 267, 1981.

5. Ulizzi, L., and L. Terrenato. Natural selection associated with birth weight. V. The secular relaxation of the stabilizing component. *Annals of Human Genetics* 51: 205, 1987.

6. Ulizzi, L., and L. Terrenato, L. Natural selection associated with birth weight. VI. Towards the end of the stabilizing component. *Annals of Human Genetics* 56: 113, 1992.

7. Ulizzi, L., and L. A. Zonta. Sex ratio and natural selection is humans: A comparative analysis of two Caucasian populations. *Annals of Human Genetics* 57: 211–219, 1993.

8. Park, E. A. The etiology of rickets. *Physiological Review* 3: 106–163, 1923.

9. Childs, B., S. Cantalino, and M. K. Dyke. Observations on sex differences in human biology. *Bulletin of the Johns Hopkins Hospital* 110: 134–144, 1962.

10. Scriver, C. R. Changing heritability of nutritional disease: Another explanation for clustering. In A. P. Simopoulos and B. Childs (eds.). *Genetic Variation and Nutrition.* Basel: Karger, 1990.

11. Boerwinkle, E. Genotype by environment interaction: It's a fact of life. In C. F. Sing and C. L. Harris (eds.). *Genetics of Cellular, Individual, Family, and Population Variability.* New York: Oxford University Press, 1993.

12. Maclachlan, A. K., J. W. Gerrard, C. S. Houston, and E. J. Ives. Familial infantile cortical hyperostosis in a large Canadian family. *Canadian Medical Association Journal* 130: 1173–1175, 1984.

13. Rowe, P. C., D. Valle, and S. W. Brusilow. Inborn errors of metabolism in children referred with Reye's syndrome. *Journal of the American Medical Association* 260: 3167, 1988.

CHAPTER 24: INFECTIONS

1. Garrod, A. E. *Inborn Factors in Disease.* Oxford, UK: Oxford University Press, 1931.

2. Childs, B., E. R. Moxon, and J. A. Winkelstein. Genetics and infectious disease. In R. A. King, J. I. Rotter, and A. G. Motulsky. (eds.). *Genetic Basis of Common Disease.* New York: Oxford University Press, 1992.

3. Anderson, R. M., and R. M. May. Population biology of infectious diseases. *Nature* 280: 361–367, 1979.

4. Lederberg, J. Medical science, infectious disease and the unity of mankind. *Journal of the American Medical Association* 260: 684–685, 1988.

5. Holland, J. J. Evolving virus plagues. *Proceedings of the National Academy of Sciences* 93: 545–546, 1996.

6. Oldstone, M. B. A. Principles of viral pathogenesis. *Cell* 87: 799–801, 1966.

7. Janeway, C. A. The immune system evolved to discriminate infections non-self from non-infectious self. *Immunology Today* 13: 11–16, 1992.

8. World Health Organization Scientific Group. Primary immunodeficiency diseases. *Clinical and Experimental Immunology* 99, suppl. 1: 2–24, 1995.

9. Sorenson, T. I. A., G. G. Nielson, P. K. Anderson, and T. W. Teasdale. Genetic and environmental influences on premature death in adult adoptees. *New England Journal of Medicine* 318: 727–732, 1988.

10. Hedlund, J. U., A. B. Ortquist, M. Kalin, G. Scalia-Tomba, and J. Gieske. Risk of pneumonia in patients previously treated in hospital for pneumonia. *Lancet* 340: 396–397, 1992.

11. Winkelstein, J. A., and B. Childs. Genetically determined variation in the immune system: implications for host defense. *Pediatric Infectious Disease Journal* 8: 531–534, 1989.

12. Biozzi, G., D. Mouton, C. Stiffel, and Y. Bouthillier. Major role of macrophages in quantitative genetic regulation of immuno-responsiveness and anti-infections immunity. *Advances in Immunology* 36: 189–234, 1984.

13. Skamene, E. *Genetic Control of Host Resistance to Infection and Malignancy.* New York: A.R. Liss, 1985.

14. McGuiness, B. J., I. N. Clarke, P. R. Lambden, A. K. Barlow, J. I. Poolman, D. M. Jones, and J. E. Heckels. Point mutation in meningococcal por-A gene associated disease. *Lancet* 337: 514–517, 1991.

15. Bloom, B. R. Games parasites play. *Nature* 279: 21–36, 1979.

16. Beverley, S. M. Hijacking the cell: Parasites in the driver's seat. *Cell* 87: 787–789, 1996.

17. Maizels, R. M., D. A. P. Bundy, M. E. Selkirk, D. F. Smith, and R. M. Anderson. Immunological modulation and evasion by helminth parasites in human populations. *Nature* 365: 797–805, 1993.

18. Pincus, S. H., P. A. Rosa, G. J. Spangrude, and G.J. Heinemann. The interplay of microbes and their hosts. *Immunology Today* 13: 471–473, 1992.

CHAPTER 25: THE MOMENT

1. Cordell, H. J., and J. A. Todd. Multifactorial inheritance in type I diabetes. *Trends in Genetics* 11: 499–504, 1995.

2. Owerbach, D., and K. H. Gabbay. The search for IDDM susceptibility genes: The next generation. *Diabetes* 45: 544–551, 1996.

3. Pugliese, G., R. Gianani, R. Moromisato, Z. L. Awdek, C. Separ, H. A. Erlich, R. A. Jackson, and G. S. Eisenbarth. HLA-DQB1*0602 is associated with dominant protection from diabetes even among islet cell antibody-positive first degree relatives of patients with IDDM. *Diabetes* 44: 608–613, 1996.

4. Ludrigsson, J., and A. O. Afoke. Seasonality of type I diabetes mellitus. *Diabetologia* 32: 84–91, 1989.

5. Karvonen, M., J. Tuomilheto, I. Libman, and R. LaPorte. A review of the recent epidemiological data on the worldwide incidence of type I (insulin dependent) diabetes mellitus. *Diabetologia* 36: 883–892, 1993.

6. Gerstein, H. C., and J. VanderMeulen. The relationship between cow's milk exposure and type I diabetes. *Diabetic Medicine* 13: 23–29, 1995.

7. Kahn, N., and J. J. Couper. Low birth weight infants show earlier onset of IDDM. *Diabetes Care* 17: 653–656, 1994.

8. Johannson, C., U. Samuelsson, and J. Ludvigsson. A high weight gain early in life is associated with an increased risk of type I (insulin dependent) diabetes mellitus. *Diabetologia* 37: 91–94, 1994.

9. Vadheim, C. M., J. I. Rotter, N. K. Maclaren, W. S. Riley, and C. E. Anderson. Preferential transmission of diabetic alleles within the HLA gene complex. *New England Journal of Medicine* 315: 1314–1318, 1986.

10. Rewers, M., T. L. Bugawan, J. M. Norris, A. Blair, M. Hoffman, R. S. McDuffie, R. F. Hamman, G. Klingensmith, G. S. Eisenbarth, and H. A. Erlich. Newborn screening for HLA markers associated with IDDM: Diabetes autoimmunity study in the young. *Diabetologia* 39: 807–812, 1996.

11. Rubinstein, P., M. Walker, F. Ginsberg, and F. Fellner. Excess of DR3/4 in type I diabetes: What does it portend? *Diabetes* 35: 985, 1986.

12. Chern, M. M., V. E. Anderson, and J. Barbosa. Empirical risk for insulin-dependent diabetes in sibs. *Diabetes* 31: 1115–1118, 1982.

13. Johnston, C., D. A. Pyke, A. G. Cudworth, and E. Wolf. HLA-DR typing in identical twins with insulin-dependent diabetes. *British Medical Journal* 286: 253–255, 1983.

14. Karjalainen, J., P. Salmela, J. Ilonen, H. M. Surcel, and M. Knip. A comparison of childhood and adult type I diabetes mellitus. *New England Journal of Medicine* 320: 881–885, 1989.

15. Wagener, D. K., R. E. LaPorte, T. J. Orchard, D. Cavender, L. H. Kuller, and A. L. Drash. The Pittsburgh diabetes study: An increased prevalence with older maternal age. *Diabetologia* 25: 82–85, 1983.

CHAPTER 26: THE LIFETIME

1. Barker, D. J. P. (ed.). *Fetal and Infant Origins of Adult Disease*. London: British Medical Journal, 1992.

2. Marmot, M. G. Early life and adult disorder: Research themes. *British Medical Bulletin* 53: 3–9, 1997.

3. Lucas, A. Programming by early nutrition in man. In *The Childhood Environmental and Adult Disease*. Ciba Foundation Symposium 156. Chichester, UK: Wiley, 1991.

4. Pettit, D. J., K. Aleck, H. R. Baird, M. J. Carraher, P. H. Bennett, and W. C. Knowler. Congenital susceptibility to NIDDM: Role of intrauterine environment. *Diabetes* 37: 622–628, 1988.

5. Valdez, R., M. A. Athens, G. H. Thompson, B. S. Bradshaw, and M. P. Stern. Birthweight and adult health outcomes in a biethnic population in the U.S.A. *Diabetologia* 37: 624–631, 1994.

6. Lithell, H. O., P. M. McKeigne, L. Borglund, R. Mohsen, J.-B. Lithell, and D. A. Leon. Relation of size at birth to non-insulin dependent diabetes and insulin concentrations in men aged 50–60 years. *British Medical Journal* 312: 406–410, 1966.

7. Leonetti, D. L., W. Y. Fujimoto, and P. W. Wahl. Early-life background and the development of non-insulin dependent diabetes mellitus. *American Journal of Physical Anthropology* 79: 345–355, 1989.

8. Gennser, G., P. Rymark, and P. E. Isberg. Low birthweight and risk of high blood pressure in adulthood. *British Medical Journal* 296: 1498–1500, 1988.

9. Law, C. M., M. deSwiet, C. Osmond, P. M. Fayers, D. J. P. Barker, A. M. Cruddas, and C. H. D. Fall. Initiation of hypertension in utero and its amplification throughout life. *British Medical Journal* 306: 24–27, 1993.

10. Edwards, C. R. W., R. Benediktsson, R. S. Lindsay, and J. R. Seckl. Dysfunction of placental glucocorticoid barriers: Link between fetal environment and adult hypertension. *Lancet* 341: 355–357, 1993.

11. Lever, A. F., and S. B. Harrap. Essential hypertension: A disorder of growth with origins in childhood. *Journal of Hypertension* 10: 101–120, 1992.

12. Elford, J., P. Whincup, and A. G. Shaper. Early life experiences and adult cardiovascular disease: Longitudinal and case-control studies. *International Journal of Epidemiology* 20: 833–844, 1991.

13. Sambrook, P. N., P. J. Kelly, N. A. Morrison, and J. A. Eisman. Genetics of osteoporosis. *British Journal of Rheumatology* 33: 1007–1010, 1994.

14. Seeman, E., J. L. Hopper, L. A. Bach, M. E. Cooper, E. Parkinson, J. McKay, and G. Jerums. Reduced bone mass in daughters of women with osteoporosis. *New England Journal of Medicine* 320: 554–558, 1989.

15. Christian, J. C., P.-L. Yu, C. W. Slemenda, and C. C. Johnston, Jr. Heritability of bone mass: A longitudinal study in aging male twins. *American Journal of Human Genetics* 44: 429–433, 1989.

16. Finkelstein, J. S., R. M. Neer, B. M. K. Biller, J. D. Crawford, and A. Klibanski. Osteopenia in men with a history of delayed puberty. *New England Journal of Medicine* 326: 600–614, 1992.

CHAPTER 27: BIOLOGICAL AND SOCIAL HISTORY, AND A VISION OF DISEASE IN THREE TIME FRAMES

1. Binstock, R. H. The oldest old. A fresh perspective, or compassionate ageism revisited. *Milbank Memorial Fund Quarterly* 63: 420–451, 1985.

2. Kunitz, S. J. The roots and ideological functions of disease concepts in three primary care specialties. *Bulletin of the History of Medicine* 57: 412–432, 1983.

CHAPTER 28: THE HUMAN GENOME PROJECT

1. Tanner, E. *Why Things Bite Back: Technology and the Revenge of Unintended Consequences.* New York: Knopf, 1996.

2. Dutton, D. B. *Worse Than the Disease: Pitfalls of Medical Progress.* New York: Cambridge University Press, 1988.

3. Cook-Deegan, R. *The Gene Wars: Science, Politics, and the Human Genome.* New York: Norton, 1994.

4. Kevles, D. J., and L. Hood. *The Code of Codes.* Cambridge, MA: Harvard University Press, 1992.

5. Boyd, C. A. R., and D. Noble. *The Logic of Life: The Challenge of Integrative Physiology.* New York: Oxford University Press, 1993.

6. Goodfellow, P., and A. M. L. Lever. Gene therapy. *British Medical Bulletin* 51: 1–242, 1997.

7. Gilbert, W. A vision of the grail. In D. J. Kevles and L. Hood (eds.). *The Code of Codes.* Cambridge, MA: Harvard University Press, 1992.

8. Goodrich, N. L. *The Holy Grail.* New York: HarperCollins, 1992.

9. Childs, B. Galton, Garrod and clinical medicine. *Yale Journal of Biology and Medicine* 46: 297–313, 1973.

10. Hoagland, H., and R. W. Burhoe (eds.). *Evolution and Man's Progress.* New York: Columbia University Press, 1962.

11. Sonneborn, T. M. (ed.). *The Control of Human Heredity and Evolution.* New York: Macmillan, 1965.

12. Handler, P. (ed.). *Biology and the Future of Man.* New York: Oxford University Press, 1970.

13. Wolstenholme, G. E. W. (ed.). *The Future of Man.* Boston: Little, Brown, 1963.

14. Roslansky, J. D. (ed.). *Genetics and the Future of Man.* New York: Appleton-Century-Crofts, 1996.

15. Vaux, K. (ed.). *Who Shall Live: Medicine, Technology, Ethics.* Minneapolis: Augsberg Fortress, 1970.

16. Changing mores of biomedical research. *Annals of Internal Medicine* 67, suppl. 7: 1–83, 1967.

17. Paterson, D. (ed.). *Genetic Engineering.* London: BBC Publications, 1969.

18. Hamilton, M. H. *The New Genetics and the Future of Man.* Grand Rapids, MI: Eerdmans, 1972.

19. Hilton, B., D. Callahan, M. Harris, P. Condliffe, and B. Berdley. *Ethical Issues in Human Genetics.* New York: Plenum, 1973.

CHAPTER 29: THE MEDICAL-GENETIC SYNTHESIS AND SOCIETY

1. Rosenberg, C. R. Toward an ecology of knowledge. In *The Organization of Knowledge in Modern America, 1860–1920.* Baltimore, MD: Johns Hopkins University Press, 1979.

2. Brandt, A. M. Emerging themes in the history of medicine. *Milbank Quarterly* 69: 199–214, 1991.

3. Burnham, J. C. America and medicine's golden age: What happened to it. *Science* 215: 1474–1479, 1982.

4. Andrews, L. B., J. E. Fullarton, N. A. Holtzman, and A. G. Motulsky. *Assessing Genetic Risks.* Washington, DC: National Academy of Sciences Press, 1994.

5. Nelkin, D., and M. S. Lindee. *The DNA Mystique: The Gene as a Cultural Icon.* New York: W. H. Freeman, 1995.

6. McInerney, J. D. Molecular biology: How can we translate the laboratory. In R. F. Weir, S. C. Laurence, and E. Fales (eds.). *Genes and Human Self-Knowledge.* Iowa City, IA: University of Iowa Press, 1994.

7. Pelikan, J. *The Idea of the University.* New Haven, CT: Yale University Press, 1992.

CHAPTER 30: A BASIS FOR MEDICAL EDUCATION

1. The goals of medicine: Setting new priorities. *Hastings Center Report* 26, suppl.: 1–27, 1996.

2. Hunter, K. M. A science of individuals: Medicine and uncertainty. *Hospital Practice:* 183–218, 1992, 15 May.

3. Lederberg, J. The interface of biology and medicine. *Mount Sinai Journal of Medicine* 59: 380–383, 1992.

Index

Page numbers in *italics* denote figures and exhibits; those in **boldface** denote tables.

case example of, 125–26; development-phenotype in, 128; environment-phenotype in, 128–29; gene-phenotype in, 127–28; genetics of, 126–27; symptoms of, 127

Diabetes mellitus, 7, 17, 226, 231; type I, 109, 212, 241, 243–47, **244**; type II, 196, 221–22, 227, 251

Diagnosis, 243, 259; of "classical case," 30, 40; history taking for, 76, 256; Oslerian, 15; specificity of, 38, 206, 208, 219–20; technology and, 20–21

Diagnosis-related groups (DRGs), 173

Diathesis, 11, 13–14

Diet, 227; fat in, 120

Diploidy, 177–83; advantages of, 179–81, 180; disadvantages of, 180, 181–82; maintenance of, 178; in prokaryotes, 177–78

Disease frequency, 185–87, 205, 205, 207, 227, 286; among abortuses, 188–89; determinants of, 186–87, 205; estimation of, 187; individuality and, 188; multiple diseases, 189; overt vs. occult disease, 188–89; variable penetrance and, 187–88

DNA, 14, 32, 33, 53, 81–82, 98, 133, 134, 138–43, 286; failure of repair of, 112; identification as genetic material, 138–39; language of, 4–5, 161; mutations of, 152–58, 209; replication of, 152, 154; structure of, 138–40, 142

Doctor-patient relationship, 20–21, 23, 276

Dominance, 179–81, 205

Drug-induced disorders, 257

Duodenal ulcer, 221

Dysautonomia, 185

Educating public about genetic medicine, 279–81

Embryogenesis, 105–6, 108–10, 155, 249, 270

Environment, 33; contributions to type I diabetes, 245; definition of, 115–16; external, 116–18; infections as environmental diseases, 234–40; interaction between genes and, 83, 114–16, 120, 123–24, 123; internal, 116; sociocultural homeostasis, 114–21; unintended ecological disruptions, 257

Epidemiological studies, 30–32, 144, 226; of disease frequency, 185–87, 227; of rickets, 229; of type I diabetes, 245–46

Epistatic genes, 115, 161

Essentialist definition of disease, 39–43

Ethology, 51

Eukaryotes, 83, 84, 153

Evolution and natural selection, 13, 14, 26–27; adaptation and, 65–72, 93; cultural, 69, 102; evolutionary synthesis, 57–58; logic of disease and, 45–46; medical thought and, 93–95; Mendelist views of, 134–35; mutations, 152–58; role in disease, 66, 93; significance of variant genes to, 209

Exons, 141–42, 160, 165

Families, 51–52, 259; distributions of disease in, 177; epidemiological studies of, 144

Feedback mechanisms, 82–83

Fertility, 102; impairment in monogenic diseases, 214

Fertilization, 143, 178

Fisher, R. A., 94, 135, 179, 181, 184–85, 213

Fitness of populations, 184–85

Flexner report, 7, 24

Founder effect, 50, 65, 97, 99

Fractures, osteoporotic, 253–55

Fragile X syndrome, 142

Galton, Francis, 135–36, 144

Garrod, Archibald, 11–16, 26, 31, 45, 59, 74, 90, 93, 97, 99, 118, 136, 137, 144, 192, 235, 237, 249, 260, 266, 289. *See also* Inborn errors

Gaucher disease, 185

Gene frequency, 184–90; disease frequency and, 185–87; interpopulation

Haploidy, 109, 178–82
Hartnup's disorder, 232
Health: continuity of disease with, 206–9; homeostatic interactions and, 123; in tribal societies, 70–71
Health industry, 2, 5
Health maintenance organizations (HMOs), 2, 31
Heart attack, 67, 99, 120, 199, 222, 231, 233
Heat shock proteins, 95–96, 105
Hemolytic anemia, 193
Hemophilia, 34–35, 280
Henderson, L. J., 78, 90–91, 114, 120
Heritability, 175, 225–33; applications of, 225–26; of birth weight, 228; coefficient of, 225; definition of, 225; educational uses of, 226–27; meaning of, in context of logic of disease, 232–33; other examples of, 232; of rickets, 229–31
Heterogeneity, 191–200; definition of, 191; genetic, 192–99; nongenetic, 199–200
Heterozygote advantage, 50, 55, 96–99, 179, 268
High blood pressure, 7, 17, 54, 148, 174, 196, 197–99, 224, 226, 251–52
Hippocratic oath, 71
History taking, 76, 256
Homeobox domains, 143
Homeostasis, 7, 25, 73–76; biology and social history, 256–58; classifying disease based on aberrations in unit steps of, 169–74; definitions of, 74, 77, 80–82, 149; developmental, 101–13; disease as outcome of incongruence with, 33, 43, 91, 172–73, 186–87, 190; of environment, 74; genetic, 74, 92–100; of immunity, 75; mutation and, 46; ontogeny of, 79; physiological, 74, 77–91; sociocultural, 79, 114–21
Homeostatic interactions, 122–30, 123, 124; case example of nephrogenic dia-

betes insipidus, 125–30; generalizations about, 129–30
Homozygosity, 55, 96
Human Genome Project, 7, 80, 90, 99, 144, 149, 189, 199, 218, 257–58, 261, 265–74, 278, 282; data: —affecting classification, 270–71; —affecting prevention, 271; —affecting treatment, 269; —on development, 270; —on polymorphism, 267–68; —on range of human disease, 268–69; humanity and, 274; medical thinking and, 271–74; outcomes of, 267–71; predictions of unintended hazards of, 266; purpose of, 274
Human identity, 20–21
Human immunodeficiency virus (HIV), 34, 236, 285
Humanities, 121
Huntington's disease, 142, 212, 222
Hypertension, 7, 17, 54, 148, 174, 196, 197–99, 224, 226, 251–52

Iatrogenic disease, 257
Immune system, 75, 86, 153, 236
Immunization, 237, 239
Immunodeficiencies, 31, 237, 240
Imprinting of parental genes, 109, 182
Inborn errors, 11–16, 90, 93, 97, 137–38, 141; allelic variation in, 192, 193; classification of, 167, 168; definition of, 11, 12, 14; discovery of, 11–12; epidemiology of, 186; Garrod's concept of, 11–14; immunodeficiencies, 237; monogenic, 170–71; multifactorial, 171–72; treatments for, 90
Inborn Factors in Disease (Garrod), 11, 13, 45, 93, 235, 260
Individuality, 29–32, 73, 259; biological and medical views of, 50–51; causes of disease and, 33–36, 76; chemical, 11–16, 74, 90, 97, 99 (see also Inborn errors); constancy of, 73–74 (see also Homeostasis); of development, 107–8; disease frequency and, 188; doctor-

evolution and, 93–95; facts and, 20; human identity and, 20–21; humanities in, 121; intellectual disjunction between preclinical and clinical years, 287–89; lessons from phylogeny, 65–72; medical-genetic synthesis as basis of, 284–90; Osler's and Garrod's views of, 15–16; philosophy of medicine, 282–84; proceeding from reduction to integration, 287; on proximate and remote causes, 35; remedies for shortcomings in, 23–27; signs of unease about, 19–20; social context for, 2–3, 21–23; textbooks for, 201–3

Medical-genetic synthesis and society, 275–83

Medical specialties, 19, 31

Medical thinking, 9; definitions of disease, 37–43; impact of Human Genome Project on, 271–74; on inborn errors and chemical individuality, 11–16; on individuality and causes, 29–36; medical practice and, 18; prevalent medical thought, 18–19; synthesis of medical and biological thought, 58–62, 116; transition from Oslerian to Garrodian medicine, 17–28

Meiosis, 143, 209, 269

Memory, phylogenetic and developmental, 104

Mendelian Inheritance in Man, 156, 214

Mendelism, 85, 134–36, 143, 192

Metabolic and Molecular Bases of Inherited Disease, The, 11–12, 14, 156, 168–72, 174, 193

"Metabolic" disease, 167, 168. *See also* Inborn errors

Methemoglobinemia, 192

Microcytosis, 232

Microorganisms, 234–36; adaptations for survival of, 238–39; genetic variations in, 236, 238–39; points of entry into human cells, 236; virulence and pathogenicity of, 235–36

Migration, 65, 97, 163, 206, 208, 220, 221

Milieu intérieur, 78, 81, 86

Mode of inheritance of disease, continuity of, 204–5, 205, 207; in monogenic disease, 212–18, 217; in multifactorial disease, 218–24

Modifying genes, 115, 161

Molecular biology, 5, 18–19, 24, 27, 33, 45–46, 271

Molecular Biology of the Cell (Alberts et al.), 45, 82, 131

Molecular genetics, 51, 57, 141–45; language of, 159–61

Monogenic diseases: age at onset of, 212, 214; burden of, 214, 217; classification of, 170–71; genetic heterogeneity in, 193–94; gradient of selective effect in, 216–18; immunodeficiencies, 237; modes of inheritance of, 212–13; monogenic and multigenic phenotypes, 195, 212, 219; mortality from, 214, 216–18; other characteristics of, 214–18; treatment outcomes for, 214–16

Monosomy, 189

Morgan, T. H., 136

Mortality, 55; circadian rhythms and, 88; distribution by age, 210, 211, 248; due to monogenic disease, 214, 216–18; intrauterine, 188–89, 217–18; perinatal, 228; smoking-related, 67–68

Muller, H. J., 61, 96, 138

Multifactorial diseases, 96, 134; age at onset of, 212, 220–21; aging and, 112–13; classification of, 171–72; continuity of modes of inheritance of, 218–24; genetic heterogeneity in, 194; gradient of selective effect in, 219–24; models for, 195–99; monogenic and multigenic phenotypes, 195, 212–13, 219; sex differences in, 220, 221; treatment outcomes for, 222

Multiple diseases, 189

Mutation, 46, 51, 66, 76, 89, 134, 152–58, 209; classical-balance controversy about, 96–97; constraints on, 203; gradient of selective effect, 95, 99–100, 155–56, 163, 209–12, 211; individual variation in mutability, 154–55; lethal, 155, 203; meaning of mutant, 159–60; in microorganisms, 236, 238–39; openness of everything to, 153–54; predictability of phenotypes, 156–57; protective effect of dominance and, 179–81; randomness of, 94–95, 98, 156, 286; vs. wild-type genes, 160, 163–65; X-linked, 182

Mutational load, 163

Myocardial infarction, 67, 99, 120, 199, 222, 231, 233

Myotonic dystrophy, 142, 222

Natural history of disease, 54

Natural obligations, 103–4

Natural selection. *See* Evolution and natural selection

Neo-Darwinism, 29, 58

Neoteny, 106–7, 111, 253

Nominalist definition of disease, 39–43

Norms of reaction, 115

Number of diseases, 205–6, 208

Nutritional diseases, 227, 232, 251, 286; rickets, 229–31

Oncogenes, 160–61

One gene–one protein principle, 137–38, 142, 143, 145, 213

Ontogeny, 26, 27, 34, 46, 53, 60, 79, 101–3, 124, 144, 203

Origins of disease, 6–8, 33–35; adaptation and, 66; aging, 112–13, 269; alternative to machine concept, 26–28, 59, 262; body-as-machine concept, 15, 18–19, 24–27, 59, 262; development as remote cause, 253; evolutionary processes, 66, 93; genetic and environmental, 33; inborn errors and chemical individuality, 11–16, 90, 93, 137–38,

141; incongruence with homeostasis, 33, 43, 91, 172–73, 186–87, 190, 203, 276–77; mutation, 46; for rare diseases, 186; social, 21–22, 186–87, 276–77

Osler, William, 14–16, 45, **59**, 167, 289

Oslerian ideal, 14, 15, 17, 18

Osteoporosis, 99, 253–55

Overt vs. occult disease, 188–89

Oxidative stress, 112

Parental effects on development, 108–9, 182

Parkinson's disease, 221

Pathogenesis, 15, 24, 33–35, 45, 58, 89, 93, 134, 141; classification of disease and, 168. *See also* Origins of disease

Pathogenicity, 236–37

Pedigree analysis, 144

Pellagra, 232

Penetrance, 187–88

Phenotype(s), 57–58, 60, 61, 96, 122, 273; as adaptation to experiences, 149; analysis in nephrogenic diabetes insipidus, 127–29; complex, 85–86; definition of, 147; differential choice of, 95; elements contributing to individuality of, 123–25, 123; gradient of selective effect and, 209–11; monogenic and multigenic, 195, 212, 219; paths: —from gene to, 143, 144, 146–50, **148**, 202; —to gene from, 149–50; predictability of, 156–57; variations evoked by foreign substances, 115

Phenylketonuria (PKU), 31, 99, 109, **148**, 168, 193, 199, 213, 253

Philosophy of medicine, 282–84

Phylogeny, 7, 26, 46, 53, 65–72, 75, 83, 95–96, 100, 105, 114, 122, 144, 166, 203, 204, 242, 256, 286

Physiological homeostasis, 74, 77–91; adaptation and, 86–87; communication for preservation of, 82–83; complexity and hierarchy of, 84–86; definitions of, 80–82; gene protein products and, 144; homeostatic interactions and, 89–90, 114, 122–30; integrity of systems, 81–82; organization of, 83–84; origins of idea, 77–80; rhythmicity and, 87–88

Pneumonia, 216, 237, 238

Polio, 236

Polygenes, 195–96

Polymorphism, 50, 66, 97–99, 109, 155, 163–64; data from Human Genome Project, 267–68; heterozygote advantage, 50, 55, 96–99, 179, 268; neutral, 97–98

Population thinking, 29–31, 40, 57, 98, 162–63, 186, 191, 201, 223, 227, 240, 265

Predictive power of genetics, 54, 60, 94, 156–57

Prevention, 118, 151, 173, 227, 259; data from Human Genome Project, 271; primacy of, 277–78

Principles and Practice of Medicine, The (Osler), 14–15, 19, 167

Principles of disease, 45–46

Progress in biology and medicine, 54–56

Prokaryotes, 83, 153; diploid stage in, 177–78

Pseudoalleles, 136

Puberty, 102, 210

"Purifying" selection, 152, 209

Randomness of mutation, 94–95, 98, 156, 286

Range of human disease, 268–69

Receptor-ligand system, 115

Recessive condition, 179, 205

Reductionist analysis of disease, 58, 80, 162, 173, 275, 289–90

Relationships between biology and medicine, 24–25, 47–56; families, 51–52; goals, 48–50, 49; individuality, 50–51; progress, 54–56; time, 53–54; uncertainty, 52–53

Reproduction, 102, 177–83

Reproductive decisions, 54

Reye's syndrome, 232

Rheumatoid arthritis, 221–22

Rhythmicity, 87–88

Rickets, 229–31

"Riddle of life," 139, 177

RNA, 139, 141–142

Rosenberg, Charles, 275

Samaritan functions, 21, 28

Schama, Simon, 116–17

Schizophrenia, 7, 109, 148

Secular change, 205, 206, 220, 221

Segregation analysis, 144

Semantics. *See* Language

Sensitivity, 86

Sex chromosomes, 178

Sex differences in disease, 205, 206, 208, 220

Sleep-wake cycles, 88

Smallpox, 239

Smoking, 67–68

Social context of medicine, 2–3, 21–23, 187; books on social consequences of genetic knowledge, 278, 279; medical-genetic synthesis and society, 275–83; medicine's points of contact with society, 281–83; primacy of prevention, 277–78; public education about genetics, 279–81; social and biological history, 256–58; social component of all disease, 276–77

Social development, 107

Sociocultural homeostasis, 79, 114–21, 123; cultural inheritance, 118–20, 227; external environment, 116–18; gene-environment interaction, 114–16, 123–24, 123

Socioeconomic status (SES), 205, 206, 208, 220, 221, 240

Species identity, 13, 63, 204

Species interdependence, 117–18, 122

Specificity, diagnostic, 38, 206, 208, 219–20

Stature, 207

The Library of Congress has cataloged the hardcover edition of this book as
follows:

Childs, Barton.
    Genetic medicine : a logic of disease / Barton Childs.
      p. cm.
    Includes bibliographical references and index.
    ISBN 0-8018-6130-6 (alk. paper)
    1. Medical genetics. 2. Medicine—Philosophy. 3. Human
evolution. I. Title.
    [DNLM: 1. Genetics, Medical. 2. Hereditary Diseases. QZ 50
C537g 1999]
    RB155.C496 1999
    616'.042—dc21
    DNLM/DLC
    for Library of Congress   99-12783

ISBN 0-8018-7442-4 (pbk.)